Multilingual Aspects of Fluency Disorders

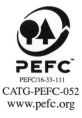

PEFC
PEFC/16-33-111
CATG-PEFC-052
www.pefc.org

COMMUNICATION DISORDERS ACROSS LANGUAGES
Series Editors: Dr Nicole Müller and Dr Martin Ball, *University of Louisiana at Lafayette, USA*

While the majority of work in communication disorders has focused on English, there has been a growing trend in recent years for the publication of information on languages other than English. However, much of this is scattered through a large number of journals in the field of speech pathology/communication disorders, and therefore, not always readily available to the practitioner, researcher and student. It is the aim of this series to bring together into book form surveys of existing studies on specific languages, together with new materials for the language(s) in question. We also envisage a series of companion volumes dedicated to issues related to the cross-linguistic study of communication disorders. The series will not include English (as so much work is readily available), but will cover a wide number of other languages (usually separately, though sometimes two or more similar languages may be grouped together where warranted by the amount of published work currently available). We envisage being able to solicit volumes on languages such as Norwegian, Swedish, Finnish, German, Dutch, French, Italian, Spanish, Russian, Croatian, Japanese, Cantonese, Mandarin, Thai, North Indian languages in the UK context, Celtic languages, Arabic and Hebrew among others.

Full details of all the books in this series and of all our other publications can be found on http://www.multilingual-matters.com, or by writing to Multilingual Matters, St Nicholas House, 31–34 High Street, Bristol BS1 2AW, UK.

COMMUNICATION DISORDERS ACROSS LANGUAGES
Series Editors: Dr Nicole Müller and Dr Martin Ball,
University of Louisiana at Lafayette, USA

Multilingual Aspects of Fluency Disorders

Edited by
Peter Howell and John Van Borsel

MULTILINGUAL MATTERS
Bristol • Buffalo • Toronto

Library of Congress Cataloging in Publication Data
Multilingual Aspects of Fluency Disorders/Edited by Peter Howell and
John Van Borsel.
Communication Disorders Across Languages: 5
1. Speech disorders in children. 2. Language disorders in children.
3. Multilingualism.
I. Howell, Peter, 1947– II. Borsel, John van.
RJ496.S7.M76 2011
618.92'855—dc22 2011000612

British Library Cataloguing in Publication Data
A catalogue entry for this book is available from the British Library.

ISBN-13: 978–1–84769–359–4 (hbk)
ISBN-13: 978–1–84769–358–7 (pbk)

Multilingual Matters
UK: St Nicholas House, 31–34 High Street, Bristol BS1 2AW, UK.
USA: UTP, 2250 Military Road, Tonawanda, NY 14150, USA.
Canada: UTP, 5201 Dufferin Street, North York, Ontario M3H 5T8, Canada.

The policy of Multilingual Matters/Channel View Publications is to use papers that
are natural, renewable and recyclable products, made from wood grown in
sustainable forests. In the manufacturing process of our books, and to further support
our policy, preference is given to printers that have FSC and PEFC Chain of Custody
certification. The FSC and/or PEFC logos will appear on those books where full
certification has been granted to the printer concerned.

Typeset by Integra Software Services Pvt. Ltd, Pondicherry, India.
Printed and bound in Great Britain by the MPG Books Group

Contents

Contributors

Professor Nan Bernstein Ratner, Department of Hearing and Speech Sciences, University of Maryland, 0100 Lefrak Hall, College Park, MD 20742, USA. nratner@hesp.umd.edu

Dr, Mônica de Britto Pereira, Speech pathology, Universidade Veiga de Almeida, 20271-020, Rio de Janeiro, Brasil. monicabp@uva.br

Dr Shelley B. Brundage, Department of Speech & Hearing Sciences, George Washington University, 2115 G Street NW., Monroe Hall of Govt., Washington, DC 20052, USA. brundage@gwu.edu

Dr Courtney T. Byrd, Communication Science and Disorders, The University of Texas at Austin, 10627 Floral Park Drive, Austin, TX 78759. courtneybyrd@mail.utexas.edu

Dr Edna J. Carlo, Speech-Language Pathology Program SHP Trailer 2B Medical Sciences Campus, University of Puerto Rico, PO Box 365067, San Juan, PR 00936-5067. edna.carlo@upr.edu

Prof. Dr. A. De Houwer, Sprachwissenschaft (Anglistik), Universität Erfurt, Nordhäuser Str. 63, D-99089 Erfur. Germany. annick.dehouwer@uni-erfurt.de

Dr Katharina Dworzynski, Research Fellow, National Clinical Guidelines Centre, Royal College of Physicians, 11 St Andrews Place, London NW1 4LW, United Kingdom. Katharina.Dworzynski@rcplondon.ac.uk

Dr Peter Howell, Division of Psychology and Language Sciences, 26 Bedford Way building, University College London, London WC1H OAP, United Kingdom. p.howell@ucl.ac.uk

Dr Hamid Karimi, Department of Speech and Language Therapy, School of Rehabilitation Sciences, Isfahan University of Medical Sciences, Isfahan, Iran. hamidkarimi_slp@yahoo.com

Dr Denise Klein, Cognitive Neuroscience Unit, Montreal Neurological Institute, McGill University, 3801 University Street, Montreal, Quebec, Canada, H3A 2B4. denise.klein@mcgill.ca

Dr Valerie Lim, Senior Principal Speech Therapist, Singapore General Hospital, Outram Road, Singapore 169608. valerie.lim.p.c@sgh.com.sg

Dr Michelle Lincoln, School of Communication Sciences and Disorders, The University of Sydney, PO Box 170, Lidcombe, NSW 1825, Australia. M.Lincoln@usyd.edu.au

Dr Ineke Mennen, ESRC Centre for Research on Bilingualism, School of Linguistics and English Language, Bangor University, 37-41 College Road, Bangor, Gwynedd, LL57 2DG, Wales. i.mennen@bangor.ac.uk

Dr Reza Nilipour, Department of Speech Therapy, University of Welfare & Rehabilitation Sciences, Kudakyar Ave, Evin, 19834 Tehran, Iran. rnilipour@gmail.com

Dr Patricia M. Roberts, School of Rehabilitation Sciences, University of Ottawa, 451 Smyth Road, Room 3072, Roger Guindon Hall, Ottawa, ON K1H 8M5, Canada. proberts@uottawa.ca

Ms Sarah Rusbridge, Division of Psychology and Language Sciences, 26 Bedford Way building, University College London, London WC1H OAP, United Kingdom. s.rusbridge@ucl.ac.uk

Dr Rosalee C. Shenker, Montreal Fluency Centre, 4626 Ste. Catherine Street West, Westmount, Quebec H3Z 1S3, Montreal, Canada. rosalee.shenker@mcgill.ca

Dr Anne-Marie Simon, French National Research Institute – in Medecine Hôpital de la Salpétrière, Paris, France. am.simon@wanadoo.fr

Ms Pei-Tzu Tsai, Department of Hearing and Speech Sciences, University of Maryland, 0100 Lefrak Hall, College Park, MD 20742, USA. ptsai@hesp.umd.edu

Professor Akira Ujihira, Institute of Liberal Arts and Science, Toyohashi University of Technology, Hibarigaoka 1-1, Tempaku-cho, Toyohashi-shi, Aichi-ken, 441-8580, Japan. ujihira@hse.tut.ac.jp

Dr John Van Borsel, Ghent University Hospital, Ghent University, Department of Logopaedics and Audiology, UZ Gent 2P1, De Pintelaan 185, B-9000 Gent, Belgium. john.vanborsel@ugent.be

Dr Kate, E. Watkins, Dept. of Experimental Psychology, University of Oxford, South Parks Road, Oxford, OX1 3UD, U.K. kate@fmrib.ox.ac.uk

Dr Jennifer B. Watson, Communication Science and Disorders, Texas Christian University Fort Worth, Texas 76129, USA. j.watson@tcu.edu

Preface

Recent years have seen considerable advances in what has been learned about stuttering. This persuaded Anne Smith in 2008 to propose the following statement on the British Stammering Association's website:

> Stuttering is a neurodevelopmental disorder involving many different brain systems active for speech – including language, motor, and emotional networks. Each infant is born with a genetic makeup that contributes to his or her probability of stuttering, however whether stuttering will develop depends upon experience. To learn to speak fluently, a child's brain must develop many different neural circuits, and these circuits must interact in very precise and rapid ways. *Stuttering emerges in childhood as a symptom that the brain's neural circuits for speech are not being wired normally.* For this reason, early intervention is critical, because by shaping the child's experience, we can affect the ongoing wiring process in the child's rapidly developing brain. The longer the stuttering symptoms persist in early childhood, the more difficult it is for us to change the brain's wiring, and stuttering becomes a chronic, usually lifelong problem.

It can be seen in this definition that language is one of the prominent, but not the only aspect involved in stuttering.

In this quotation, Smith uses the word 'involving', perhaps as a way of avoiding having to be specific about the role language and the other factors play. Is a language deficit a factor necessary for stuttering to start, is it one of many mutually exclusive causes, does a child who starts to stutter operate within the margins of 'fluent speech' but the pressures of producing language (at language, motor and emotional levels) occasionally tip the child into bouts of non-fluency that can become established as incipient and later chronic stuttering? This small selection of the many questions that might be raised and the plurality of answers that could be given to each of them lead to a multiplicity of informal and formal theories about how stuttering should be explained.

Smith goes on to highlight the fact that a child's genetic endowment influences risk for stuttering and hints at the way in which this might affect developing neural circuits. She finishes off by highlighting her view that catching stuttering early and intervening are advisable. This makes accurate early diagnosis important. Once that is done, early interventions can be tried and their efficacy assessed.

Both the editors have a particular interest in language diversity and stuttering and they were honoured to be asked by the series editors (Nicole Müller and Martin Ball) to edit a collection of papers about multilingualism and fluency disorders. This led to the chapters in this book that focus mainly on language factors. Motor and emotional factors that Smith included in her definition are not discussed in detail in most chapters. This should not be taken to indicate that these are less important than language, it is merely a reflection of the topic of this volume.

The chapters are organized in three parts. The first is about procedures, methods and findings for studying language and its disorders. We were delighted that two authorities on multilingualism and child language (De Houwer and Mennen) agreed to write chapters highlighting different perspectives about bilingualism and language development. The chapters take psycholinguistic and linguistic approaches that tend to reflect cognitive and phonological processes respectively. Dworzynski was the lead author in a recent seminal paper that used twin methodology to estimate heritability of stuttering and she is able to talk informatively about genetics and methodology more generally. In her chapter, she describes the current state of the art on genetics and language, detailing not only work on stuttering, but also specific language impairment and speech disorder in a classic and well-studied family with a genetic speech disorder (the KE family). She explains the methods involved in this work, highlights how the link between genetics and brain structures have been mapped in the KE family (a step Smith's definition indicates will be necessary) and warns of some of the pitfalls in interpreting the link between genes, behaviour and CNS mechanisms. Our understanding of brain processes involved in language and its disorders has accelerated since scanning technologies have been available for research purposes. The two authors of Chapter 4 are authorities in the use of scanning data to document how the brain operates during stuttering (Watkins) and in bilinguals (Klein). They review the methods and procedures used in these areas. They point out that the regions of the brain that operate differently in stuttering and bilingualism correspond and consider ways in which this might affect risk for stuttering.

Part 2 addresses how language structure affects stuttering. The chapter by Howell and Rusbridge has two main aims. It attempts to: (1) show the state of our current knowledge about the pattern of stuttering in English; and (2) highlight some of the differences in language structure between English and the other languages of the world. Obviously these are mammoth tasks and fraught with difficulties. With respect to the first aim, the work is reviewed from a particular point of view (authors of other chapters offer different perspectives). With regard to the second aim, only the major considerations are highlighted, specifically those which might have relevance to stuttering and some of the main online resources that will facilitate cross-linguistic research are indicated. In some ways the role undertaken with respect to the second aim might have been more appropriate for Part 1. Chapters follow that examine Japanese, Spanish, Portuguese and Farsi (as well as other languages spoken in Iran). Some of these languages have markedly different structure to English and offer a testbed about which factors are and are not universal which will influence future accounts of stuttering. The authors of some of these chapters are leading authorities in their own country whose work is not known about in the West. The last chapter in this part is not about language per se. It concerns animism, which is widespread in Africa, and how this affects beliefs about stuttering in the family and at large. The picture painted about approaches to treatment offer a salutary lesson about how the introduction of new languages and cultures through colonial influences has not impacted at all levels of society.

Part 3 examines stuttering in bilingual speakers. Although stuttering and bilingualism have implications for theory (as seen in the first two chapters in Part 1, Van Borsel's review in this part, the proposal in Lim and Lincoln's, and Tsai *et al.*'s chapters), the main topic that most of the chapters address is about treatment of stuttering in bilingual speakers. One of the main topics in the work reviewed in Part 2 was how stuttering should be defined and this has an effect on many aspects of stuttering (theories of how language affects stuttering, as well as applied aspects like diagnosis and treatment). This topic is thrown into prominent relief by the chapters in this part where alternative symptoms were used to classify children as stutterers. This topic and the related issue of language features and symptoms of stuttering seen at different ages is returned to in the final chapter (Howell and Van Borsel). Although there is a diversity of perspectives about how language features and stuttering symptoms link together, everyone in the field is in agreement about their importance. More attention to the role of symptom specification for assessing fluency in bilinguals and their age-dependency would be useful for research into bilingualism in general and its impact on stuttering in particular.

It has been our pleasure working with the authors of these chapters, the series editors and the publishing staff. We hope that the topic of this volume will be revisited in a few years time to see which of the issues have been resolved, what new ones have been raised and how this has advanced our understanding of fluency disorders and language diversity.

Peter Howell and John Van Borsel
July 2010

Part 1

Procedures, Methods and Findings for Language and Its Disorders

Chapter 1

The Speech of Fluent Child Bilinguals

ANNICK DE HOUWER

Summary

This chapter discusses preliterate bilingual children's language development and issues of fluency. In doing so, it distinguishes between children with bilingual input from birth (Bilingual First Language Acquisition; BFLA) and children who added a second language to a first (Early Second Language Acquisition; ESLA). While many patterns of language development are similar for both these kinds of bilingual children, others are quite different. It is emphasized that an assessment of young bilingual children's language behavior needs to take into account the length of time of exposure to each language and children's levels of production proficiency in each language. These can vary greatly amongst bilingual children and are crucial in helping to determine whether any disfluencies are likely to be developmental in nature or not.

It is established that so far, there is no evidence for the claim that early bilingualism may be a cause of abnormal disfluencies. Rather than disfluent, the speech of young bilinguals is generally quite fluent. Disfluencies that do appear in bilingual children show the same patterns as have been identified in young monolinguals.

1 Introduction

In 1937, the influential French psychoanalyst and linguist Edouard Pichon published a book on stuttering with a speech therapist (Pichon & Borel-Maisonny, 1937) in which they claimed that early child bilingualism was a risk factor for stuttering. Pichon and Borel-Maisonny proposed that having to choose a word from the proper language amongst two alternatives each from a different language slowed down the speech production process and made it much more laborious and difficult, resulting in a higher chance of stuttering. In the same year, Travis, Johnson and Shover claimed to have shown a correlation between bilingualism and stuttering in nearly 5000 school children ranging from 4 to 17 years of age. Lebrun and Paradis (1984) criticized this work for failing to point out that one group of monolinguals in the Travis *et al.* (1937) study (the so-called 'Black monolinguals') presented proportionally more stutterers than the 'White or Oriental bilinguals' or 'White or Oriental multilinguals'. Lebrun and

3

Paradis (1984) thus suggested that instead of bilingualism, a racial factor might be relevant. Recent empirical evidence, however, shows that there is no basis for assuming that there is anything like racially determined stuttering (Proctor *et al.*, 2008). Lebrun and Paradis' (1984) point, though, that early bilingualism is not a causal factor for stuttering has recently been supported by Howell *et al.* (2009). Howell *et al.* showed that the proportion of diagnosed child bilingual stutterers in a sample of 317 children who stuttered in the greater London area (69 out of 317, or 21.8%) was in fact smaller than the proportion of child bilingual speakers in London schools (28.4%). This again calls into question the idea that bilingual children stand a higher chance of stuttering than monolingual ones.

The notion that early bilingualism might be a risk factor for stuttering, though, continues to be a concern to many parents and educators and, indeed, scholars: Karniol (1992) has gone as far as to suggest that early bilingualism should be avoided. She based this opinion on another view, viz. that acquiring two languages in early childhood increases cognitive load, and by implication increases the chance of stuttering. This is in line with Pichon and Borel-Maisonny's (1937) earlier claim that having to choose the proper word among two alternatives slows down the language production process.

The 'bad press' for early child bilingualism continues to exist. Yet, if a bilingual language learning situation really were to slow down the language production process, child bilinguals should be slower to develop speech than monolinguals. In fact, they are not. In spite of having to learn two languages rather than just one, bilingual children reach specific developmental milestones within the same age ranges as children who hear just one language (for overviews, see De Houwer, 2002, 2005, 2009, and below). In addition, reports of bilingual children's speech usually show them to be generally quite fluent in their speech production (I return to this point below; see also Mennen, this volume). Transcripts of actual bilingual child speech (see, e.g. the bilingual transcripts available through CHILDES (e.g. MacWhinney, 1991) as summarized in De Houwer, 2009) fail to show any general evidence of difficulties with speech production.

Until quite recently, however, there was no direct evidence that could either refute or substantiate the claim that in comparison to early child monolingualism, early child bilingualism increases cognitive load and thereby slows down learning. Recent research has shown that if there is an issue of slower learning, it is the monolingual children who are learning at a slower pace, and it is the bilingual children who have a cognitive advantage. Compared to age-matched bilingual infants, monolinguals have a much smaller comprehension lexicon (De Houwer *et al.*, 2006, in preparation), are much less able to suppress a previously learned response when needed (Kovács & Mehler, 2009a), exhibit less inhibitory control (Ibáñez *et al.*, 2009), cannot learn multiple structural regularities (Kovács & Mehler, 2009b), are less able to identify their native language in situations of high speaker variability (Polka *et al.*, 2010) and are less able to learn similar-sounding words (Fennell & Byers-Heinlein, 2010). Other research has found that bilingual and monolingual infants perform similarly on cognitive and language-related tasks (e.g. Albareda-Castellot *et al.*, 2010; Byers-Heinlein & Werker, 2010).

Clearly, bilingual infants show a cognitive and linguistic advantage over monolingual infants at best or perform similarly at worst. For somewhat older children, Grech and Dodd (2008) found that children growing up bilingually develop phonology faster than monolinguals. There is thus no empirical basis for earlier claims of a cognitive or linguistic disadvantage for young bilinguals. This, of course, does not imply that some bilingual children cannot develop fluency disorders. If they do, however, this should not be attributed to the fact that they are developing bilingually. Other factors will be playing a role.

In order to be able to assess whether children are developing any sort of language or speech disorder, it helps to know the facts about children who are developing according to expectations. In the following I will briefly summarize what those expectations are for hearing children under age 6 who have had experience with more than one language. The cut-off point of 6 years was chosen because the interest in this chapter is on bilingual children's speech as they acquire it in a non-instructed setting. Prior to age 6, few children get literacy instruction. Once formal literacy instruction is started, children's speech may be influenced by this literacy instruction (e.g. Gillis & De Schutter, 1996), thus adding an important variable that needs to be controlled for, especially in a bilingual setting, but that is beyond the scope of this chapter.

2 Experience with More Than One Language under Age 6

There are two main setting in which young children may gain experience with more than one language: the family, or more institutional settings such as day-care centers and nursery schools. Typically, when children hear two or more languages at home they will be hearing these languages from birth, and will be growing up in a Bilingual First Language Acquisition or BFLA setting (De Houwer, 1990, 2009; Swain, 1976). These children are acquiring two (or more) first languages.

Children who come into contact with a second language in a day-care setting or nursery school will have first been growing up monolingually, but soon after regular contact with a second language has become part of their lives they will be growing up bilingually as well. These children are then growing up in an Early Second Language Acquisition or ESLA setting (De Houwer, 1990, 2009; Letts, 1991; Li & Hua, 2006; Nicholas &

Lightbown, 2008; Pfaff, 1992; Vilke, 1988; a recent issue of the *German Journal of Linguistics* was devoted to ESLA, see Stark *et al.*, 2009).

Note that the difference between BFLA and ESLA refers only to the time of first regular exposure to a particular language[1]. It does not say anything about the reason why children start to hear two languages rather than one.

As I have argued elsewhere (e.g. De Houwer, 1998, 1999, 2009), a bilingual upbringing is usually a necessity, not a 'free' choice. This is true both for more wealthy families and for poor immigrant families.

So far there is no evidence suggesting that the difference between BFLA and ESLA is at all correlated with differences in socioeconomic background. However, it is important to distinguish between BFLA and ESLA for several other reasons. The dynamics, expectations and emotional demands are different in both settings. BFLA families will want children to learn to understand and speak two languages from the beginning (Language A (LA) and Language Alpha (LAlpha), no chronologically first or second language in this case) and there will be an emotional connection with both languages. In ESLA families there will generally be much more of an emotional connection with the first, home, language (L1) than with the second language that children are learning through day-care or preschool (L2).

The differences in learning settings for BFLA and ESLA imply that language use patterns will also be quite different in BFLA versus ESLA. Children in BFLA families will generally be expected to speak two languages at home and switch between them according to addressee or topic, whereas in ESLA, families will often expect monolingual L1 language use at home. In ESLA, parent–child communication patterns will often be disrupted if children start to speak the L2 at home (e.g. Wong Fillmore, 1991): parents may have insufficient comprehension proficiency in the L2 to allow full communication with their children.

Despite the expectation of bilingual language use in BFLA families, BFLA children may speak only a single language. This single language usually is the environmental language. Also in ESLA, children may end up speaking only the L2 (the environmental language). Unlike for ESLA families, BFLA children's use of only the environmental language does not usually disrupt parent–child communication to the extent that meaning exchange is no longer possible. However, there may be emotional consequences that impede harmonious communication within the family (De Houwer, 2009).

The fact that bilingual children may speak only a single language in spite of having regular contact with two languages is fairly common (about a quarter of bilingual families is in this situation; see De Houwer, 2007). To assume speech production in two languages in young bilinguals is thus unrealistic, although in three-quarters of the cases, children will in fact speak two languages to some degree. This is, however, a far cry from the 100% language transmission in monolingual cases where no language learning problems exist.

I defined BFLA and ESLA as relating to different acquisitional settings. There are also some important differences between BFLA and ESLA children that show up in the course of language development for each (in addition to similarities). This development is the focus in the next section.

3   A Brief Overview of the Course of Language Development in BFLA and ESLA: Focus on Speech Production

Like monolingual children, BFLA children start to produce single words in at least a single language at around the age of 12 months. Future ESLA children who are, at this point in time, still learning only a single language will also be saying some single words. Infants differ a lot from each other, however, in, for instance, how many different single words they say, and how fast they learn to say new words. This does not depend on how many languages children speak: children just vary a lot from each other in how fast they learn to talk. Some children produce 100 different words by the time they are 18 months old, others only 5 or 6 (De Houwer, 2009).

All BFLA children studied so far produce single words in both their languages in the second year of life. Some BFLA children produce their first words in two languages on the very same day, while it takes others a little more time to start saying words in LA in addition to LAlpha. The maximum time lag reported so far between children's first production of a word in LA and their production of a word in LAlpha is 3.8 months (De Houwer, 2009).

Since many future ESLA children are still in a monolingual environment when they say their first word, there is, compared to BFLA, generally a much wider gap between the ages at which an individual ESLA child produces her first word in the L1 and her first word in the L2. For instance, some ESLA children may speak their first L1 words at the age of 13 months, but will start to say L2 words only at the age of 50 months (4 years and 2 months), which is 37 months later. For ESLA children the point at which they start to say words in their L2 (in addition to their L1) is highly variable. Some ESLA children start to speak their L2 3 months after they first started to regularly hear it. Other children may start to speak in the L2 only after a year or even longer (Tabors, 2008). It appears that there is no absolute effect of age of first regular exposure here. On the whole, however, the earlier that ESLA children regularly come into contact with their L2, the sooner they will start to say words in their L2.

By the time children are 2 years of age, they typically start to produce utterances consisting of two words. Some children will have started to do so much earlier, but by their second birthdays, most children will have started to use these two-word utterances. There is no difference in the age range at which one can normally expect to hear two-word utterances from monolingual versus BFLA children (Patterson, 1998, 2000). This is yet another important milestone in speech production, then, where monolingual and bilingual children show no difference.

In the course of the third year of life, BFLA children (like monolinguals) start to produce three- and four-word utterances. Once children start to say utterances with three or four words, these utterances contain bound morphemes if the languages they are speaking employ them. However, the total number of different bound morphemes used by both BFLA and monolingual children will still be quite restricted in comparison to adult speech.

Length of utterance for children under age 6 is an important indication of the grammatical complexity of their speech. Gradually, BFLA and monolingual children's utterances will be so long that they can incorporate dependent clauses, different sentence moods and much more (Clark, 2009; De Houwer, 2009).

As previously indicated, when monolingual children start to regularly be in an environment where they hear another language (L2), they typically first say nothing in that L2. As noted before, this 'silent period' may be quite long. Once the previously monolingual but now ESLA children start to say words in the L2, these words may be used by themselves, or as part of formulaic utterances (Tabors, 2008). These are longer fixed phrases that might sound entirely error free, but which show little variation. The formulae often are imitations of other children's or the teacher's speech. Gradually, as ESLA children start to hear more of their L2 and want to use it more in interaction, they start to build utterances that are less fixed. This is when they start to make grammatical errors as well. The time lapse between ESLA children's first use of formulaic utterances and more constructed utterances varies greatly from child to child. As ESLA children use more and more novel, constructed utterances they usually show some structural influence from their L1 (in the domain of morphosyntax). This influence is most commonly shown through word order errors (Genesee *et al.*, 2004), although agreement errors (both within noun and verb phrases) are common, too.

There is a lot of variation between ESLA children in how fast they develop in their L2. A 6-year-old ESLA child who has had 3 years of intense exposure to an L2 may speak that L2 at the level of an age-matched monolingual child who has had input to that language as L1 for 6 years. At the same time, there are 6-year-old ESLA children with 3 years of intense L2 input whose level of language use in the L2 is more like that of a monolingual 3-year-old. Very little is known about the development of ESLA children's L1.

In contrast to ESLA children, BFLA children hardly show any structural morphosyntactic influence from one of their languages on the other. Quite to the contrary, as soon as BFLA children start to say multiword utterances, they follow the morphosyntactic rules of each of their two languages (De Houwer, 1990, 2009; Meisel, 2001). This is captured by the Separate Development Hypothesis or SDH, which states that 'the morphosyntactic development of the one language does not have any fundamental effect on the morphosyntactic development of the other' (De Houwer, 1990: 66). In spite of occasional reports of some BFLA children's speech production that may suggest that there is cross-linguistic transfer at play, the SDH appears to be very robust. An overview of nearly 50 BFLA children who as a group were acquiring 17 different language combinations, including typologically very distinct languages such as Basque and Spanish, as well as languages that are structurally much more similar, such as French and German, shows all of them to support the SDH (De Houwer, 2009, Appendix G).

The fact that BFLA children develop language according to the SDH does not imply that BFLA children speak their two languages at the same level of proficiency: there might, in fact, be quite a large difference between both (De Houwer, 2009). Some BFLA children speak one of their languages very well, and the other one at a level that reminds one of a much younger child. In this respect, BFLA and ESLA children resemble each other. However, there are most likely proportionally many more BFLA children under age 6 who speak both their languages with ease and at similar levels of proficiency than there are ESLA children who speak both their L1 and their L2 with ease and at similar levels of proficiency.

Speaking of course involves producing sounds. Relative to morphosyntactic development, we know fairly little about phonological and phonetic development in young BFLA and ESLA children (but see, e.g. Ronjat, 1913; Leopold, 1970; Johnson & Lancaster, 1998, for BFLA and the studies in Hua & Dodd, 2006a, for ESLA). We know even less of the variation in that development in relation to the variation amongst and within bilingual children as regards their overall use of a language, and their overall proficiency in it. One major finding for ESLA children, though, is that patterns of phonological and phonetic development differ in function of the specific languages that are being acquired. Thus, a Cantonese/English ESLA child will show different patterns of phoneme substitution or other kinds of errors than a Spanish/English ESLA child, for instance (Hua & Dodd, 2006b).

For BFLA, it is not clear to what extent the separate development that is in evidence for morphosyntax also applies to phonetics and phonology. There appears to be a great deal of variation between BFLA children in whether they approach their two input languages as phonetically and phonologically distinct. Also, there may be signs of differentiation for one particular aspect, such as syllable structure, but much less differentiation on the phoneme level (for an overview, see Chapter 5 in De Houwer, 2009). At issue is where this large variation between children comes from. One source may be the specific environment in which BFLA children grow up: it often happens that only a single person acts as a language model for a BFLA child to learn from. In BFLA phonetic and phonological development, the characteristics of this individual speech model may be a very strong guide for a particular BFLA child. In this case, peculiarities of a child's pronunciation may be explicable by the precise nature of the model.

In spite of the variation that is clear amongst BFLA children, they typically use the same kinds of phonological processes that have been found in monolingual children (De Houwer, 2009). ESLA children make abundant use of such phonological processes as well (see the contributions in Hua & Dodd, 2006a). Depending on the languages that are being acquired, the process through which children learn to correctly pronounce phonological segments may not be fully completed until children are well into the school years.

By the time they are 6, both BFLA and ESLA children are generally understandable to strangers and will generally be able to tell a connected story and use complex sentences.

4   Bilingual Children's Language Repertoires and Determinants of Which Language to Use

There are fundamentally two language use patterns for bilingual children under age 6 (Table 1.1). After a period of time in which they are just listening to a language but not yet actively speaking it, they start to speak two languages and continue to do so throughout their lives (see Pattern 1(a) for BFLA and Pattern 1(b) for ESLA). They are bilingual speakers. The other pattern is the one where, in spite of bilingual input, bilingual children eventually stop speaking one of their languages, and are now effectively monolingual speakers (see Pattern 2(a) for BFLA and Pattern 2(b) for ESLA).

Bilingual children who speak two languages have the option of saying utterances with words from just a single language (unilingual utterances) and utterances with words from two languages (mixed utterances). Bilingual children who are bilingual speakers are able to smoothly switch from one language to the other. The language repertoire of BFLA and ESLA children who speak just a single language is limited to unilingual utterances and, possibly, mixed utterances as well.

At age 6, most children have a well-developed metalinguistic ability which allows them to reflect on their own and other people's language use. This implies they will have some degree of awareness of how they

Table 1.1 Language use patterns for bilingual children under age 6

Pattern 1(a)	BFLA: child speaks two languages from the second year of life on, and continues to do so
Pattern 1(b)	ESLA: child speaks L1 from the second year of life on and continues to do so; child starts to speak L2 some time before age 6 and continues to do so
Pattern 2(a)	BFLA: child speaks two languages from the second year of life on, but stops speaking the non-environmental language some time before age 6
Pattern 2(b)	ESLA: child speaks L1 from the second year of life on; child starts to speak L2 some time before age 6 and continues to do so; child stops speaking L1 some time after the child has developed some speaking proficiency in L2

and others are speaking. For bilingual children, this awareness starts at a young age. Already in the third year of life, bilingual children make comments on what languages other people speak, or what languages they themselves speak (De Houwer, 1990, 2009). These comments show that for many bilingual children, the specific language(s) that people use is an important issue from early on. Consider, for instance, the case of Orren, a boy who lived in Israel who heard Hebrew and English from birth in the family, and Hebrew at daycare (Karniol, 1992). Orren heard English from his parents, who addressed each other in Hebrew. His parents spoke Hebrew and English to his older sister, who was instructed to speak only English to him. Hungarian relatives who visited spoke English to the child but not to his parents and sister. Thus, Orren was the only one in his family to be exclusively addressed in English. All the other family members shared something he was not part of at home: Hebrew (this is my interpretation of Karniol's description). Prior to age 2, Orren spoke English and Hebrew fluently. After age 2, Orren became more and more reluctant to speak English, complained that he was not addressed in Hebrew, and often begged his parents not to talk to him in English. After several months the parents did indeed decrease their use of English to Orren and started to address him in Hebrew as well. Orren stopped speaking English, and continued speaking in Hebrew (but also understanding English, as he overheard it mainly when his parents spoke it to his sister). This example shows how the use of a particular language in a bilingual family is something that can be negotiated and has strong emotional components.

Bilingual children who are also bilingual speakers will always have to select among their communicative options. In conversations with other bilingual speakers, children have the option of using unilingual utterances in each of two languages. Whether this option will be used, or whether children will use just one particular language, will depend on the interactional history that has been built up between the child and the bilingual speaker. This interactional history in turn will have been shaped by the specific discourse strategies that the bilingual speaker has used (Lanza, 1997). In bilingual settings, speakers can negotiate a monolingual discourse setting by not responding to utterances in a second language, or by asking for translations of utterances in a second language, or by asking for clarification, and, of course by using only utterances in a single language. These are monolingual interaction strategies. Bilingual interaction strategies allow the use of two languages within a conversation. Bilingual children are very sensitive to whether their bilingual conversational partners use monolingual or bilingual discourse strategies, and will build up expectations for which language should be used based on these discourse strategies (see also De Houwer, 2009, Chapter 4). It is likely that bilingual speakers who use bilingual interaction strategies with young bilingual children create a situation in which it is no longer necessary for a bilingual child to actually speak two languages. Combined with other factors such as input frequency, the use of bilingual interaction strategies may be a major explanation for why so many BFLA children end up speaking just a single language (De Houwer, 2009, Chapter 4).

In conversations with monolinguals, bilingual children who are also bilingual speakers will typically use only the language that their monolingual conversational partner understands. Bilingual children who are monolingual speakers can of course only effectively communicate with people who understand the one language they speak. ESLA children who only speak their L2 at home with family members who speak only the L1 will be able to do so with communicative effect only if their family understands the L2. This is not always the case, or at least, not sufficiently so. Especially as children grow older, family communication in this case becomes very difficult, with bad effects for all involved. As Tseng and Fuligni (2000: 473) found in their study: 'Adolescents who conversed with their parents in different languages felt more emotionally distant from them and were less likely to engage in discussions with them than were youths who shared the same language with their parents.' In BFLA settings, the monolingual speaker status of a child may create problems in communication with extended family members who do not understand the language the child speaks. The nature of bilingual children's language repertoires, then, is an important factor in their overall development (see also De Houwer, 2009, Chapter 8).

5 Developmental Disfluencies

Researchers investigating monolingual child speech have studied young children's speech errors in their own right (e.g. Bernstein

Ratner & Costa-Sih, 1987) and as a window into the beginnings of metalinguistic awareness (e.g. Clark, 1978, 1982). The notion 'speech error' refers to 'one-time error[s] in speech production planning (...) so that the production is at odds with the plan' (Jaeger, 2005: 2).

Speech errors may be repaired or just ignored. If they are repaired, a hesitation occurs, together with a reformulation (or, indeed, a repetition). Repairs or self-corrections, then, constitute a disruption of the flow of speech. Like other normal disfluencies, such as phrase repetitions, filled pauses and prosodic features, self-corrections must be distinguished from stuttering (see also Proctor *et al.*, 2008).

Young children often present with speech disfluencies (Jaeger, 2005; Wijnen, submitted). These are particularly common in 2- to 3-year-olds (Yairi, 1982), but gradually get less and less common. Children also differ quite a lot from each other in the extent to which they show speech disfluencies (Wijnen, submitted; Yairi, 1982).

The proportion of speech disfluencies is about four to five times higher in young children than in adults (Wijnen, 1992). This has much to do with the fact that in young children, speech production is far less automatized than in adults (Elbers & Wijnen, 1992; Wijnen, 1992). Speech production, after all, requires a great deal of effort at the beginning (see also Clark, 2009). Children need practice before they can become fully fluent.

Children's speech disfluencies may show difficulties with encoding language at different levels (Bernstein Ratner & Costa-Sih, 1987; Jaeger, 2005). As such, children's speech disfluencies cannot be examined without giving due attention to children's level of language development (e.g. Colburn & Mysak, 1982). Problems with both grammatical and phonological encoding have been specifically identified as giving rise to children's disfluencies (e.g. Wijnen, submitted; however, see Howell and Rusbridge, this volume, for a review of this work that draws a different conclusion).

Most of young children's disfluencies are developmental in nature and disappear after some time. The evidence suggests that about four in five children stop exhibiting a lot of disfluencies without any treatment (Curlee & Yairi, 1997; Rommel, 2001; Schulze & Johannsen, 1986; Yairi & Ambrose, 1999; Yairi *et al.*, 1993). Hence the term 'developmental disfluencies'.

There have been very few research studies of young bilingual children which have considered their fluency in speaking. The first one was the longitudinal Kate study by De Houwer (1990). Kate was a Dutch-English-speaking bilingual child who was recorded in natural interactions at home between the ages of 2 years and 7 months (2;7) and 3 years and 4 months (3;4). This put Kate right at the age where one would expect to hear a fair number of disfluencies. Kate presented with disfluencies in the form of self-corrections throughout the study. In general, the more she spoke, the higher the proportion of self-corrections (De Houwer, 1990: 312). In the recordings made between the ages of 3;2 and 3;4, however, there was a surge in self-corrections in both languages, with self-repaired utterances constituting 3.7% of all English utterances, and 3.8% of all Dutch utterances. The self-corrections or repairs were grouped into five categories: lexico-semantic repairs, morpho-lexical repairs, morphological repairs, syntactic repairs and phonological repairs. Phonological and morpho-lexical repairs were the most frequent in both languages (a morpho-lexical repair involved a change in the choice of a closed class lexical item). More than half of the self-corrections in each language were improvements over the first form produced (De Houwer, 1990: 317).

It has been suggested that young children mainly repair those elements that they are in the process of acquiring (Clark & Andersen, 1979). The Kate data contained a sizeable number of errors that were not repaired (De Houwer, 1990: 318), suggesting that Kate was not yet ready to repair these errors. It may be possible that repairs are in fact more frequent on those elements that children have just acquired, rather than on those they are still working on (De Houwer, 1990: 319).

In some unpublished tape recordings of Kate's speech when she was 4.5 years old, disfluencies were quite rare (again supporting the notion that many disfluencies in early child speech are developmental in nature). It should be noted, however, that Kate was one of those BFLA children who stopped speaking one of her languages (Kate stopped speaking Dutch after the family had moved from Dutch-speaking Belgium to the United States). Kate is now a mature multilingual adult with no history of stuttering.

Another BFLA child who stopped speaking one of his languages is the boy Orren who was mentioned earlier (Karniol, 1992). His speech contained a high level of disfluencies between the ages of 2;1 and 2;10. Orren was quite disfluent in both languages (given that data collection proceeded through the diary method, no proportions of disfluent vs. fluent utterances were given). At age 2;1, Orren was a proficient speaker of both English and Hebrew, and the examples of some of his utterances suggest that Orren was linguistically quite advanced for his age. There were no more disfluencies after age 2;10, once again confirming the notion that often disfluencies in early child speech are developmentally determined. Apart from a few exceptions, Orren stopped speaking English soon after that age. At around age 3;3, Orren started speaking English again after having been at a summer camp in Canada, and after some weeks in Canada, he stopped talking Hebrew. There were no disfluencies in Orren's English other than for some mid-sentence whole word repetitions with pauses in between.

A third longitudinal study that has focused on disfluencies in a bilingual setting is the one by Gut (2000), who focused on the acquisition of intonation in three German-English-speaking BFLA children between the ages of 2 and 4. The two girls in the study, Hannah and Laura, often paused between words as they started to produce longer utterances (Gut, 2000: 146–147, 150–153). Real disfluencies were more apparent when the children were older and were producing complex sentences. Thus, at age 3;10, the boy in the study, Adam, suddenly started to speak with lots of restarts, stuttering and interruptions. This happened in both languages. The pauses that Adam inserted, however, were not random. For instance, he did not insert pauses between a determiner and a noun (Gut, 2000: 157). Since there are no later data, we do not know how Adam's language development continued. Still, the types of disfluencies that he produced were very similar to those common in monolingual children.

Finally, my own longitudinal diary notes of my Dutch-English BFLA daughter Susan show that between the ages of 3;6 and 3;8 she went through a period of many hesitations and restarts as she attempted to formulate complicated ideas. Afterwards, she again became quite fluent, as she had been before.

Shenker *et al.* (1998) present a clinical case study of a French-English BFLA child who had started to stutter at age 2;5. The goal of the study was to see whether treatment in one language (English) would also benefit the other language. Treatment started when the girl was aged 2;11. Stuttering started to substantially decrease in English after 20 weeks of treatment, soon to be followed by a reduction in French (the untreated language) as well. The authors see this as evidence that this early stuttering could be successfully treated, even in a bilingual environment, but the possibility exists that what was defined as stuttering was in fact normal developmental disfluency, which would have decreased even without an intervention program.

To my knowledge, for ESLA children under age 6 there has so far been only a single study that has focused specifically on fluency. Carias and Ingram (2006) examined patterns of disfluency in two Spanish-English bilingual 4-year-old boys, M1 and M3, during a single therapy session with a speech and language clinician. M1 had been referred to speech and language therapy due to his preschool teacher's concerns about fluency and vocal quality. M1 had started to hear two languages at age 2 (it is not mentioned which was his L1). M3 had been diagnosed with language delay and was being treated for language disorder (his treatment did not focus on fluency). There is no information on M3's language learning history, so M3 might either be a BFLA or an ESLA child.

Carias and Ingram analyzed the types of disfluencies that occurred in the boys' speech samples in both their languages. The types of disfluencies identified were very similar to those found for monolingual children (repetitions, insertions, prolongations, pauses and repairs). Both children showed very different disfluency patterns, and whereas M1 used similar proportions of the various types of disfluencies in both of his languages, M3 tended to use repetitions mostly in Spanish but prolongations and insertions mostly in English. Both boys showed different proportions of disfluencies in both languages (M1 was most disfluent in the language that he also said the longest utterances in, i.e. Spanish; M3 was most disfluent in English, although the average length of his multiword utterances was fairly similar in both languages).

Since the sample sizes in this study were quite small (a total of 61 multiword utterances for M1 and even fewer – 49 – for M3) and concern only a single data point, it is too early to generalize these findings. However, findings from older Spanish-English bilingual children confirm the finding that disfluency patterns may differ across an individual child's two languages (see Carias & Ingram, 2006, for a 9-year-old boy and a 10-year-old girl; see Howell *et al.*, 2004, for a nearly 12-year-old boy).

Further empirical studies on fluency in pre-literate ESLA children appear to be lacking. One might expect issues of fluency to be discussed in connection with early phonological development and/or problems in phonological development. However, in the only volume on phonological development and phonological disorders in young ESLA children acquiring a range of languages to date (Hua & Dodd, 2006a) there is no mention of disfluencies. This may indicate that there weren't many. However, many testing situations that were used in the book did not necessarily tap into speech production.

The evidence so far, then, suggests that patterns of developmental disfluencies noted for bilingual children are similar to those found for monolingual children. Like monolingual children, bilingual children usually speak quite fluently. Periods with increased disfluencies are common, but short-lived and without noticeable effect on speech production later on, except that as bilingual children get older, their speech production becomes more automatized and more fluent still. We can concur with Shenker (2002) that so far, 'No evidence has been found to suggest that speaking two languages [by children] causes stuttering'.

6 Conclusion

What counts as speaking fluently will be different from one speech community to the next (e.g. Bernstein Ratner, 2004). There is also considerable cross-linguistic variation in the types of normal disfluencies that are used across different speech communities (e.g. Andersen *et al.*, 1999). In addition, the importance attributed to speaking fluently is culturally determined (Bernstein Ratner, 2004).

In spite of these important considerations, which are particularly relevant to a bilingual setting, where norms from two speech communities are combined, the fact remains that speech fluency has much to do with speech automaticity. Speech automaticity is gained after a lot of practice in speaking a particular language. For bilingual children, then, any assessment of the nature of their speech production in terms of fluency must take into account how long and how much they have been speaking a particular language.

ESLA children who have started to hear their L2 at age 4, say, may have only started to produce spontaneous, non-imitative speech in L2 at the age of 4 years and 8 months. If such a child is assessed at age 5, and found to speak very hesitatingly, a conclusion that the child is suffering from a fluency disorder would be premature. Any disfluencies may in fact be developmental in nature, and may disappear as the child gains more practice with the new language (see also Mattes & Omark, 1984, who warned against confusing disfluency that results from limited proficiency with a clinical fluency disorder).

Similarly, BFLA children who have unlearned one of their languages but who have started to speak them again may present with developmental disfluencies as well, even when they are already quite a bit older (age 5, say). Also, BFLA children who speak one of their languages much less frequently than the other, and, as an implication, usually also at a much lower level of proficiency (the weaker language) may also present with disfluencies in that language that are not present in their other language (the stronger language). The reason most likely is that the children in question have not yet had the opportunity to become quite as 'automaticized' in the weaker language. They might be going through developmental stages in that language which are typical of younger children. Such younger children might, at the same time of linguistic development, have shown normal developmental disfluencies as well.

For some BFLA children, the weaker language may be the environmental language: they may indeed have heard the environmental language and another language at home from birth, but may have had very little input to the environmental language at home (or what is called impoverished input, i.e. input from beginning second language learners). Thus, they may hardly speak the environmental language (but parents would say 'yes' to the question whether their child spoke the environmental language at school entry). Only when they start to attend pre-school or school may these children have a chance to develop their skills in the environmental language more fully. These kinds of BFLA children may have constituted a large proportion of the group of the 23 older BFLA child stutterers studied by Howell *et al.* (2009)[2].

Assuming that indeed level of automaticity is an important factor that helps explain developmental disfluency, it is important to control for actual speech practice in both a bilingual child's two languages. For bilingual children who have had a lot of experience with actually speaking in two languages there is no reason to assume that they will present with more than the normal developmental disfluencies at around the expected ages. However, like for monolingual children, considerable individual variation is to be expected. Unfortunately, for both monolingual and bilingual children, there are insufficient data on the length of the period of time that developmental disfluencies can still be considered within the normal range. This makes it difficult to assess whether a child at, say, age 5, who presents with a high proportion of false starts and repetitions is showing the beginnings of a fluency disorder. This is the case for both monolingual and bilingual children.

Indeed, the chance of developing a fluency disorder would seem to be the same for monolingual and bilingual children. There is nothing in the research literature on bilingual children under age 6 to suggest that there might be more chance of a fluency disorder in a bilingual than in a monolingual setting. This does not preclude the existence of wide variation within the large, heterogeneous group of bilingual children. In a unique study that takes into account stuttering bilingual children's language learning history, Howell *et al.* (2009) suggest that ESLA (or, in their terminology, LE) children have less of a chance of developing a fluency disorder than BFLA (or, in their terminology, BIL) children (they do not explain why this might be the case, though). They come to this conclusion on the basis of the fact that (1) in their group of bilingual stutterers, there happened to be more (N = 23) BFLA than ESLA children (N = 15); (2) in a matched group of bilingual non-stutterers, there happened to be more (N = 28) ESLA than BFLA children (N = 10), and (3) that the recovery rate of the ESLA children in the stuttering group was better than that of the BFLA children. More convincing evidence would come from a large group study of BFLA children on the one hand and age- and gender-matched ESLA children on the other, controlling for actual speech production in two languages and amount and regularity of input in the two languages within each group. If for a large cohort of, say, 6-year-olds, indeed statistically significant group differences were found for the incidence of stuttering, there would be sufficient proof. It then would still need to be explained why such a difference could be found. It seems more intuitive to expect more disfluencies in ESLA children, at least in their new second language, than in BFLA children who usually (in 3/4 of the cases; see above) have had experience with speaking two languages from early on.

In conclusion, in the assessment of possible disfluency disorders in young bilingual children under age 6, the length of time of exposure to each language and children's levels of proficiency in each language are to be taken into account. These can vary greatly amongst bilingual children and are crucial in helping to determine whether any disfluencies are likely to be developmental in nature or not. Rather than disfluent, however, the speech of young bilinguals is generally quite fluent. At present, there is no convincing evidence for the frequent claim that a bilingual childhood increases the chances of developing a fluency disorder.

Notes

1. The terms BFLA and ESLA are more precise than the perhaps at first sight similar terms 'simultaneous' and 'successive' or 'sequential' bilingualism. However, these are often used with different meanings. Often, 'simultaneous bilingualism' is used to refer to situations where children under age 3 have begun to acquire two languages, thus disregarding the crucial difference between acquiring two languages from birth and after. The term 'successive/sequential bilingualism' also applies to teens or adults who are acquiring a second language, and usually no distinction is made between children at pre-literacy ages and older children. For a terminological critique, see De Houwer (1990). See also more recently Verhelst (2009).
2. Howell *et al.* (2009) found that proportionally fewer of some of the BFLA children in their sample had recovered from stuttering by around age 12 than either ESLA or monolingual children. This is in contrast to findings reported by Shenker (2004), who reports that BFLA children on average needed fewer clinic visits than monolingual children to reach a point where they were no longer considered to be stuttering.

References

Albareda-Castellot, B., Pons, F. and Sebastián-Gallés, N. (2010) Acquisition of phonetic categories in bilingual infants: New insights from the anticipatory eye movements procedure, Paper presented at the 2010 International Conference on Infant Studies, Baltimore, MD, USA, 11–14 March.

Andersen, E.S., Brizuela, M., Dupuy, B. and Gonnerman, L. (1999) Cross-linguistic evidence for the early acquisition of discourse markers as register variables. *Journal of Pragmatics* 31, 1339–1351.

Bernstein Ratner, N. (2004) Fluency and stuttering in bilingual children. In B. Goldstein (ed.) *Bilingual Language Development and Disorders in Spanish-English Speakers* (pp. 287–308). Baltimore: Paul H. Brooks.

Bernstein Ratner, N. and Costa Sih, C. (1987) Effects of gradual increases in sentence length and complexity on children's dysfluency. *Journal of Speech and Hearing Disorders* 52, 278–287.

Byers-Heinlein, K. and Werker, J.F. (2010) How bilingual experience shapes early word learning, Paper presented at the 2010 International Conference on Infant Studies, Baltimore, MD, USA, 11–14 March.

Carias, S. and Ingram, D. (2006) Language and disfluency: Four case studies on Spanish-English bilingual children. *Journal of Multilingual Communication Disorders* 4, 149–157.

Clark, E.V. (1978) Awareness of language: Some evidence from what children say and do. In A. Sinclair, R. Jarvella and W. Levelt (eds) *The Child's Conception of Language* (pp. 17–43). Berlin: Springer-Verlag.

Clark, E.V. (1982) Language change during language acquisition. In M. Lamb and A. Brown (eds) *Advances in Developmental Psychology. Volume 2* (pp. 171–195). Hillsdale, NJ: Lawrence Erlbaum Associates.

Clark, E.V. (2009) *First Language Acquisition.* Cambridge: Cambridge University Press.

Clark, E.V. and Andersen, E. (1979) Spontaneous repairs: Awareness in the process of acquiring language. *Papers and Reports on Child Language Development* 16, 1–12.

Colburn, N. and Mysak, E.D. (1982) Developmental disfluency and emerging grammar I. Disfluency characteristics in early syntactic utterances. *Journal of Speech and Hearing Research* 25, 414–420.

Curlee, R. and Yairi, E. (1997) Early intervention with early childhood stuttering: A critical examination of the data. *American Journal of Speech-Language Pathology* 6, 8–18.

De Houwer, A. (1990) *The Acquisition of Two Languages from Birth: A Case Study.* Cambridge: Cambridge University Press.

De Houwer, A. (1998) Two or more languages in early childhood: Some general points and some practical recommendations. *AILA Newsletter* 1(1), 15–18.

De Houwer, A. (1999) Two or more languages in early childhood: Some general points and some practical recommendations. *ERIC Digest.* EDO-FL-99-03, July 1999, ERIC Clearinghouse on Languages and Linguistics. Center for Applied Linguistics, Washington, USA; http://www.cal.org/ericcll/digest/earlychild. html (sponsored by the U.S. Dept. of Education).

De Houwer, A. (2002) Comparing monolingual and bilingual acquisition. *Alkalmazot Nyelvtudomány [Hungarian Journal of Applied Linguistics]* II, 5–19.

De Houwer, A. (2005) Early bilingual acquisition: Focus on morphosyntax and the Separate Development Hypothesis. In J. Kroll and A. de Groot (eds) *The Handbook of Bilingualism* (pp. 30–48). Oxford: Oxford University Press.

De Houwer, A. (2007) Parental language input patterns and children's bilingual use. *Applied Psycholinguistics* 28(3), 411–424.

De Houwer, A. (2009) *Bilingual First Language Acquisition.* Bristol: Multilingual Matters.

De Houwer, A., Bornstein, M. and Putnick, D. (2006) Bilingual infants know more words: A monolingual-bilingual comparison of lexical development at 13 months using the CDI. Presentation at the Language Acquisition and Bilingualism Conference, Toronto, Canada, 4–7 May.

De Houwer, A., Bornstein, M. and Putnick, D. (in preparation) A bilingual-monolingual comparison of young children's word comprehension and production. Manuscript.

Elbers, L. and Wijnen, F. (1992) Effort, production skill, and language learning. In C. Ferguson, L. Menn and C. Stoel-Gammon (eds) *Phonological Development: Models, Research, Implications* (pp. 337–368), Parkton, MD: York Press.

Fennell, C. and Byers-Heinlein, K. (2010) Cues to a word's language boost bilingual infants' learning of minimal pairs. Paper presented at the 2010 International Conference on Infant Studies, Baltimore, MD, USA, 11–14 March.

Genesee, F., Paradis, J. and Crago, M. (2004) *Dual Language Development & Disorders. A Handbook on Bilingualism & Second Language Learning.* Baltimore, MD: Paul Brookes Publishing.

Gillis, S. and De Schutter, G. (1996) Intuitive syllabification: Universals and language specific constrains. *Journal of Child Language* 23, 487–514.

Grech, H. and Dodd, B. (2008) Phonological acquisition in Malta: A bilingual language learning context. *International Journal of Bilingualism* 12(3), 155–171.

Gut, U. (2000) *Bilingual Acquisition of Intonation: A Study of Children Speaking German and English*. Tübingen: Max Niemeyer Verlag.

Howell, P., Davis, S. and Williams, R. (2009) The effects of bilingualism on speakers who stutter during late childhood. *Archives of Disease in Childhood* 94, 42–46.

Howell, P., Ruffle, L., Fernández-Zúñiga, A., Gutiérrez,R., Fernández, A. H., O'Brien, M.L., Tarasco, M., Vallejo-Gomez, I. and Au-Yeung, J. (2004) Comparison of exchange patterns of stuttering in Spanish and English monolingual speakers and a bilingual Spanish-English speaker. In A. Packman, A. Meltzer and H.F.M. Peters (eds) *Theory, Research and Therapy in Fluency Disorders* (pp. 415–422). Nijmegen: Nijmegen University Press.

Hua, Z. and Dodd, B. (eds) (2006a) *Phonological Development and Disorders in Children. A Multilingual Perspective*. Clevedon: Multilingual Matters.

Hua, Z. and Dodd, B. (2006b) Towards developmental universals. In Z. Hua and B. Dodd (eds) *Phonological Development and Disorders in Children. A Multilingual Perspective* (pp. 431–449). Clevedon: Multilingual Matters.

Ibáñez Lillo, A., Pons Gimeno, F., Costa, A. and Sebastián Gallés, N. (2009) Inhibitory control in 8-month-old monolingual and bilingual infants: Evidence from an anticipatory eye movement task. 15th Annual Conference on Architectures and Mechanisms for Language Processing (AMLaP), Barcelona, Spain.

Jaeger, J. (2005) *Kids' Slips: What Young Children's Slips of the Tongue Reveal about Language Development*. Mahwah: Lawrence Erlbaum Associates.

Johnson, C. and Lancaster, P. (1998) The development of more than one phonology: A case study of a Norwegian-English bilingual child. *International Journal of Bilingualism* 2(3), 265–300.

Karniol, R. (1992) Stuttering out of bilingualism. *First Language* 12, 255–283.

Kovács, Á. and Mehler, J. (2009a) Cognitive gains in 7-month-old bilingual infants. *Proceedings of the National Academy of Sciences of the United States of America* 106(16), 6556–6560.

Kovács, Á. and Mehler, J. (2009b) Flexible learning of multiple speech structures in bilingual infants, *Science* 325(5940), 611.

Lanza, E. (1997) *Language Mixing in Infant Bilingualism. A Sociolinguistic Perspective*. Oxford: Clarendon Press.

Lebrun, Y. and Paradis, M. (1984) To be or not to be an early bilingual? In Y. Lebrun and M. Paradis (eds) *Early Bilingualism and Child Development* (pp. 9–18). Amsterdam: Swets and Zeitlinger.

Leopold, W. (1970) *Speech Development of a Bilingual Child. A Linguist's Record*. New York: AMS Press. (Original work published 1939–1949).

Letts, C.A. (1991) Early second language acquisition: A comparison of the linguistic output of a preschool child acquiring English as a second language with that of a monolingual peer. *International Journal of Language and Communication Disorders* 26, 219–234.

Li, W. and Hua, Z. (2006) The development of code-switching in early second language acquisition. *BISAL* 1, 68–81.

MacWhinney, B. (1991) *The CHILDES Project. Tools for Analyzing Talk*. Hillsdale, NJ: Lawrence Erlbaum Associates.

Mattes, L. and Omark, D. (1984)*Speech and Language Assessment for the Bilingual Handicapped*. Boston: College-Hill Press.

Meisel, J. (2001). The simultaneous acquisition of two first languages. Early differentiation and subsequent development of grammars. In J. Cenoz and F. Genesee (eds) *Trends in Bilingual Acquisition* (pp. 11–41). Amsterdam/Philadelphia: John Benjamins.

Nicholas, H. and Lightbown, P. (2008) Defining child second language acquisition, defining roles for L2 instruction. In J. Philp, R. Oliver and A. Mackey (eds) *Second Language Acquisition and the Younger Learner* (pp. 27–52). Amsterdam/Philadephia: John Benjamins.

Patterson, J. (1998) Expressive vocabulary development and word combinations of Spanish-English bilingual toddlers. *American Journal of Speech-Language Pathology* 7, 46–56.

Patterson, J. (2000) Observed and reported expressive vocabulary and word combinations in bilingual toddlers. *Journal of Speech, Language and Hearing Research* 43, 121–128.

Pfaff, C. (1992) The issue of grammaticalization in early German second language. *Studies in Second Language Acquisition* 14, 273–296.

Pichon, E. and Borel-Maisonny S. (1937) *Le bégaiement. Sa nature et son traitement.* Paris: Masson et Cie Editeurs.

Polka, L., Valji, A. and Mattock, K. (2010) Language listening preferences: Bilingual infants are more selective than their monolingual peers. Paper presented at the 2010 International Conference on Infant Studies, Baltimore, MD, USA, 11–14 March.

Proctor, A., Yairi, E., Duff, M.C. and Zhang, J. (2008) Prevalence of stuttering in African American preschoolers. *Journal of Speech, Language and Hearing Research* 51(6), 1465–1479.

Rommel, D. (2001) Die Bedeutung der Sprache für den Verlauf des Stotterns im Kindesalter. *Sprache Stimme Gehör* 25, 25–33.

Ronjat, J. (1913) *Le développement du langage observé chez un enfant bilingue.* Paris: Champion.

Schulze, H. and Johannsen, H.S. (1986) *Stottern bei Kindern im Vorschulalter. Theorie – Diagnostik – Therapie.* Ulm: Verlag Phoniatrische Ambulanz der Universität Ulm.

Shenker, R.C. (2002) *Stuttering and the Bilingual Child.* Memphis, TN: The Stuttering Foundation. Brochure for parents.

Shenker, R.C. (2004) Bilingualism in early stuttering: Empirical issues and clinical implications. In A.K. Bothe (ed.) *Evidence-based Treatment of Stuttering: Empirical Bases and Clinical Applications* (pp. 81–96). Mahwah: Lawrence Erlbaum Associates.

Shenker, R.C., Conte, A., Gringras, A., Courcy, A. and Polomeno, L. (1998) The impact of bilingualism on developing fluency in a preschool child. In E.C. Healy and H.F. Peters (eds) *Proceedings of the Second World Congress on Fluency Disorders* (pp. 200–204). Nijmegen, The Netherlands: Nijmegen University Press.

Stark, E., Bisang, W., von Heusinger, K., Grijzenhout, J., Geilfuss-Wolfgang, J. and Stiebels, B. (eds) (2009) *Early Second Language Acquisition/ Früher Zweitspracherwerb*, Special Issue, *Zeitschrift für Sprachwissenschaft* 28(1).

Swain, M. (1976) Bilingual first-language acquisition. In W. von Raffler-Engel and Y. Lebrun (eds) *Baby Talk and Infant Speech* (pp. 277–280). Amsterdam: Swets & Zeitlinger.

Tabors, P.O. (2008) *One Child, Two Languages* (2nd edn). *A Guide for Early Childhood Educators of Children Learning English as a Second Language*. Baltimore: Paul Brookes.

Travis, L.E., Johnson, W. and Shover, J. (1937) The relation of bilingualism to stuttering: A survey in the East Chicago, Indiana, schools. *Journal of Speech Disorders* 2, 185–189.

Tseng, V. and Fuligni, A.J. (2000) Parent-adolescent language sse and relationships among immigrant families with East Asian, Filipino, and Latin American backgrounds. *Journal of Marriage and the Family* 62(2), 465-476.

Van Borsel, J., Maes, E. and Foulon, S. (2001) Stuttering and bilingualism: A review. *Journal of Fluency Disorders* 26, 179–205.

Verhelst, M. (ed.) (2009) *Framework of Reference for Early Second Language Acquisition*. Language Policy Division, Council of Europe. Den Haag/The Hague: Nederlandse Taalunie.

Vilke, M. (1988) Some psychological aspects of early second-language acquisition. *Journal of Multilingual and Multicultural Development* 9, 115–128.

Wijnen, F. (1992) Incidental word and sound errors in young speakers. *Journal of Memory and Language* 31, 734–755.

Wijnen, F. (submitted) Disfluent speech in children: Encoding trouble and monitoring at different levels. Manuscript under review.

Wong Fillmore, L. (1991) When learning a second language means losing the first. *Early Childhood Research Quarterly* 6, 232–346.

Yairi, E. (1982) Longitudinal studies of disfluencies in two-year-old children. *Journal of Speech and Hearing Research* 25, 155–160.

Yairi, E. and Ambrose, N. (1999) Early childhood stuttering I: Persistency and recovery rates. *Journal of Speech, Language and Hearing Research* 42, 1097–1112.

Yairi, E., Ambrose, N. and Niermann, R. (1993) The early months of stuttering. A developmental study. *Journal of Speech and Hearing Research* 36, 521–528.

Chapter 2

Speech Production in Simultaneous and Sequential Bilinguals

INEKE MENNEN

Summary

Many children grow up in a bilingual or multilingual environment. Most of these children will learn to speak their two (or more) languages without any obvious difficulties. Even so, their speech may not be the same as that of children growing up in a monolingual environment. This chapter reviews the literature in the field of bilingual speech production. It will show how simultaneous and sequential bilingual children and adults produce the sound system of their two languages, and will focus on the similarities and differences of their productions with those of monolingual children. It will try to give an insight into the various steps bilingual children go through before developing the sound system of their languages from the preverbal stage towards actual acquisition of segments and prosody. From this review we can conclude that the child's brain is as able to cope with two (or even more!) sound systems as it is with one. The rate and path of sound acquisition in bilingual children appears to broadly follow that of monolingual acquisition. However, the two language systems of bilingual children tend to interact depending on a number of factors (such as age and manner of acquisition) and this causes slight differences between monolingual and bilingual children in their realisation of speech sounds and prosody in each language.

1 Introduction

Just as some monolingual children may develop fluency problems, so may simultaneous and sequential bilingual children. It is therefore important to have an understanding of the speech of typically developing bilingual children, as this will allow identification of atypical or disordered speech production or development. This chapter will therefore provide a description of typical speech and speech development in simultaneous and bilingual children.

Most bilinguals who started learning a second language (L2) later in life (i.e. in adolescence or adulthood) end up speaking the L2 with some kind of foreign accent. Such foreign accents can even be evident in the

L2 of bilinguals when exposure to the L2 started as young as 2 years of age (Flege *et al.*, 1995). More intriguingly, research suggests that even when bilinguals are exposed to two languages from birth, their speech production differs to some extent to that of monolingual speakers in each language (e.g. Kehoe, 2002). Just as we would not expect bilinguals to behave like two perfect monolinguals with proficiency levels equal to monolinguals in each of their languages (due to the fact that they use their languages for different purposes and in different situations and hence will have different needs and uses of the two languages, Grosjean, 1989), we also would not expect them to behave like two perfect monolinguals with respect to their sound systems. Many studies have shown that the degree to which the sound systems of bilingual speakers differ to those of monolingual speakers in each language depends to a large extent on whether exposure to both languages was from birth (simultaneous or childhood bilingualism) or whether the exposure was sequential (first one language, then the other), and in the latter case on the age of exposure to the L2 (Kehoe, 2002, Flege *et al.*, 1995; Piske *et al.*, 2001). This chapter will address the question of how simultaneous and sequential bilinguals manage two (possibly competing) sound systems, and to what extent and at which level they differ from monolinguals. It will present research pertaining to this question in healthy bilinguals (i.e. those without a speech or fluency disorder) both at the segmental or sound level (i.e. phonemes and allophones) and at the prosodic level (such as rhythm and intonation). It will also discuss some of the prerequisites a child needs to possess at the preverbal stage to enable him or her to acquire the sound system of two languages.

2 Towards the Development of a Sound System

This section gives a brief overview of some of the abilities bilingual children develop during the early stages of learning (i.e. the preverbal stage, before the child has reached the stage where they produce one-word utterances) and the steps they go through before ultimately acquiring the sound systems of their two languages.

2.1 Language discrimination

In order for bilingual children to acquire their two languages, they first need to be able to distinguish them from one another. One possible source for distinguishing their two languages is through cross-language phonetic differences. For bilingual children or infants to use this source of information, they have to be able to perceive these differences, remember them and distinguish them from other types of variation, such as regional, social or stylistic variation. Research shows that infants do indeed possess these abilities. Infants as young as 2 months of age show a preference for their surrounding language (i.e the one spoken by their parents) and one way they are able to discriminate it from other languages is by using the prosodic cues (in particular rhythm) that are available to them in the speech input (Mehler *et al.*, 1988). Bilingual infants were shown to have this same ability as monolingual children to discriminate their two languages on the basis of rhythm (Bosch & Sebastián-Gallés, 2001).

Other cross-language differences children may perceive are differences in their phonetic inventories and their fine-phonetic realisation of individual sounds. Very little is known about the abilities of bilingual children to discriminate the phonetic categories of each language when they are exposed to the phonetic segments of two languages from birth. What we do know from the limited evidence is that by the end of the first year of life, simultaneous bilingual children are able to discriminate both vowel and consonant categories in each language (Bosch & Sebastián-Gallés, 2001; Burns *et al.*, 2003, 2007). As for sequential bilinguals, discrimination may be poorer for some phonetic distinctions in the second language, as evidenced by a large body of research (see Strange, 1995, 2007).

In summary, we can conclude that simultaneous bilingual children appear to have the capacity to discriminate and remember language-specific characteristics of their two languages, which means that they possess at least some of the critical prerequisites to acquire these features in production.

2.2 Babbling

When does the speech of children start to resemble that of the ambient language(s) that they hear? Infants' early vocalizations are not thought to be language-specific, and infants appear to use sounds which could be from many different kinds of languages. Once they start babbling, either canonical or reduplicated, the sounds children make start to be combined in ways that could be conceived of as resembling real words. Research in monolingual infants has shown that the sounds produced during the babbling stage start to resemble aspects of the target sound system during the second half of the first year (Boysson-Bardies & Vihman, 1991; Boysson-Bardies *et al.*, 1984; Levitt & Utman, 1992; Whalen *et al.*, 1991). These studies showed differences in the distribution of certain phonetic characteristics, such as the use of fewer stops in French infants than in Swedish infants (Boysson-Bardies & Vihman, 1991), the greater proportion of closed syllables in English children as compared to French children (Levitt & Utman, 1992), or the larger proportion of rising than falling intonation in French children as compared to English children (Whalen *et al.*, 1991), reflecting differences in the adult target languages.

A few studies have investigated babbling in bilingual children. For instance, Oller *et al.* (1997) compared the time course of babbling in bilingual and monolingual children, and found that the onset of canonical babbling was the same for the bilingual and monolingual children in their study. Other studies investigated whether bilingual children phonetically adapt to the language they are babbling in, and found both evidence for as well as against. Maneva and Genesee (2002) found rhythmic differences between the babbling of a bilingual French-English boy (between the ages of 10–15 months) depending on whether he was interacting with his French-speaking father or his English-speaking mother. However, no reliable language-specific differences were found in the babbling of French-English bilinguals of a similar age by Poulin-Dubois and Goodz (2001). As there are only two studies investigating ambient language effects on phonetic features in bilingual children, it is too early to come to any firm conclusions as to whether the bilingual child's sound productions start to resemble that of adults in each language during the babbling stage. The next sections of this chapter deal with the actual production of language-specific features of the two languages of simultaneous and sequential bilinguals, and whether and how they differ from those produced by monolingual children and adults.

3 Bilingual Speech Segments

Traditionally, research into the acquisition of bilingual speech was mostly restricted to investigations of speech segments and in particular those produced by sequential bilinguals (i.e. L2 learners). This is reflected in L2 speech models such as Flege's Speech Learning Model (Flege, 1995, 2003) and Best's Perceptual Assimilation Model (Best, 1995; Best *et al.*, 2001) which without exception have yet to attempt to account for prosodic aspects of speech learning. Languages are known to differ in their phoneme inventories and their prosody (see Section 4), but even those phonemes that are judged 'similar' across languages may show subtle differences in the way they are phonetically realised, in their phonotactic distribution and they may even show 'systematic social and stylistic differences' (Khattab, 2002b: 336) (giving rise to many interesting discussions as to what should be considered similar, see for example Bohn, 2002). Such differences – alongside more global differences in the language-specific way the speech apparatus is used (for an overview, see Mennen *et al.*, 2010) – have to be learned by bilingual speakers. This section gives a general overview of the production of phonemes and language-specific allophonic realisation in the speech of simultaneous and sequential bilinguals.

3.1 Bilingual phoneme acquisition

The first question to ask is whether phonemes are acquired at the same rate and manner as in monolingual acquisition, or whether bilingual children show signs of delay or deviation in one or both of their languages. In order to answer that question there needs to be consensus on what it means to have 'acquired' a phoneme. Given the discussion above about the various levels of cross-language differences in sound systems, it follows that there are various levels of 'accurateness' of phonological acquisition, such as the level of the phoneme, fine-phonetic detail (i.e. phonetic implementation or realisation), distribution and sociophonetic variation. However, little consensus is found in existing studies on child bilingual phonological acquisition, making findings difficult to interpret, and there are hardly any studies investigating phonological acquisition at the distributional level or the level of sociophonetic variation (with the exception of Khattab, 1999, 2002b). For this reason, discussion is restricted to phonological acquisition at the level of the phoneme (this section) and the level of fine-phonetic detail (Section 3.2), but as the number of studies is small and the methodologies are different, care needs to be taken when interpreting the results.

Much of the research on child bilingual phonological acquisition has been concerned with the question of whether or not these children have one or two phonological systems at the start of phonological acquisition. It begs the question, though, whether we can actually talk about a phonological 'system' at the earliest stages of learning, and therefore the question of 'one versus two' does or should not actually arise (Vihman, 2002). What is perhaps more important is whether or not bilingual children acquire the phonologies of their two languages in the same way and at the same rate as monolinguals do. The majority of research has shown that this is generally the case. Bilingual children acquire the phonologies of their two languages with phonological patterns largely consistent with those of monolingual children (Genesee *et al.*, 2004; Ingram, 1981; Johnson & Lancaster, 1998; Lleo & Kehoe, 2002; Navarro *et al.*, 1995; Paradis, 1996, 2001). Nevertheless, some studies also show some level of interaction between the two systems. For example, Gildersleeve-Neumann *et al.* (2008) found a lower intelligibility, more segmental errors and more uncommon or atypical phonological errors in Spanish-English 3-year-olds when compared to age-matched monolingual children in each language. Goldstein and Washington (2001) also found that Spanish-English 4-year-olds were less accurate than monolingual children in their production of certain sound classes, yet overall accuracy levels were similar for bilingual and monolingual speakers. Similarly, Paradis (2001) found some differences in the truncation patterns of structurally ambiguous items by 30-month-old French-English bilingual children as compared to monolingual children. However, as pointed out by Goldstein (2005), the majority of phonological errors found in bilingual children are also commonly found in monolingual children. This suggests that the general path of child bilingual phonological acquisition follows that of monolingual acquisition, but with the possibility of some atypical patterns occurring due to the interaction of the two languages.

Much the same appears to be true for the phonological acquisition in sequential bilingual children. Holm and Dodd (1999) conducted a longitudinal study of two Cantonese-English children. The children were between the ages of 2 and 3, and were recorded at regular intervals starting at 3 months after their first exposure to English. Holm and Dodd (1999) concluded that their phonological systems for each language developed in similar ways to those of their monolingual peers, but that they also produced some atypical 'error' patterns and that there were differences in the rate and order of acquisition of some sound classes. These differences were attributed to language interaction. Results from a larger study (Tin, 2005) investigating phonological acquisition in Cantonese-English sequential bilingual children showed a faster rate of acquisition of phonemes that were common to both languages and that acquisition was faster in the dominant language (Cantonese). Differences were also found in the order of acquisition of some sound classes and in the prevalence of phonological processes produced.

3.2 Bilingual production of language-specific differences in fine-phonetic detail

Most studies of phoneme acquisition reviewed in the previous section rely on phonetic transcriptions of speech. In contrast, studies on child or adult bilingual production of fine-phonetic detail usually rely on acoustic measures. One of the most commonly studied acoustic measures is that of voice onset time (VOT). The seminal study by Caramazza *et al.* (1973) was the first to exploit cross-language differences in VOT patterns in order to investigate productions of these language-specific patterns in French-English bilingual speakers. Since, many studies have followed suit, including studies of bilingual children speaking French and English (Hazan & Boulakia, 1993; Watson, 1995), Spanish and English (Deuchar & Clark, 1996; Deuchar & Quay, 2000; Flege & Eefting, 1987b; Konefal & Fokes, 1981), German and English (Deuchar & Clark, 1996; Deuchar & Quay, 2000; Flege & Eefting, 1987a; Konefal & Fokes, 1981), English and Japanese (Johnson & Wilson, 2002), German and Spanish (Kehoe *et al.*, 2004), and Arabic and English (Khattab, 2000). Although the bilingual children investigated in these studies were mostly simultaneous bilinguals (Deuchar & Clark, 1996; Deuchar & Quay, 2000; Johnson & Wilson, 2002; Kehoe *et al.*, 2004; Khattab, 2000; Sundara *et al.*, 2006; Watson, 1990; Whitworth, 2000), a few presented results from sequential bilingual children (Flege & Eefting, 1987a, 1987b; Hazan & Boulakia, 1993; Konefal & Fokes, 1981). The gist of the findings is that simultaneous bilingual children are able to produce language-specific differences in their productions of stops, but that they differ from monolinguals in their phonetic implementation or realisation of these stops (particularly in the case of voiceless stops where VOT values are often different from monolingual values but the voicing contrast is maintained). Similar conclusions were made about the production of voicing contrast in *adult* simultaneous bilingual speakers (Sundara *et al.*, 2006).

There have been several studies that have investigated the acquisition of the voicing contrast in adult *sequential* bilingual acquisition (Caramazza *et al.*, 1973; Flege & Eefting, 1987a, 1987b; Flege *et al.*, 1995, 2003; Grosjean & Miller, 1994; Hazan & Boulakia, 1993; Mack, 1989). Results for this group confirm the findings for the simultaneous bilingual children in that these adults were able to produce language-specific differences in voicing, but their implementation was different to that of monolingual speakers with VOT values which are often reported to be intermediate to monolingual speakers in each language. Interestingly, when adult simultaneous bilingual speakers were compared to adult sequential bilingual speakers, the difference appeared to be in their similarities to monolingual speakers. It was found that although both groups were able to differentiate the voicing patterns of their languages, the sequential bilingual speakers differed from the monolingual speakers whereas the simultaneous adult bilinguals did not (Sundara *et al.*, 2006). This suggests that early learners have an advantage over late learners, as is also found in other aspects of speech production (see below).

Not all studies on the phonetic implementation of segment production in bilingual speakers were concerned with the acquisition of the voicing contrast. The number of studies of child bilingual acquisition that have investigated aspects other than VOT, such as the production of vowels (Gordeeva, 2005; Kehoe, 2002; Khattab, 1999), and liquids (Khattab, 2002a, 2002b), are however rather few. As with the production of the voicing contrast by simultaneous bilingual children, results of these studies show both a degree of language differentiation and systematic language interaction patterns. Simultaneous bilingual children are able to differentiate their languages with respect to the production of certain (but not necessarily all) language-specific sound structures, yet they differ from monolinguals in one or both of their languages (Gordeeva, 1995). The direction and extent of this interaction might to a large extent be dependent on the amount of exposure and is known to decrease over time (Gordeeva, 1995). This suggests that, as reported for VOT (Sundara *et al.*, 2006), once simultaneous bilingual children reach adulthood, there should be little or no difference between their sound production and that of monolingual adults and differentiation is then thought to be (near) complete. The vast body of work on sound production in sequential bilingual adults shows that this is indeed the case, with evidence for a milder foreign accent (Flege *et al.*, 1995, 1999b), and a more native-like production of vowels (Flege *et al.*, 1999a, 2003; Munro *et al.*, 1996; Piske *et al.*, 2002) and consonants (Flege, 1991; Flege *et al.*, 1995) in early than in late bilinguals. As we saw above, the evidence points to the fact that for sound production earlier is indeed better if the aim is to sound like a native speaker. Alongside age of learning, many other factors are thought to affect the degree of foreign accent in sequential bilingual adults, ranging from genetic make-up (e.g. neural networks), personality traits and attitudes (e.g. motivation, empathy, extraversion) to biographical factors (e.g. age of learning, length of residence or amount of L1 and L2 use) (see Piske *et al.*, 2001 for an overview). Of course, these factors would not only influence the degree of success in learning to accurately produce the segments of an L2, but also L2 prosody (as will be shown in Section 4).

4 Bilingual Prosody

In linguistics, prosody refers to aspects of speech such as its rhythm, tempo, loudness, stress, voice quality and intonation. Research into bilingual production of prosody is extremely limited, and the little available research, with a few notable exceptions, is mainly concerned with prosody in *sequential* bilinguals. As most studies have focused on bilingual intonation or rhythm, these are the prosodic aspects this section focuses on.

4.1 Bilingual intonation

Intonation has many important functions in communication; it conveys linguistic information such as whether a sentence is a question or a statement or which words in a sentence group together, it also provides the listener with information about the speaker, including aspects of their identity (gender, age), emotional or affective state (e.g. whether the speaker is happy, sad, angry), general health and social roles (e.g. Munson *et al.*, 2006; Scherer, 1986). Languages are known to differ in how these aspects of intonation are implemented in speech. Bilingual speakers who have access to two languages will therefore have to acquire the language-specific aspects of each intonational system.

There is a general belief that children acquire prosody and in particular intonation very early on in life, even before they have acquired their first words (Cruz-Ferreira, 2006; Snow, 2006; Snow & Balog, 2002) Indeed, when listening to babies babbling, one clearly gets the impression that the child is talking in a particular language by the baby's use of a language-appropriate melody. Yet, using a language-appropriate melody does not mean that the child has fully acquired the language's intonation system, including its rich inventory of structural elements (i.e. pitch accents and boundary tones), how these elements combine into intonational tunes (i.e.

phonotactics), and in particular the language-specific phonetic realisation of these tunes and pitch accents (i.e. the timing or height of peaks or valleys).

To my knowledge, there are just three studies that have investigated the acquisition of intonation in simultaneous bilinguals, namely Cruz-Ferreira (2003, and more detail is given in Cruz-Ferreira, 2006), Grichkovtsova (2006) and Gut (2000). Cruz-Ferreira (2006) followed her own Portuguese-Swedish bilingual children between the ages of 0;7 and 1;9 and found that even when they were still at the stage of canonical babbling and were not using words as yet, the intonation of their utterances sounded like Portuguese or Swedish depending on the language of the interlocutors. This suggests that the children varied their intonation patterns in a language-appropriate way, even though they might still be some distance away from full mastery of the intonation system of each language.

Grichkovtsova (2006) investigated the production of affective prosody (such as happiness, sadness, anger) by seven Scottish-English/French bilingual children between the ages of 7 and 10. She measured some of the acoustic correlates involved in the production of affective prosody in these two languages and found that the bilingual children were able to produce affective prosody in a language-specific manner (as each affective state was identified correctly by adult native listeners), even though there were some differences between their productions of affective states and those produced by monolingual children in each language. Interestingly, she reports that affective states had a higher recognition rate in the bilingual children than in the monolingual children, suggesting that the bilingual children might have exaggerated the differences between the two languages, perhaps in order to maintain differences across affective states both within and across languages (in line with observations at the segmental level by Mack 1990).

Gut (2000) investigated the intonational acquisition of three German-English bilingual children between the ages of 2;1 and 5;5. Her study focused on three aspects of intonation, i.e. nucleus placement, pitch and intonational phrasing, and each of these areas was investigated at both the phonetic and phonological level. Gut's results show that these bilingual children had a different rate of development in their two languages in all three aspects of investigation. Furthermore, the bilingual children were able to produce some cross-language differences, although these were not produced consistently and varied between the three children.

We now turn to the production of intonation in sequential bilinguals. The intonation systems of languages can differ along four dimensions of intonation (Ladd, 1996) and the cross-language differences in each of these dimensions need to be learned by bilingual speakers. These dimensions of intonation are, according to Ladd (1996: 119): (1) the inventory of structural elements (i.e. boundary tones and pitch accents); (2) the phonetic implementation or realisation of these elements; (3) their distribution (phonotactic differences); and (4) functionality (i.e. how they are used to signal certain functions such as marking interrogativity or focus). Most research into the intonation production of sequential bilinguals employs a 'target deviation' or 'error analysis' approach which uses the monolingual production of the target language as a yardstick against which certain aspects of L2 intonation are measured. As such, most of the above-mentioned dimensions of intonation have been investigated, albeit usually not within a single study. The exceptions are Chen and Mennen (2008); Mennen, Chen & Karlsson (2010), which investigated the intonation system of sequential bilinguals along all four of Ladd's dimensions.

Willems (1982) investigated the *inventory* and *distribution* of pitch accents and found that Dutch-English sequential bilinguals produced rises where monolingual English speakers would use falls. Similar findings of differences in the type and/or distribution of pitch accents and boundary tones between bilinguals and monolinguals were found by Adams and Munro (1978), Backman (1979), Huang and Jun (2009), Jenner (1976), Jilka (2000) and Lepetit (1989). The dimension of *phonetic realisation* appears to be particularly susceptible to mutual influences from the sound systems of sequential bilinguals (Mennen, 2004; Mennen, Chen & Karlsson 2010). Examples are differences in the slope of a pitch rise (e.g. Backman, 1979; Ueyama, 1997; Willems, 1982) or the timing of phonologically identical rising pitch accents (Mennen, 2004). Another example of phonetic realisation is pitch register (i.e. the overall height of someone's voice) and global pitch range (i.e. pitch variation during speech), both of which have often been reported to differ between monolingual and bilingual speakers (Backman, 1979; Braun, 1994; Gfroerer & Wagner, 1995; Jenner, 1976; Jilka, 2000; Mennen, 2007; Scharff-Rethfeldt *et al.*, 2008; Willems, 1982). Studies concerning the *functional use* of intonation in sequential bilinguals investigated amongst other things the use of intonation in focus marking (Ueyama & Jun, 1998) and turn taking (Cruz-Ferreira, 2003, 2006; Wennerstrom, 1994). As with the other dimensions of intonation, differences were found between the functional use of intonation in sequential bilinguals as compared to monolinguals, including the use of different cues to signal focus (such as differences in f0 excursion, duration, or intensity) and realisational differences in the signalling of topic shift.

In summary, it is clear from the above studies that the intonation system of sequential bilingual speakers does not necessarily resemble that of monolingual speakers in every single detail. Furthermore, the research suggests that it may differ from the system of monolingual speakers in each of the four dimensions of intonation, although differences might be most obvious in the distribution of structural elements and their phonetic realisation (e.g. Mennen, 2004; Mennen, Chen & Karlsson, 2010). As for simultaneous bilinguals, there are currently too few studies to come to conclusions as to how childhood bilinguals deal with two intonation systems and to what extent they differ from monolingual children. However, just as with speech segments, it appears that age of exposure may exert an effect on overall success in acquiring L2 intonation. Thus, Huang and Jun (2009) found that individuals who were exposed to two languages from childhood (with age of arrival between 5 and 9 years of age) performed better in L2 intonation than individuals who arrived in early adolescence or adulthood.

4.2 Bilingual rhythm production

The idea that languages can be classified according to whether they are 'stress-timed' or 'syllable-timed' has been around for a very long time (Abercrombie, 1967; Pike, 1945). In so-called 'syllable-timed' languages (such as French) syllables were thought to be of equal duration, whereas in 'stress-timed' languages (such as English or German) it was thought that it was the inter-stress intervals that were of equal duration. Instrumental support for a language dichotomy based on syllable-based or stress-based isochrony has, however, not been found. Yet, adults (Dupoux *et al.*, 2003) and even newborns (Nazzi *et al.*, 1998, 2000) can discriminate utterances according to their global rhythmic properties and are thus sensitive to rhythm classes. More recently, various timing metrics have been suggested to quantify these perceptual cross-language differences in rhythm. Specifically, various metrics that exploit cross-language differences in syllable complexity, final lengthening and vowel reduction have been proposed, such as the pairwise variability indices (PVI) and interval measures (see White & Mattys, 2007 for a discussion). These metrics segment speech into vocalic and intervocalic (consonantal) intervals, thus exploiting structurally determined differences between stress-timed and syllable-timed languages (such as for example the fact that in stress-timed languages there is a larger differences in vowel duration between stressed and unstressed syllables).

The above-described metrics have been used in a number of studies to investigate the acquisition of speech rhythm in monolingual and bilingual children and adult L2 learners. For example, Grabe *et al.* (1999a) showed for monolingual children, that both French and British English-speaking 4;3- to 5;0-year-olds had similar PVI values at the syllable-timed end of the spectrum, even though the PVI values of the target languages (French and English) spoken by monolingual adults differ (with values more at the stress-timed end in English and more at the syllable-timed end in French). As acquisition progressed, the values for rhythmic patterns of children started to diverge, with English-speaking children developing more stress-timed rhythm and French-speaking children remaining more at the syllable-timed end of the spectrum. This suggests that children may go through a first stage of syllable-timed rhythm before developing a more target-like rhythm, although more research with carefully controlled materials is needed to ensure that this is not an artefact of cross-language differences in syllable structure.

Whitworth (2002) used PVI measures to examine the acquisition of rhythm by six simultaneous German-English bilingual children varying in age from 5;0 to 13;2. Both German and English are usually considered stress-timed languages, although due to differences in syllable structure and stress patterns they are placed at different places on the continuum with German more towards the higher end of stress-timed languages than English (Grabe & Low, 2002; Grabe *et al.*, 1999b). Whitworth (2002) found that children were able to produce separate rhythmic patterns for the two languages, but that these patterns differed from adult monolingual patterns. She also found support for Grabe *et al.*'s (1999b) finding that children proceed from a more syllabic rhythmic pattern (despite the fact that they are acquiring two languages that are considered stress-timed) to a more target-like pattern during the acquisition process; Whitworth's results suggest that this process might not be complete until around the age of 11.

Bunta and Ingram (2007) investigated the acquisition of rhythm by Spanish-English simultaneous bilingual 4- and 5–year-olds. The sample group in this study is relatively large, compared to prior investigations of rhythm acquisition, with a total of 30 children (10 monolingual American English children, 10 monolingual Mexican Spanish children and 10 Spanish-English bilingual children) and 18 adults (6 American English monolinguals, 6 Mexican-Spanish monolinguals, and 6 Spanish-English bilingual adults) investigated. In line with Grabe *et al.* (1999b), the results showed an early bias for syllable-timed rhythm. However, as Bunta and Ingram (2007) point out, it is not possible to ascertain whether this bias is due to an acquisitional process that makes children start out with syllable-timed rhythm before acquiring target-like rhythm or whether it is due to Spanish dominance (given that all children were Spanish dominant). Nevertheless, children at 4 years of age were able to differentiate the rhythm patterns of their languages in production, although their English rhythm patterns were not identical to that of their monolingual peers. In other words, although they produced distinct rhythm patterns for the two languages, there was some interference from Spanish rhythm in their production of English rhythm (which also confirmed that they were Spanish dominant). The results for the 5-year-old bilingual children were similar to that of the 4-year-olds, except that at this age the differences between the bilingual children and their monolingual English peers had diminished somewhat. This finding suggests that bilingual children over time acquire the language-specific rhythm for both languages. This is further confirmed by the results for the bilingual adults, which showed that they were able to produce similar rhythm patterns to their monolingual peers in each language.

A number of studies have used rhythm metrics to investigate the acquisition of rhythm of the L2 in sequential bilinguals (Carter, 2005; Grenon & White, 2008; Gut, 2003; Lin & Wang, 2005, 2007; Low *et al.*, 2000; White & Mattys, 2007), with a variety of target languages (including American English, British English, Canadian English, Castellano Spanish, Dutch, German, Japanese and Singapore English) and source languages (Castellano Spanish, Chinese, Dutch, French, Italian, Japanese, Mexican Spanish, and Romanian). The general finding is that L2 rhythm values are usually intermediate between those of monolingual speakers of the L1 and L2.

In summary, the limited studies on bilingual rhythm acquisition suggest that simultaneous bilinguals may have a better chance than sequential bilinguals at achieving native-like values for the rhythm patterns in both their languages, but that learning the language-specific rhythm may take up to 10 years to acquire (Whitworth, 2002). Sequential bilinguals, on the other hand, may never acquire native patterns of speech rhythm and end up with values intermediate between the L1 and L2.

5 Summary and Conclusion

Despite the challenge of acquiring the two (often competing) sound systems of their languages, bilingual children appear to achieve this with remarkable ease. Although some aspects of sound structure may take longer than others, overall it appears that when children acquire two languages simultaneously they are able to differentiate language-specific sounds and over time the differences between their sound productions and those of monolingual children will diminish. Interaction between the sound systems of the two languages should be seen as a normal phenomenon and is usually particularly prominent at the beginning stages of learning. As with other aspects of bilingual acquisition, the earlier learning starts the better the prospects of achieving nativeness. This applies to segmental as well as prosodic acquisition. It is clear that children are perfectly well equipped to acquire two languages (or more), as the rate and manner of sound acquisition broadly follows that of monolingual acquisition. Nevertheless, the differences that have been observed between monolingual and bilingual acquisition are very interesting as they provide a source of information about how sound systems interact and what their phonetic/phonological representation is. They certainly deserve to be studied much more than they currently are, and studies examining cross-language differences in speech production in bilingual children with fluency or other speech disorders would shed further light on the interaction of speech systems, particularly since some of these differences are still present at the age when children usually begin to stutter.

Acknowledgements

The support of the Economic and Social Research Council (ESRC), the Higher Education Funding Council for Wales and the Welsh Assembly Government, is gratefully acknowledged. This work was part of the programme of the Centre for Bilingualism in Theory and Practice. I would also like to thank Dr Mikhail Ordin for his valuable input to this chapter.

References

Abercrombie, D. (1967) *Elements of General Phonetics.* Edinburgh: Edinburgh University Press.

Adams, C. and Munro, R. (1978) In search of the acoustic correlates of stress: Fundamental frequency, amplitude, and duration in the connected utterances of some native and non-native speakers of English. *Phonetica* 35, 125–156.

Backman, N. (1979) Intonation errors in second language pronunciation of eight Spanish speaking adults learning English. *Interlanguage Studies Bulletin* 4(2), 239–266.

Best, C. (1995) A direct realist view of cross-language speech perception. In W. Strange (ed.) *Speech Perception and Linguistic Experience: Theoretical and Methodological Issues* (pp. 171–204). Timonium, MD: York Press.

Best, C., McRoberts, G. and Goodell, E. (2001) American listeners' perception of nonnative consonant contrasts varying in perceptual assimilation to English phonology. *Journal of Acoustical Society of America* 1097, 775–794.

Bohn, O. (2002) On phonetic similarity. In P. Burmeister, T. Piske and A. Rohde (eds) *An Integrated View of Language Development: Papers in Honor of Henning Wode* (pp. 191–216). Verlag, Trier: Wissenschaftlicher.

Bosch, L. and Sebastián-Gallés, N. (2001) Evidence of early language discrimination abilities in infants from bilingual environments. *Infancy* 2(1), 29–49.

Boysson-Bardies, B. and Vihman, M.M. (1991) Adaptation to language: Evidence from babbling and first words in four languages. *Language* 67, 297–319.

Boysson-Bardies, B., Sagart, L.M. and Durand, C. (1984) Discernible differences in the babbling of infants according to target language. *Journal of Child Language* 11(1), 1–15.

Braun, A. (1994) Sprechstimmlage und Muttersprache. *Zeitschrift für Dialektologie und Linguistik* LXI(2), 170–178.

Bunta, F. and Ingram, D. (2007) The acquisition of speech rhythm by bilingual Spanish- and English-speaking four- and five-year-old children. *Journal of Speech, Language, and Hearing Research* 50, 999–1014.

Burns, T.C., Werker, J. and McVie, K. (2003) Development of phonetic categories in infants raised in bilingual and monolingual environments. In *Proceedings of the 27th Annual Boston University Conference on Language Development.*

Burns, T.C., Yoshida, K.A., Hill, K. and Werker, J.F. (2007) The development of phonetic representation in bilingual and monolingual infants. *Applied Psycholinguistics* 28(3), 455–474.

Caramazza, A., Yeni-Komshian, G.H., Zurif, E. and Carbone, E. (1973) The acquisition of a new phonological contrast: The case of stop consonants in French-English bilinguals. *Journal of the Acoustic Society of America* 54(2), 421–428.

Carter, P.M. (2005) Prosodic variation in SLA: Rhythm in an urban North Carolina Hispanic community. *Penn Working Papers in Linguistics* 11(2), 59–71.

Chen, A. and Mennen, I. (2008) Encoding interrogativity intonationally in a second language. In *Speech Prosody 2008*, Campinas, Brazil.

Cruz-Ferreira, M. (2003) Two prosodies: Two languages: Infant bilingual strategies in Portugese and Swedish. *Journal of Portugese Linguistics* 2, 45–60.

Cruz-Ferreira, M. (2006) *Three Is a Crowd?: Acquiring Portuguese in a Trilingual Environment (Child Language and Child Development)* (illustrated edition). Clevedon: Multilingual Matters.

Deuchar, M. and Clark, A. (1996) Early bilingual acquisition of the voicing contrast in English and Spanish. *Journal of Phonetics* 24(3), 351–365.

Deuchar, M. and Quay, S. (2000) *Bilingual Acquisition: Theoretical Implications of a Case Study.* Oxford: Oxford University Press.

Dupoux, E., Kouider, S. and Mehler, J. (2003) Lexical access without attention? Explorations using dichotic priming. *Journal of Experimental Psychology: Human Perception and Performance* 29(1), 172–184.

Flege, J.E. (1991) Age of learning affects the authenticity of voice onset time (VOT) in stop consonants produced in a second language. *Journal of Acoustical Society of America* 89(1), 395–411.

Flege, J.E. (1995) Second language speech learning: Theory, findings, and problems. In W. Strange (ed.) *Speech Perception and Linguistic Experience: Theoretical and Methodological Issues* (pp. 233–277). Timonium, MD: York Press.

Flege, J.E. (2003) Assessing constraints on second-language segmental production and perception. In A. Meyer and N. Schiller (eds) *Phonetics and Phonology in Language Comprehension and Production, Differences and Similarities* (pp. 319–355). Berlin: Mouton de Gruyter.

Flege, J.E. and Eefting, W. (1987a) Cross-language switching in stop consonant perception and production by Dutch speakers of English. *Speech Communication* 6, 185–202.

Flege, J.E. and Eefting, W. (1987b) Production and perception of English stops by native Spanish speakers. *Journal of Phonetics* 15, 67–83.

Flege, J.E., MacKay, I.R. and Meador, D. (1999a) Native Italian speakers' perception and production of English vowels. *Journal of Acoustical Society of America* 106(5), 2973–2987.

Flege, J.E., Munro, M. and MacKay, I.R. (1995) Effects of age of second-language learning on the production of English consonants. *Speech Communication* 16(1), 1–26.

Flege, J.E., Schirru, C. and MacKay, I.R. (2003) Interaction between the native and second language phonetic subsystems. *Speech Communication* 40, 467–491.

Flege, J.E., Takagi, N. and Mann, V. (1995) Japanese adults can learn to produce English /r/ and /l/ accurately. *Language and Speech* 38(1), 25–55.

Flege, J.E., Yeni-Komshian, G. and Liu, S. (1999b) Age constraints on second-language acquisition. *Journal of Memory and Language* 41(1), 78–104.

Genesee, F., Paradis, J. and Crago, M. (2004) *Dual Language Development and Disorders: A Handbook on Bilingualism and Second Language Learning.* Communication and Language Intervention Series. Baltmore, MD: Brookes Publishing Company.

Gfroerer, S. and Wagner, I. (1995) Fundamental frequency in forensic speech samples. In A. Braun and J. Koester (eds) *Studies in Forensic Phonetics* (pp. 41–48). Trier: Wissenschaftlicher Verlag Trier.

Gildersleeve-Neumann, C., Kester, E., Davis, B. and Peña, E. (2008) English speech sound development in preschool-aged children from bilingual English–Spanish environments. *Language, Speech, and Hearing Services in Schools* 39(3), 314–328.

Goldstein, B. (2005) Substitution patterns in the phonology of Spanish-speaking children. *Journal of Multilingual Communication Disorders* 3(2), 153–168.

Goldstein, B. and Washington, P. (2001) An initial investigation of phonological patterns in typically developing 4-year-old Spanish-English bilingual children. *Language, Speech, and Hearing Services in Schools* 32(3), 153–164.

Gordeeva, O. (1995) *Language Interaction in the Bilingual Acquisition of Sound Structure: A Longitudinal Study of Vowel Quality, Duration and Vocal Effort in Pre-School Children Speaking Scottish English and Russian*. PhD thesis, Queen Margaret University College, Edinburgh, United Kingdom.

Gordeeva, O. (2005) Acquisition of vowel duration conditioning in Russian-Scottish English bilingual children. Presented at the 5th International Symposium on Bilingualism, Universitat Politècnica de Catalunya.

Grabe, E. and Low, L. (2002) Acoustic correlates of rhythm class. In C. Gussenhoven and N. Warner (eds) *Laboratory Phonology* 7 (pp. 515–546). New York: Mouton de Gruyter.

Grabe, E., Post, B. and Watson, I. (1999a) The acquisition of rhythmic patterns in English and French. In *Proceedings of the International Congress of Phonetic Sciences*, San Francisco.

Grabe, E., Gut, U., Post, B. and Watson, I. (1999b) The acquisition of rhythm in English, French and German. In *Current Research in Language and Communication: Proceedings of the Child Language Seminar*. London: City University.

Grenon, I. and White, L. (2008) Acquiring rhythm: A comparison of L1 and L2 speakers of Canadian English and Japanese. In *Proceedings of the 32nd Boston University Conference on Language Development* (pp. 155–166). Boston.

Grichkovtsova, I. (2006) *A Cross-linguistic Study of Affective Prosody Production by Monolingual and Bilingual Children*. PhD thesis, Queen Margaret University College, Edinburgh, United Kingdom.

Grosjean, F. (1989) Neurolinguists, beware! The bilingual is not two monolinguals in one person. *Brain and Language* 36(1), 3–15.

Grosjean, F. and Miller, J. (1994) Going in and out of languages: An example of bilingual flexibility. *Psychological Science* 5(4), 201–206.

Gut, U. (2000) *Bilingual Acquisition of Intonation*. Linguistische Arbeiten. Tübingen: Niemeyer.

Gut, U. (2003) Prosody in second language speech production: The role of the native language. *Fremdsprachen Lehren und Lernen* 32, 133–152.

Hazan, V. and Boulakia, G. (1993) Perception and production of a voicing contrast by French-English bilinguals. *Language and Speech* 36(1), 17–38.

Holm, A. and Dodd, B. (1999) A longitudinal study of the phonological development of two Cantonese–English bilingual children. *Applied Psycholinguistics* 20, 349–376.

Huang, B. and Jun, S. (2009) Age effect on the acquisition of second language prosody. In *Online Supplement to the Proceedings of the 33rd Boston University Conference on Language Development*, Boston.

Ingram, D. (1981) The emerging phonological system of an Italian-English bilingual child. *Journal of Italian Linguistics* 2, 95–113.

Jenner, B. (1976) Interlanguage and foreign accent. *Interlanguage Studies Bulletin* 1(2–3), 166–195.

Jilka, M. (2000) *The Contribution of Intonation to the Perception of Foreign Accent*. Doctoral Dissertation, Arbeiten des Instituts für Maschinelle Sprachverarbeitung (AIMS), University of Stuttgart.

Johnson, C. and Lancaster, P. (1998) The development of more than one phonology: A case study of a Norwegian-English bilingual child. *International Journal of Bilingualism* 2(3), 265–300.

Johnson, C. and Wilson, I. (2002) Phonetic evidence for early language differentiation: Research issues and some preliminary data. *International Journal of Bilingualism* 6(3), 271–289.

Kehoe, M. (2002) Developing vowel systems as a window to bilingual phonology. *International Journal of Bilingualism* 6(3), 315–334.

Kehoe, M.M., Lleó, C. and Rakow, M. (2004) Voice onset time in bilingual German-Spanish children. *Bilingualism: Language and Cognition* 7(01), 71–88.

Khattab, G. (1999) A socio-phonetic study of English-Arabic bilingual children. *Leeds Working Papers in Linguistics & Phonetics* 7, 79–94.

Khattab, G. (2000) VOT Production in English and Arabic bilingual and monolingual children. *Leeds Working Papers in Linguistics & Phonetics* 8, 95–122.

Khattab, G. (2002a) /r/ production in English and Arabic bilingual and monolingual speakers. *Leeds Working Papers in Linguistics & Phonetics* 9, 91–129.

Khattab, G. (2002b) /l/ production in English-Arabic bilingual speakers. *International Journal of Bilingualism* 6(3), 335–353.

Konefal, J. and Fokes, J. (1981) Voice onset time: The development of Spanish-English distinction in normal and language disordered children. *Journal of Phonetics* 9, 437–444.

Ladd, D.R. (1996) *Intonational Phonology*. Cambridge Studies in Linguistics (1st edn). Cambridge: Cambridge University Press.

Lepetit, D. (1989) Cross-linguistic influence in intonation: French/Japanese and French/English. *Language Learning* 39(3), 397–413.

Levitt, A. and Utman, A. (1992) From babbling towards the sound systems of English and French: A longitudinal two-case study. *Journal of Child Language* 19(1), 19–49.

Lin, H. and Wang, Q. (2005) Vowel quantity and consonant variance: A comparison between Chinese and English. Presented at the Between Stress and Tone, Leiden.

Lin, H. and Wang, Q. (2007) Mandarin rhythm: An acoustic study. *Journal of Chinese Language and Computing* 17(3), 127–140.

Lleo, C. and Kehoe, M. (2002) On the interaction of phonological systems in child bilingual acquisition. *International Journal of Bilingualism* 6(3), 233–237.

Low, L., Grabe, E. and Nolan, F. (2000) Quantitative characterizations of speech rhythm: Syllable-timing in Singapore English. *Language and Speech* 43(4), 377–401.

Mack, M. (1989) Consonant and vowel perception and production: Early English-French bilinguals and English monolinguals. *Perception & Psychophysics* 46(2), 187–200.

Mack, M. (1990) Phonetic transfer in a French-English bilingual child. In P. Nelde (ed.) *Language Attitudes and Language Conflict* (pp. 107–124). Bonn: Dümmler.

Maneva, B. and Genesee, F. (2002) Bilingual babbling: Evidence for language differentiation in dual language acquisition. In *Proceedings of the 26th Boston University Conference on Language Development* (pp. 383–392). Somerville, MA: Cascadilla Press.

Mehler, J., Jusczyk, P., Lambertz, G., Halsted, N., Bertoncini, J. and Amiel-Tison, C. (1988) A precursor of language acquisition in young infants. *Cognition* 29(2), 143–178.

Mennen, I. (2004) Bi-directional interference in the intonation of Dutch speakers of Greek. *Journal of Phonetics* 32(4), 543–563.

Mennen, I. (2007) Phonological and phonetic influences in non-native intonation. In J. Trouvain and U. Gut (eds) *Non-Native Prosody. Phonetic Description and Teaching Practice* (pp. 53–76). Amsterdam: Mouton de Gruyter.

Mennen, I., Chen, A. and Karlsson, F. (2010) Characterising the internal structure of learner intonation and its development over time. In *Proceedings of New Sounds 2010:The Sixth International Symposium on the Acquisition of Second Language Speech*. Poznan, Poland.

Mennen, I., Scobbie, J., De Leeuw, E., Schaeffler, S. and Schaeffler, F. (2010) Measuring language-Specific phonetic settings. *Second Language Research* 26(1), 13–41.

Munro, M., Flege, J.E. and MacKay, I.R. (1996) The effects of age of second language learning on the production of English vowels. *Applied Psycholinguistics* 17(3), 313–334.

Munson, B., McDonald, E., DeBoe, N. and White, A. (2006) The acoustic and perceptual bases of judgments of women and men's sexual orientation from read speech. *Journal of Phonetics* 34(2), 202–240.

Navarro, A., Pearson, B., Cobo-Lewis, A. and Oller, D. (1995) Early phonological development in young bilinguals: Comparison to monolinguals. Presented at the American Speech, Language and Hearing Association Conference.

Nazzi, T., Bertoncini, J. and Mehler, J. (1998) Language discrimination by newborns. Towards understanding of the role of rhythm. *Journal of Experimental Psychology: Human Perception and Performance* 24, 1–11.

Nazzi, T., Jusczyk, P. and Johnson, E. (2000) Language discrimination by English-Learning 5-month-olds: Effects of rhythm and familiarity. *Journal of Memory and Language* 43(1), 1–19.

Oller, K., Akahane-Yamada, R., Urbano, R. and Cobo-Lewis, A. (1997) Development of precursors to speech in infants exposed to two languages. *Journal of Child Language* 24(2), 407–425.

Paradis, J. (1996) Phonological differentiation in a bilingual child: Hildegard revisited. In *Proceedings of the 20th Boston University Conference on Language Development*, Somerville, MA: Cascadilla Press.

Paradis, J. (2001) Do bilingual two-year-olds have separate phonological systems? *International Journal of Bilingualism* 5(1), 19–38.

Pike, K. (1945) *Intonation of American English*. Ann Arbor, MI: University of Michigan Press.

Piske, T., MacKay, I. and Flege, J.E. (2001) Factors affecting degree of foreign accent in an L2: A review. *Journal of Phonetics* 29(1), 191–215.

Piske, T., Flege, J., Grenon, I. and Meador, D. (2002) The production of English vowels by fluent early and late Italian-English bilinguals. *Phonetica* 59(1), 49–71.

Poulin-Dubois, D. and Goodz, N. (2001) Language differentiation in bilingual infants: Evidence from babbling. In J. Cenoz and F. Genesee (eds) *Trends in Bilingual Acquisition* (pp. 95–106). Amsterdam: John Benjamins Publishing Company.

Scharff-Rethfeldt, I., Miller, N. and Mennen, I. (2008) Unterschiede in der mittleren Sprechtonhöhe bei Deutsch/Englisch bilingualen Sprechern. *Sprache Stimme Gehör* 32(1), 123–128.

Scherer, K. (1986) Vocal affect expression: A review and a model for future research. *Psychological Bulletin* 99(2), 143–165.

Snow, D. (2006) Regression and reorganization of intonation between 6 and 23 months. *Child Development* 77(2), 281–296.

Snow, D. and Balog, H. (2002) Do children produce the melody before the words? A review of developmental intonation research. *Lingua* 112(12), 1025–1058.

Strange, W. (1995) Cross-language studies of speech perception: A historical review. In W. Strange (ed.) *Speech Perception and Linguistic Experience: Issues in Cross-language Research* (pp. 3–45). Timonium, MD: York Press.

Strange, W. (2007) Cross-language phonetic similarity of vowels: Theoretical and methodological issues. In O-S. Bohn and M.J. Munro (ed.) *Language Experience in Second Language Speech Learning: In Honor of James Emil Flege* (pp. 35–55). Amsterdam: John Benjamins Publishing Company.

Sundara, M., Polka, L. and Baum, S. (2006) Production of coronal stops by simultaneous bilingual adults. *Bilingualism: Language and Cognition* 9(1), 97–114.

Tin, C.Y. (2005) *Description of Bilingual Phonology in Cantonese-English Preschooler* (Bachelor of Science (Speech and Hearing) thesis. University of Hong Kong.

Ueyama, M. (1997) The phonology and phonetics of second language intonation: The case of Japanese English. In *Proceedings of the fifth European Conference on Speech Communication and Technology* (pp. 2411–2414). Presented at the EUROSPEECH-1997, Rhodos.

Ueyama, M. and Jun, S. (1998) Focus realization in Japanese English and Korean English intonation. *Japanese and Korean Linguistics* 7, 629–645.

Vihman, M.M. (2002) Getting started without a system: From phonetics to phonology in bilingual development. *International Journal of Bilingualism* 6(3), 239–254.

Watson, I. (1990) Acquiring the voicing contrast in French: A comparative study of monolingual and bilingual children. In J.N. Green and W. Ayers-Bennett (eds) *Variation and Change in French: Essays Presented to Rebecca Posner on the Occasion of Her Sixtieth Birthday* (pp. 37–60). London: Routledge.

Watson, I. (1995) The effect of bilingualism on the acquisition of perceptual categories underlying the voicing contrast. In K. Elenius and P. Branderud (eds) *Proceedings of the 13th International Congress of Phonetic Sciences*, Vol. 2 (pp. 710–713). Stockholm: KTH & Stockholm University.

Wennerstrom, A. (1994) Intonational meaning in English discourse: A study of non-native speakers. *Applied Linguistics* 15(4), 399–420.

Whalen, D., Levitt, A. and Wang, Q. (1991) Intonational differences between the reduplicative babbling of French- and English-learning infants. *Journal of Child Language* 18(3), 501–516.

White, L. and Mattys, S. (2007) Calibrating rhythm: First language and second language studies. *Journal of Phonetics* 35(4), 501–522.

Whitworth, N. (2000) Acquisition of VOT, and vowel length by English-German bilinguals: A pilot study. *Leeds Working Papers in Linguistics & Phonetics* 8, 1–16.

Whitworth, N. (2002) Speech rhythm production in three German-English bilingual families. *Leeds Working Papers in Linguistics & Phonetics* 9, 175–205.

Willems, N. (1982) *English Intonation from a Dutch Point of View*. Netherlands phonetic archives. Dordrecht: Foris Publications.

Chapter 3
Genetics and Language

KATHARINA DWORZYNSKI

Summary

There are many misconceptions about the contributions of genes to complex behavioural traits such as language and speech abilities. In this chapter, I start by examining the relationship between genes and such behaviours from a 'top-down' approach that goes from similarities within families (particularly those that have twins) through to genes (whose impact on behaviour is often misinterpreted). The top-down part starts with univariate genetic twin analyses (i.e. analysing heritability of a single trait – language or speech impairments) and then explores multivariate twin methods (in other words investigating the genetic and environmental influences between different language and/or speech traits). This approach not only provides insights into heritability of single abilities or difficulties in those abilities, but also shows the etiological relationship between different linguistic traits, e.g. contrasting genetic and environmental influences on grammar and articulation and the relationship between stuttering and other non-fluencies. The methods (linkage and association analysis) that delve deeper into these familial patterns to identify areas of the genome that might be related to the target behaviours are then outlined.

In the latter part of the chapter, the focus is on a 'bottom-up' approach of genetic influences. In this section it is explained how, having identified a particular gene (exemplified by the *FOXP2*[1] gene), the route can then be traced backwards. This second path starts with the gene going on to the protein it codes, then to its relationship with other genes and how this can eventually lead to changes in the brain and thus behaviour. Both these different approaches give some answers to our understanding of how genes influence our ability to communicate with each other. However, most of this chapter highlights questions that will need to be clarified to piece together the complexities of the relationship between language/speech and genes.

1　Introduction – Where is the Evidence that Genes Contribute to Language and Speech-fluency Development?

Language is a complex trait involving many physical (the parts of the body that need to be controlled to produce speech – articulators), cognitive (how we plan the content of what we want to convey and how we understand what other people tell us – expressive and receptive language) and linguistic components (such as grammar, meaning and speech sounds – syntax, semantics and phonology). Language is, therefore, a network of skills working together to help us to exchange ideas in communication. There are vast individual differences in language abilities (as well as the way that people use and apply different aspects of language) and also many different ways in which people experience difficulties with the acquisition as well as possible loss of linguistic skills. Children may fall behind in the way they develop expressive skills, they may have trouble understanding what has been said to them or they may have difficulties in the actual production of speech (for instance, in the stoppages and prolongations seen in stuttering). Adults, too, may experience medical conditions in which their language abilities are affected (acquired neurological and other medical conditions associated with language impairments, though these are outside the scope of the current chapter).

Two types of language difficulties are focused on here. One is specific language impairment (SLI) which is a disorder where language development lags significantly behind non-verbal cognitive abilities for a particular age group. SLI occurs when physical difficulties which might be related to language skills are absent (hearing loss, brain damage etc.). The second is stuttering (also called stammering) which is characterised by stoppages and prolongations that interrupt speech fluency. Aspects of individual differences in language across the whole continuum of abilities will also be touched on. The causes of each of these disorders have not been clearly identified. So the main question is how can we link the extraordinary complexities and variety of this observed behaviour (the phenotype) to the possible genetic causes of this trait (the genotype)? To investigate the genetic aetiology of behavioural traits we have to adopt scientific designs that are genetically informative.

Making our way from behaviour downwards we can look for genetic influences in speech and language development using family, adoption and twin studies. In such studies the status of family members of affected individuals is compared with the status of control families (i.e. families where none of the children experience language difficulties). If the probability of being affected is significantly higher in families for a person suffering from language/speech problems compared to control families (or the population rate of a disorder), this is then suggestive of genetic influences. There have been a number of studies in the 1990s showing familial aggregation in stuttering, speech delay and SLI (Ambrose *et al.*, 1993; Felsenfeld *et al.*, 1995; Tallal *et al.*, 2001).

Adoption studies can also address the issue of genetic influences where adopted children of biological parents with a given condition should be at increased risk for displaying this condition. Felsenfeld and Plomin (1997) carried out an adoption study of speech disorder and found evidence that children adopted away from relatives were indeed at a higher risk for developing speech disorders themselves. However, evidence from these types of family design are not entirely convincing since, in familial aggregation studies, family members share environment as well as genes. In adoption studies it is also difficult to disentangle genetic and environmental effects. Twin data can address this question better since they can separately assess the role of genes as well as two different types of environmental influences on a given trait.

2 Heritability of Language Traits – Twin Studies

This design makes use of the fact that twin pairs could stem either from one fertilised ovum (monozygotic – MZ) in which case they have identical genetic make-up or from the fertilisation of two ova (dizygotic – DZ) and therefore show the same level of genetic similarity as other siblings (i.e. 50%). If the behavioural similarity between two twins is greater for MZ than for DZ pairs it indicates the role of genes in a trait. If we investigate a particular diagnostic impairment in a categorical way we can look at the concordance between twins (i.e. what is the probability of developing a disorder if your co-twin is affected). Another important factor in twin studies is that they allow the environmental effects to be assessed. The fact that MZ twins who are genetically identical are usually not 100% identical on any measured trait points to unique environment influences (effects that make children growing up in the same family different). Whereas when DZ twins are more than half as similar in a trait compared to identical twins, this implicates shared environmental factors (effects that make children growing up in the same family similar) (Figure 3.1).

2.1 Univariate twin studies of speech and language disorders

Reviews of twin studies in SLI have shown mid to large estimates of heritability (i.e. the proportion of variance in a trait is attributable to genetic factors) between 0.5 and 0.75 in children (for reviews, see e.g. Bishop, 2002; Stromswold, 2001). Environmental influences were mainly due to non-shared effects, i.e. those that make children growing up in the same family different.

Twin studies in stuttering have also shown high estimates of heritability of 0.7 in adults (Andrews *et al.*, 1991; Felsenfeld *et al.*, 2000) and 0.6 for 4-year-old twins from the Twins Early Development Study

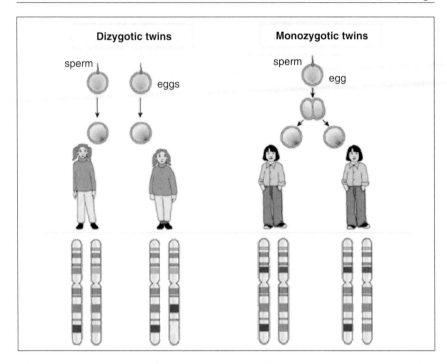

Figure 3.1 The premise of the twin design is that fraternal (dizygotic – DZ) twins share on average 50% of their DNA code whereas identical (monozygotic – MZ) twins are assumed to share 100% of their genetic make-up. If identical twins are more alike in language and speech traits compared to fraternal twins it suggests that genes contribute to this behaviour
Source: © carolguze.com.

(Dworzynski *et al.*, 2007) and 0.8 for Japanese twins with a mean age of 11.5 (Ooki, 2005). Here again, as for SLI, all studies showed that the environmental effects on stuttering were mainly due to unique environmental influences without substantial contributions of shared environmental effects (Figure 3.2).

Interestingly it was recently reported that the heritability estimates for a language disorder such as SLI also depended on the type of diagnostic classification (Bishop & Hayiou-Thomas, 2007). The authors reported that heritability estimates were substantially higher when SLI was defined in terms of referral to speech and language services (estimates of 0.96) as compared to negligible genetic influences when SLI was defined by the performance on language tests alone without referral (non-significant with confidence intervals between 0 and 0.45). Furthermore referral did not depend on severity of language difficulties, but rather was related to tests measuring a speech component on which children who had been

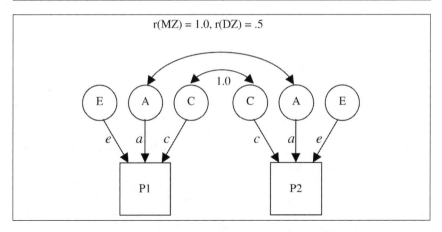

Figure 3.2 A univariate ACE twin model. A path diagram of a univariate ACE model (A = Additive genetic factors, C = shared of common environmental factors, E = non-shared environmental effects) in which the three latent independent variables influence variation (indicated by single-headed arrows) in a particular behaviour (such as language abilities for instance) or phenotype (P; P1 for twin 1 and P2 for twin 2). MZ = monozygotic; DZ = dizygotic. Partial regression coefficients (letters *a*, *c* and *e*) reflect the degree of relationship between the latent variables and the phenotype. Double-headed arrows indicate the correlations among variables

referred to services did less well. This led the authors to suggest that the hunt for genes implicated in language disorders would benefit if we defined the phenotype more in terms of speech rather than language impairments.

2.2 Beyond single trait heritability – multifactorial studies of individual differences in twins

Traditionally twin studies have been used to study heritabilities of distinct disorders. More recently twin studies have also been used to investigate the genetic underpinning of the relationship between disorders and also to investigate individual differences in diverse skills across the whole range of abilities (individual differences) and how they are aetiologically related to each other. Since deciding on the specific characteristic of the diagnostic category seems to influence heritability estimates, this provides an alternative approach by which individual differences in abilities that have been implicated in playing an important causal role in SLI can be studied. Such underlying skills, i.e. those considered 'half way' between the full set of behavioural characteristics (phenotype) under investigation and the genetic aetiology (genotype), are referred to as endophenotypes.

2.2.1 Diverse language skills

1600 twins from the Twins Early Development Study (TEDS), a UK-based longitudinal population-based sample, were tested at home on a large battery of language tests when they were 4 .5 years old. This was a subsample of children with a large proportion being at risk of developing language problems as indicated by an earlier measure of vocabulary. Since TEDS is a longitudinal project the twins have since been regularly assessed on their language and literacy attainments (Oliver & Plomin, 2007; Trouton *et al.*, 2002). Reviewing relationships between the linguistic components and literacy in TEDS, Hayiou-Thomas (2008) concluded that genetic factors influence individual variation in young children's speech and that these genetic factors also account for the relationship between speech and reading skills. However, shared environmental influences played a more dominant role in broader language skills and their relationship to later reading abilities. This highlights contrasting effects on and between speech/articulation and reading performance as compared to other linguistic skills (such as grammar, semantics and receptive language skills for instance).

2.2.2 Speech fluency abilities

A recent twin study investigated the bivariate relationship between probable stuttering (prolongations and blocks) and high non-fluency (repetitions of parts of sentences or individual words for instance), as assessed by parental report for 10,683 5-year-old twin pairs (van Beijsterveldt *et al.*, 2010). In contrast to the previous twin studies on stuttering their results showed both phenotypes to be moderately heritable but also that shared environmental effects played a role (in both about 0.4 for genetic and also 0.4 for shared environmental contributions without significant sex differences). There was a high phenotypic correlation between stuttering and high non-fluency (0.72) an association that was due to both overlapping genetic and environmental influences.

2.2.3 Endophenotype

To get a bit closer to an intermediate skill between the full phenotype and genotype, language research has also adopted an endophenotype approach. One prominent endophenotype proposed for SLI is the non-word repetition task in which subjects are asked to repeat nonsense words (such as 'brufid') that they have just heard. This is an ability that depends on a system for holding verbal information in memory for short periods of time (i.e. phonological short term memory). The underlying theory is that SLI can be caused by impairment in phonological short-term memory. The majority of children with SLI perform poorly on this task and it is often seen as a clinical marker (Conti-Ramsden *et al.*, 2001). A twin study of non-word repetition has shown that this ability is also highly heritable (Bishop *et al.*, 1996).

In sum twin research has established that language and speech abilities along the whole spectrum of skills are heritable, but that language skills are influenced by more shared environmental components than speech/articulation performance. Language impairment as a categorical trait is also moderately to highly heritable, but again there is evidence that the aetiological genetic effects are higher when a speech difficulty is involved. Twin studies of stuttering have reported high estimates for genetic effects with, on the whole, little evidence for shared environment. However, a recent bivariate analysis of the relationship between probably stuttering and high non-fluency did report both moderate genetic and shared environmental influences and also overlapping genetic and environmental contributions accounting for the association between these two characteristics.

Therefore we have supporting evidence for the genetic aetiology of speech and language skills, but how do we get from heritability estimates to genes at the molecular level?

3 What is a Gene Anyway?

As highlighted by Fisher (2005a, 2005b, 2006) one particular topic that still causes confusion is the concept of the gene, its role and function and how it relates to DNA, chromosomes and genomes. Mendelian patterns of inheritance are still those that are most widely understood by the public. This is another cause of misunderstanding of genetics leading to statements that there might be a 'gene *for* language' or *for* any other complex traits such as reading or cognitive ability. This stems from the time when a gene was defined by the overall symptoms or impairments related to its loss or mutation (mainly in the autosomal dominant/recessive fashion) (Figure 3.3).

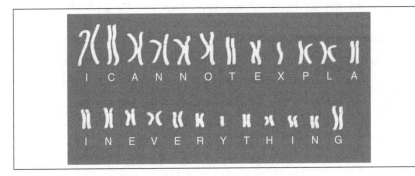

Figure 3.3 We should be cautious about the inferences that can be drawn from genetic studies in language and speech research
Source: © European Molecular Biology Organization (2007).

3.1   Mendelian laws

There are two laws in Mendel's theory of heredity. According to the first, the law of segregation, a gene may exist in two or more different forms (called alleles). During gamete formation, the two different alleles separate (segregate) and one is inherited from each parent. In the inheritance of the characteristics in pea plants that Mendel studied, he also noticed that one trait was not influenced by inheritance of the other. This pattern formed the basis of his second law, the law of independent assortment. These two laws can explain a dominant pattern of inheritance, where only one parent has to be affected to cause the disorder to be inherited (such as is the case in Huntington Disease). A recessive pattern, such as sickle cell anaemia, can also be explained whereby none of the parents need to show the disorder and it only occurs in the children when both forms of the alleles are inherited. There are many other genetic disorders that do not conform to these two laws. For some of these, the mode of inheritance has since been established due to advances in molecular genetics.

3.2   Complex traits

In a branch of genetics called quantitative genetics, the idea is that multiple gene effects lead to quantitative traits (i.e. traits like cognitive skills, such as linguistic abilities, which show wide variability). If genetic factors affect a quantitative trait, phenotypic similarity of relatives should increase with increasing degrees of genetic relatedness. The results from twin studies about language skills, described above, indicate that genetic factors play a major role in familial resemblance. The pattern of inheritance for complex disorders such as, for instance, stuttering and continuous dimensions like expressive language skills is different from that seen for single-gene traits, because multiple genes are involved. However, each individual gene is itself still inherited according to Mendel's laws.

3.3   Family pedigrees

The study of an inherited trait in many individuals of several generations of the same family is called pedigree analysis. This makes use of Mendel's law to determine the mode of inheritance. In language research the most famous pedigree is the KE family (see Figure 3.4). This is a British multi-generation family where affected members show a disorder involving deficits in both speech (severe speech motor difficulty) and language (problems with grammatical features) (Vargha-Khadem *et al.*, 1998). It can be seen on examination of the ratio of affected to unaffected individuals in each generation that about half of each generation suffer from the speech and language impairments which suggests an autosomal dominant disorder according to Mendel's description. Even though

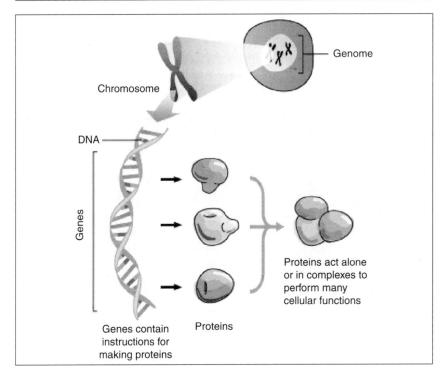

Figure 3.4 Through the processes of transcription and translation information is used from genes to make proteins. Each sequence of three bases, called a codon, codes for a particular building block of a protein, i.e. an amino acid. The assembly of further amino acids continues until a 'stop' codon is encountered (a three base pair sequence that does not code for an amino acid)

the pattern of inheritance suggested that just one gene may account for these problems, the search for the culprit took over a decade. It was then discovered that all affected family members had inherited a muta-tion in a gene now known as *FOXP2* (Lai *et al.*, 2001). Other families and cases have since been reported with different *FOXP2* mutations, but these are very rare occurrences (MacDermot *et al.*, 2005). The media and some parts of the research community widely speculated and misinter-preted the meaning of this finding for language research (such as 'gene for language' etc.).

4 DNA and Genes

In Watson and Crick's Nobel prize winning article 'Molecular Structure of Nucleic Acids' (1953), a compact article published in *Nature* about one page in length, the authors made several, now famous, understatements. For instance, 'This structure has novel features which are of considerable biological interest', and at the end of their article they mention, 'It has not escaped our notice that the specific pairing we have postulated immediately suggests a possible copying mechanism for the genetic material.'

Since the structure of DNA was identified, there has been an exponential growth in molecular genetics in both the conceptual and technological understanding of how complex human traits can be investigated. The Human Genome Project, which received a huge amount of publicity, was initiated in the early 1990s and set out to report the order of the entire four-letter nucleotide sequence (Adenine, Guanine, Cytosine and Thymine) which determines which genes and proteins are present in human cells. The genome, which is the complete string of nucleotide letters that make up the DNA sequence in our cells (in other words the full set of 'instructions' on how to build and maintain the organism), contains more than 3 billion letters. Results from this project were published in 2001 (see the special issues in *Nature* as well as *Science* Feb 2001). As a consequence of the publicity many people are now familiar with some genetic concepts. It is recognised that genetic information is encoded in DNA, that almost every cell has its own copy of the genome to refer to, that DNA is packaged (with proteins and other molecules) into forms that are called chromosomes and that human cells contain two sets of 23 chromosomes two of which are the sex chromosomes. Despite this upsurge in public understanding, there are also many misconceptions that the rapid advances and surrounding media interest in this field have caused.

In contrast to describing genes by particular dysfunctions, on a molecular genetic level it is relatively complex to define the hereditary unit of a gene. A gene is a segment of DNA that is involved in producing a polypeptide chain (i.e. a string of amino acids) in a specific protein. In addition to this, it may also include regions preceding and following this coding segment as well as introns (bits of DNA in a gene that get removed before translation of messenger RNA) between the exons (coding DNA for protein synthesis). The three-dimensional structure of the resulting protein is linked to the function it will fulfil, some of which could be enzymes, signalling factors, channels etc. The whole genome also includes information about which genes are switched on or off and where in the organism genes should be activated. It is therefore a process that changes over time (when they are switched on and off) and location within the body (where they are activated). DNA shows only little variation between unrelated humans (0.2% or 1 in 500 bases, i.e. letters). Due to random mutations some sequences do vary and such allelic variants could change

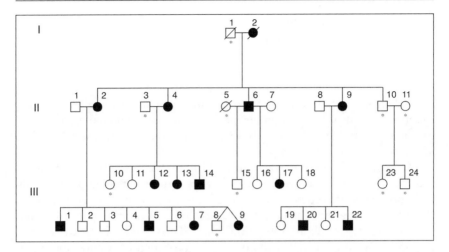

Figure 3.5 The three generations of the KE family. Squares represent male family members and circle female. Filled black shapes represent individuals who have a complex speech and language impairment which is caused by the *FOXP2* gene (Lai *et al.* 2001; Fisher *et al.* 2003)

gene function and lead to differences in (or the complete absence of) the protein or differences in structure/type (Figure 3.5).

5   Methods to Identify Genes

5.1   Linkage studies in complex traits

There is a positional strategy called linkage analysis that is used to help identify genes of major effect. This allows researchers to home in on a chromosomal region that may harbour a gene or genes involved in a trait. In this type of analysis the inheritance pattern of different chromosomal regions in families affected by a particular trait is being investigated. It is more likely that segments of DNA that are close together are also inherited together rather than those further apart. Some parts of the DNA can act as markers from which we can deduce whether a portion of DNA was inherited from the mother or father. At the outset, pairs of siblings are investigated both of whom show the particular trait or disorder. Then for a pair of alleles at a given position (termed locus) it can be worked out whether 0, 1 or 2 alleles are inherited from the same parent ('identical by descent' – IBD). When we then compare the observed IBD pattern to a pattern predicted randomly we can locate stretches of DNA that are co-inherited by affected individuals at above chance level. In this way a marker linked to a quantitative trait (i.e. such as individual differences in language abilities) will show greater than expected allele sharing for siblings who are more similar for the trait. With just a few hundred DNA markers the linkage approach is used to scan the genome systematically to look for violations of Mendel's law of independent assortment between a disorder and a marker. These particular regions are then likely to be close to genes important for this trait. When, or if, a region has been found to be linked to a particular marker more detailed analysis of genes in this segment can be carried out to identify allelic differences between affected and unaffected people.

SLI linkage studies have been carried out by the SLI Consortium which is a multi-site UK study of a large group of families affected by SLI. This uses both epidemiological and clinical samples. Three types of phenotypic traits were investigated: (1) expressive; and (2) receptive language abilities; (3) a non-word repetition task. There was linkage between a region on the long arm of chromosome 16 (all human chromosomes have two arms, the long and short arm separated by the centromere) with the non-word repetition task and between a region on the long arm of chromosome 19 and expressive language skills (SLI Consortium, 2002). Even though linkages to these two regions were replicated (Falcaro *et al.*, 2008; SLI Consortium, 2004) this finding was not shown to be linked to the same chromosomal regions in another study, but rather implicated an area on chromosome 13 instead (Bartlett *et al.*, 2002).

For stuttering, significant linkage has been reported to chromosome 12 in a study of stuttering in 46 consanguineous families from Pakistan (Riaz *et al.*, 2005). The main regions in another study were on chromosomes 9 and 15 with evidence for sex-specific linkage regions on chromosomes 7 and 21 (Suresh *et al.*, 2006) and a meta analysis revealed significant linkage only to chromosome 2.

It has to be kept in mind that linkage only implicates a chromosome region and that this, however, does not allow the identification of a specific gene related to the disorder. The region may contain many different genes and therefore after linkage a more fine-grained approach should be used to follow up the results and narrow down the search.

Linkage analyses in language research have been fruitful in identifying some regions of interest. However, replication of linkage results in most complex traits has generally not been very successful as has been shown, for example, in a review of 101 linkage studies of 31 human diseases (Altmuller *et al.*, 2001). As demonstrated above for SLI and stuttering, it is all too common that different linkage studies of the same disorder do not find evidence for the same regions or even the same chromosomes. This could be due to a number of factors such as the use of different phenotypic measures, differences in sample populations or even the types of statistical analysis techniques involved. Due to the vast number of tests that need to be carried out for each linkage false positive findings could also play a role, even when statistical procedures are employed to account for this.

5.2 Association analysis

An alternative to linkage analysis, which is most useful when looking for genes with small effects, is association analysis. The advantage of association is that it simply compares allelic frequencies for groups such as individuals with the disorder (cases) versus controls or low-scoring versus high-scoring individuals on a quantitative trait (Sham, 2001). In association studies individual markers need to be, if not directly in a given gene, very close to the locus which means that a very dense network of markers has to be used to detect an association. Recently it has become economically possible to carry out genome wide association studies, which require use of hundreds of thousands of markers, for disorders, and also for quantitative traits. Association analysis can also be used when significant linkage has been reported to tag, if possible, all or most candidate genes that may be located in this region. Due to the fact that a highly significant region was detected on chromosome 16 for non-word repetition in the SLI Consortium families, researchers decided to analyse this region with a high-density association scan (Newbury *et al.*, 2009). They identified two genes in this region: one known as *ATP2C2* and the other as *CMIP* that contributed to the susceptibility to SLI. Interestingly, the effects of these genes were detected in two samples of language-impaired individuals. However, in a large unselected sample (i.e. a sample with language measures across the entire spectrum of abilities) no association was detected between variants of these two genes and phonological short-term memory. This last point is important since it highlights a possible etiological discontinuity between abilities in the normal range from those with more serious language impairments.

As highlighted above, Riaz and co-workers studied stuttering in a group of Pakistani pedigrees and reported linkage to an area on chromosome 12. Genetic results from one particular large family (PKST72) from this sample was revisited and after a confirmation of linkage to chromosome 12 with additional family members, an association analysis was carried out on the linkage region of the long arm of chromosome 12 (Kang *et al.*, 2010). The study scanned promoter, exons and untranslated regions of 45 genes in several affected individuals, using DNA sequencing. In this way they identified a missense mutation, i.e. a single base pair substitution that changes the code for one amino acid to another, in the *GNPTAB* gene. Their study went on to screen for this and other mutations in the *GNPTAB* gene in unrelated Pakistani persons including one affected member of each of the 46 families that they had studied previously and 96 matched unrelated Pakistani control subjects. In addition they screened the same region in 270 unrelated affected individuals, from

North America and Britain as well as 276 unaffected North American control subjects. They identified five additional affected people with the same
homozygous or heterozygous mutation on the same locus of *GNPTAB*.
Only 1 of the 96 Pakistani control subjects carried this variant as well
as another one in the group of 270 North American and British people
who stuttered, but not in the 276 North American control subjects. They
detected three other *GNPTAB* mutations before they chose to screen the
genes *GNPTG* and *NAGPA* since they fit into the same functional genetic
pathway as *GNPTAB*. The authors then identified three mutations in the
GNPTG and also three in the *NAGPA* gene.

6   Going Back from Genes to Brain to Behaviour?

As described above, two genes *ATP2C2* and *CMIP* were identified
as being associated with impaired phonological memory in individuals
with predominantly expressive language difficulties, while variants of the
GNTAB, *GNPTG* and *NAGPA* genes were implicated in stuttering in a subset of people who stutter. Moreover, aetiological mutations of the *FOXP2*
gene have been found in families with a monogenic disorder impacting
on multiple aspects of speech motor and language simultaneously. It was
also established above that there is no such thing as a 'gene for language'
or a 'gene for stuttering'. In this case what do these genes actually tell us
about the disorders they are associated with?

By looking at *FOXP2* mutation in detail, Fisher and colleagues are making progress in bridging the gap. *FOXP2* contains a stretch of sequence
that is called a forkhead-box, a part of a protein involving 80–100 amino
acids which allow it to bind to DNA. When *FOXP2* binds to DNA the
function of certain target genes can be activated or repressed. A protein
that can switch other genes on or off is called a transcription factor. Vernes
et al. (2008) reasoned that even though *FOXP2* is only involved in a small
number of cases of speech and language disorder, it regulates other genes
that are necessary for the development of neural pathways associated
with language processing in the brain. One of their goals was to assess
whether genes that are switched on or off by binding to *FOXP2* could
then also be linked to cases of SLI that are more frequent than the rare
speech/language disorder first studied in the KE family. They carried out
genomic screening and found that *FOXP2* binds to and down-regulates
(i.e. decreases the quantity of the output from) *CNTNAP2*, a gene that
encodes a neurexin, a type of membrane protein known to be important in
neural development. They then used the SLI Consortium families to investigate whether *CNTNAP2* was also implicated in more common forms
of language difficulties and detected significant quantitative associations
between genomic variants at the locus and performance on the non-word
repetition task (described here earlier as an endophenotype of SLI).

However, presence of the particular risk version of the *CNTNAP2* gene does not by itself lead to bad non-word repetition performance since many of those who performed below average did not have this variant whereas some of those with good skills had one or both versions of it. Using animal studies the functions of particular genes can be traced back to animal's brain circuitry and then also the resulting behaviour when certain genes are 'knocked out'. In 'knock out' mice's brains (in other words when the function of the *FOXP2* homologue stopped) there is decreased brain plasticity (Groszer *et al.*, 2008) and these mice showed impaired motor function. When mice have two non-functional *Foxp2* alleles they produce much fewer ultrasonic vocalisations than their wild-type littermates (Fujita *et al.*, 2008; Shu *et al.*, 2005). It has to be pointed out that these animals suffer from severe developmental deficits and die around 3 weeks after birth, and therefore may not represent specific effects of Foxp2 on mouse vocalisations. However, in zebra finches with decreased FOXP2 functioning there are problems in the acquisition of bird songs (Haesler *et al.*, 2007). The birds had difficulties in accurately learning songs from an adult tutor and their vocal output became jumbled: they contained the same components (similar to syllables in speech production) as the songs of their tutors, but with parts rearranged, left out, repeated incorrectly or sung at the wrong pitch.

With regards to the rare mutations in the three genes (*GNPTAB, GNPTG* and *NAGPA*) that have been reported by Kang and colleagues for stuttering in their Pakistani families/cases, there are interesting hints of what possible biological pathways may be involved. These genes are involved in lysosome processes. The lysosome contains enzymes which help to recycle substances, such as food particles etc., into material that the cell can utilise. Two rare inherited disorders, mucolipidosis types II and III (two types of lysosomal storage disease), are directly related to mutations in *GNPTAB* and *GNPTG* and show the severe effects that lysosomal dysfunction can cause. Individuals with these disorders not only have predominantly skeletal, cardiac and ocular impairments, but they also have motoric problems and developmental delay. It needs to be highlighted that there were people in the sample who carried the mutation and were not affected by stuttering (geneticists call this incomplete penetrance) and on the other hand there were individuals who stuttered without any of these mutations (what is referred to as phenocopy).

7 Further Pieces of the Puzzle

The vast neuroimaging literature in language research will not be discussed in detail here. Members of the KE family have been scanned and certain relevant brain areas were identified. A further interesting aspect of the *FOXP2* gene is its evolutionary development. Enard and coworkers

(2002) discovered that the human version of the *FOXP2* protein has undergone accelerated evolution. The human version differs from those of chimpanzees by two amino acids and from that of mice by three. It means that humans have had two further changes since their lineage split from the lineage leading to chimpanzees. When Krause (Krause *et al.*, 2007), one of Enard's colleagues, later reported that Neanderthals have an identical gene the popular press widely speculated about their language abilities.

The genetic studies of stuttering have also posed some further questions. In an editorial to the issue in which Kang and colleagues' paper about stuttering appeared, Fisher (2010) stressed that it is now important to use their findings in a similar way and directly test the properties of the putative risk forms of the GNPT (encoded by the *GNPTAB* and *GNPTG* genes) and NAGPA enzymes using biochemical methods. With the investigation of these proteins/enzymes it is possible that progress could be made in a similar manner to *FOXP2* to understand their function and dysfunction in relation to speech ability and stuttering.

8 Genes and Interventions

Another issue that has received a lot of media coverage and controversy is the relationship between genetic susceptibility to a disorder and treatment/intervention. It is often wrongly assumed that having a version of a particular gene that may put you at risk of developing a particular disorder means that this means people have a lifelong condition. Again it is important to highlight that for many genes there is incomplete penetrance, i.e. not all people with the risk gene develop the disorder. Early intervention even in single gene disorders is often extremely important. The case of phenylketonuria (PKU) is probably the most often cited one in this respect. PKU is a single gene recessive disorder and leads to moderate cognitive disorders (IQs often are below 50). When the genetics of PKU were studied a mutation was found in the gene (*PAH*) that codes for the enzyme phenylalanine hydroxylase. When the gene is mutated, the encoded enzyme does not work properly, and it is less efficient in catalysing the breakdown of phenylalanine. Phenylalanine comes from food, especially red meats; and if it cannot be broken down properly, it builds up and damages the developing brain. This is where the early treatment is vital. In fact, all newborns in most countries are screened for elevated phenylalanine levels in their blood, because early diagnosis of PKU can help parents prevent retardation by serving low-phenylalanine diets to their affected children.

The studies reported above may have some putative paths that could be explored for the purpose of interventions. The genetic mutations recently reported for stuttering by Kang and colleagues open up possibilities about the metabolic lyosomal enzymes. In other words, like the enzyme phenylalanine hydroxylase in PKU, there might be a way of preventing such forms of genetic stuttering (notably only 5% of people who stuttered had these variants in this study). It is possible that other such strategies might be developed when the genetic pathways and interactions of genes linked to complex traits (such as language and speech) are uncovered. With regards to *FOXP2* it is the case that this gene is highly similar in vertebrate species and the mouse Foxp2 differs from the human by only three substitutions. As mentioned previously, Grozer and colleagues showed that mice with the same point mutation to that of the KE family had abnormal synaptic plasticity in striatal and cerebellar neural circuits. These overlap with those regions/structures shown to be altered in neuroimaging studies of the KE family (Watkins *et al.*, 2002). Research such as this shows potential for the development of drugs that target the appropriate circuits to somehow rescue the reduced plasticity.

However, these mutations are very rare and affect only certain aspects of language skills/difficulties. In the majority of cases of complex language abilities/impairments where many interacting genes are involved as risk (or protective) factors it will be a lot more challenging to develop effective treatments.

9 Summary and Future Directions

The journey from language to brain to genes is a complex story which sheds some light on the basis of this trait, but throws up more questions than answers. This chapter has started with similarities amongst twins and the inferences we can draw about receptive, expressive and speech skills. Evidence was highlighted that heritability appears higher in developmental language disorders when speech rather than language understanding abilities are affected. Furthermore, there was evidence for high heritability for stuttering and other non-fluent speech. Molecular studies of families have shown which areas of the genome can be linked to language disorders and speech impairments and a number of candidate genes have now been discovered. The example of *FOXP2* shows how functional analyses of susceptibility genes can begin to bridge gaps from gene to brain to behaviour. It is now important to go down the same road for stuttering as has been taken for those genes that have been implicated in language impairments. Many genes as well as environmental influences have to work in concert to create a trait as complex as human language. Gene–gene and gene–environment interaction studies are needed to better characterise these effects.

Acknowledgements

The author likes to thank Prof Peter Howell for the constructive discussions about this chapter and his own chapter on genetic aspects of dysfluencies (Howell, 2010). The author is also very grateful for the helpful comments and suggestions by Dr Simon Fisher and Dr Dianne Newbury.

Note

1. When writing about the genetic material (DNA or RNA) the convention is to use italics (*FOXP2*). The gene is coding a protein by the same name but which is then written without italics (FOXP2). The lower case *Foxp2* (and again without italics for the protein) is used for the nonhuman homologue.

References

Altmuller, J., Palmer, L.J., Fischer, G., Scherb, H. and Wjst, M. (2001) Genomewide scans of complex human diseases: True linkage is hard to find. *American Journal of Human Genetics* 69(5), 936–950.

Ambrose, N.G., Yairi, E. and Cox, N. (1993) Genetic aspects of early childhood stuttering. *Journal of Speech and Hearing Research* 36(4), 701–706.

Andrews, G., Morris-Yates, A., Howie, P. and Martin, N.G. (1991) Genetic factors in stuttering confirmed. *Archives of General Psychiatry* 48(11), 1034–1035.

Bartlett, C.W., Flax, J.F., Logue, M.W., Vieland, V.J., Bassett, A.S., Tallal, P., *et al.* (2002) A major susceptibility locus for specific language impairment is located on chromosome 13q21. *American Journal of Human Genetics* 71, 45–55.

Bishop, D.V.M. (2002) Putting language genes in perspective. *Trends in Genetics* 18(2), 57–59.

Bishop, D.V.M. and Hayiou-Thomas, M.E. (2007) Heritability of specific language impairment depends on diagnostic criteria. *Genes, Brain and Behavior* 7, 365–372.

Bishop, D.V.M., North, T. and Donlan, C. (1996) Nonword repetition as a behavioural marker for inherited language impairment: Evidence from a twin study. *Journal of Child Psychology and Psychiatry and Allied Disciplines* 37(4), 391–403.

Conti-Ramsden, G., Botting, N. and Faragher, B. (2001) Psycholinguistic markers for Specific Language Impairment (SLI). *Journal of Child Psychology & Psychiatry* 42(6), 741–748.

Dworzynski, K., Remington, A., Rijsdijk, F., Howell, P. and Plomin, R. (2007) Genetic etiology in cases of recovered and persistent stuttering in an unselected, longitudinal sample of young twins. *American Journal of Speech-Language Pathology* 16(2), 169–178.

Enard, W., Przeworski, M., Fisher, S.E., Lai, C.S., Wiebe, V., Kitano, T., *et al.* (2002) Molecular evolution of FOXP2, a gene involved in speech and language. *Nature* 418(6900), 869–872.

Falcaro, M., Pickles, A., Newbury, D.F., Addis, L., Banfield, E., Fisher, S.E., *et al.* (2008) Genetic and phenotypic effects of phonological short-term memory and grammatical morphology in specific language impairment. *Genes, Brain and Behavior* 7(4), 393–402.

Felsenfeld, S. and Plomin, R. (1997) Epidemiological and offspring analyses of developmental speech disorders using data from the Colorado Adoption Project. *Journal of Speech, Language, and Hearing Research* 40(4), 778–791.

Felsenfeld, S., McGue, M. and Broen, P.A. (1995) Familial aggregation of phonological disorders: Results from a 28-year follow-up. *Journal of Speech and Hearing Research* 38(5), 1091–1107.

Felsenfeld, S., Kirk, K.M., Zhu, G., Statham, D.J., Neale, M.C. and Martin, N.G. (2000) A study of the genetic and environmental etiology of stuttering in a selected twin sample. *Behavior Genetics* 30(5), 359–366.

Fisher, S.E. (2005a) Dissection of molecular mechanisms underlying speech and language disorder. *Applied Psycholinguistics* 26, 111.

Fisher, S.E. (2005b) On genes, speech, and language. *New England Journal of Medicine* 353(16), 1655–1657.

Fisher, S.E. (2006) Tangled webs: Tracing the connections between genes and cognition. *Cognition* 101(2), 270–297.

Fisher, S.E. (2010) Genetic susceptibility to stuttering. *New England Journal of Medicine* 362(8), 750–752.

Fujita, E., Tanabe, Y., Shiota, A., Ueda, M., Suwa, K., Momoi, M.Y. and Momoi, T. (2008) Ultrasonic vocalization impairment of Foxp2 (R552H) knockin mice related to speech-language disorder and abnormality of Purkinje cells. *Proceedings of the National Academy of Sciences of the United States of America* 105, 3117–3122.

Groszer, M., Keays, D.A., Deacon, R.M., de Bono, J.P., Prasad-Mulcare, S., Gaub, S., *et al.* (2008) Impaired synaptic plasticity and motor learning in mice with a point mutation implicated in human speech deficits. *Current Biology* 18(5), 354–362.

Haesler, S., Rochefort, C., Georgi, B., Licznerski, P., Osten, P. and Scharff, C. (2007) Incomplete and inaccurate vocal imitation after knockdown of FoxP2 in songbird basal ganglia nucleus Area X. *PLoS Biology* 5(12), e321.

Hayiou-Thomas, M.E. (2008) Genetic and environmental influences on early speech, language and literacy development. *Journal of Communication Disorders* 41(5), 397–408.

Howell, P. (2010) *Recovery from Stuttering*. New York: Psychology Press.

Kang, C., Riazuddin, S., Mundorff, J., Krasnewich, D., Friedman, P., Mullikin, J.C., *et al.* (2010) Mutations in the lysosomal enzyme-targeting pathway and persistent stuttering. *New England Journal of Medicine* 362(8), 677–685.

Krause, J., Lalueza-Fox, C., Orlando, L., Enard, W., Green, R.E., Burbano, H.A., *et al.* (2007) The derived FOXP2 variant of modern humans was shared with Neandertals. *Curr Biology* 17(21), 1908–1912.

Lai, C.S., Fisher, S.E., Hurst, J.A., Vargha-Khadem, F. and Monaco, A.P. (2001) A forkhead-domain gene is mutated in a severe speech and language disorder. *Nature* 413(6855), 519–523.

MacDermot, K.D., Bonora, E., Sykes, N., Coupe, A.M., Lai, C.S., Vernes, S.C., *et al.* (2005) Identification of FOXP2 truncation as a novel cause of developmental speech and language deficits. *American Journal of Human Genetics* 76(6), 1074–1080.

Newbury, D.F., Winchester, L., Addis, L., Paracchini, S., Buckingham, L.L., Clark, A., *et al.* (2009) CMIP and ATP2C2 modulate phonological short-term memory in language impairment. *American Journal of Human Genetics* 85(2), 264–272.

Oliver, B.R. and Plomin, R. (2007) Twins' Early Development Study (TEDS): A multivariate, longitudinal genetic investigation of language, cognition and behavior problems from childhood through adolescence. *Twin Research and Human Genetics* 10(1), 96–105.

Ooki, S. (2005) Genetic and environmental influences on stuttering and tics in Japanese twin children. *Twin Research and Human Genetics* 8(1), 69–75.

Riaz, N., Steinberg, S., Ahmad, J., Pluzhnikov, A., Riazuddin, S., Cox, N.J., *et al.* (2005) Genomewide significant linkage to stuttering on chromosome 12. *American Journal of Human Genetics* 76(4), 647–651.

Sham, P. (2001) Shifting paradigms in gene-mapping methodology for complex traits. *Pharmacogenomics* 2(3), 195–202.

Shu, W., Cho, J.Y., Jiang, Y., Zhang, M., Weisz, D., Elder, G.A., Schmeidler, J., De Gasperi, R., Sosa, M.A., Rabidou, D. *et al.* (2005) Altered ultrasonic vocalization in mice with a disruption in the Foxp2 gene. *Proceedings of the National Academy of Sciences of the United States of America* 102, 9643–9648.

S. L. I. Consortium (2002) A genomewide scan identifies two novel loci involved in specific language impairment. *American Journal of Human Genetics* 70, 384–398.

S. L. I. Consortium (2004) Highly significant linkage to the SLI1 locus in an expanded sample of individuals affected by specific language impairment. *American Journal of Human Genetics* 74(1225), 1238.

Stromswold, K. (2001) The heritability of language: A review and metaanalysis of twin, adoption, and linkage studies. *Language* 77(4), 647–723.

Suresh, R., Ambrose, N., Roe, C., Pluzhnikov, A., Wittke-Thompson, J.K., Ng, M.C., *et al.* (2006) New complexities in the genetics of stuttering: Significant sex-specific linkage signals. *American Journal of Human Genetics* 78(4), 554–563.

Tallal, P., Hirsch, L.S., Realpe-Bonilla, T., Miller, S., Brzustowicz, L.M., Bartlett, C., *et al.* (2001) Familial aggregation in specific language impairment. *Journal of Speech, Language, and Hearing Research* 44(5), 1172–1182.

Trouton, A., Spinath, F.M. and Plomin, R. (2002) Twins early development study (TEDS): A multivariate, longitudinal genetic investigation of language, cognition and behavior problems in childhood. *Twin Research* 5, 444–448.

Van Beijsterveldt, C.E., Felsenfeld, S. and Boomsma, D.I. (2010) Bivariate genetic analyses of stuttering and nonfluency in a large sample of 5-year old twins. *Journal of Speech, Language, and Hearing Research* 53, 609–619.

Vargha-Khadem, F., Watkins, K.E., Price, C.J., Ashburner, J., Alcock, K.J., Connelly, A. *et al.* (1998) Neural basis of an inherited speech and language disorder. *Proceedings of the National Academy of Sciences of the United States of America* 95(21), 12695–12700.

Vernes, S.C., Newbury, D.F., Abrahams, B.S., Winchester, L., Nicod, J., Groszer, M., *et al.* (2008) A functional genetic link between distinct developmental language disorders. *New England Journal of Medicine* 359(22), 2337–2345.

Watkins, K.E., Vargha-Khadem, F., Ashburner, J., Passingham, R.E., Connelly, A., Friston, K.J., *et al.* (2002) MRI analysis of an inherited speech and language disorder: Structural brain abnormalities. *Brain* 125(Pt 3), 465–478.

Watson, J.D. and Crick, F.H. (1953) The structure of DNA. *Cold Spring Harbor Symposia on Quantitative Biology* 18, 123–131.

Chapter 4

Brain Structure and Function in Developmental Stuttering and Bilingualism

KATE E. WATKINS AND DENISE KLEIN

Summary

Brain imaging studies of developmental stuttering are starting to reach some consensus regarding the underlying neural mechanisms. Here, we provide some background to the different methods used to obtain and analyse brain imaging data. We review the findings from such studies in people who stutter that show, relative to fluent-speaking controls, overactivity in the right hemisphere centered on the right inferior frontal gyrus (homologue of Broca's area), underactivity of auditory areas in the temporal lobe and abnormal activation of subcortical structures involved in the control of movement, namely the cerebellum and the basal ganglia. Structural abnormalities in the frontal and temporal lobes and the white matter connections between them are also commonly reported in people who stutter and may be related to the functional abnormalities. Although there are many behavioural studies on stuttering in bilinguals, to our knowledge there are no reports of neuroimaging in such individuals. Findings in each field separately, however, might inform the other. For example, studies in bilinguals have debated the relative involvement of the left and right hemispheres in processing first and second languages and incomplete cerebral dominance for speech and language is a candidate theory to explain stuttering. In addition, recent work in bilingualism has implicated the basal ganglia in regulating language output control. This idea is in agreement with proposals that stuttering is caused by dysfunction in the basal ganglia, which leads to timing problems with speech production. Brain imaging studies of developmental stuttering and bilingualism will inform our understanding of the neural bases of speech, vocal learning, auditory-motor integration and the development of language representation in the bilingual brain. Moreover, the questions of whether and in what way learning a second language might interact with or affect stuttering should shed light on optimal strategies for the treatment of stuttering both in monolingual and in bilingual children.

1   Introduction

The specific neurobiological basis of developmental stuttering (DS) is unknown. Unlike other disorders of speech and language, either acquired or developmental, there appear to be no *post mortem* studies that have examined the brain either micro- or macro-scopically. The available data are obtained *in vivo*, therefore, using modern brain imaging methods. Due to the wide availability of brain scanners and increasing sophistication in analysis methods, there is a growing set of studies that have examined brain structure and function in people who stutter (PWS). These studies are starting to show some consensus with respect to the functional and structural abnormalities associated with DS. Here, we first introduce some background to the methodology of brain imaging studies and then review some of the growing body of findings from both structural and functional imaging studies in DS.

To our knowledge, there are no reports of imaging investigations of stuttering in bilingualism. This fact is somewhat surprising as there is an interesting overlap in the brain areas investigated in bilingualism and some of the brain areas showing abnormality in DS. For example, different nuclei of the basal ganglia are activated differently in first (L1) and second (L2) language processing; abnormal function of these nuclei is also reported in DS. Researchers have also proposed that a second language might be differently lateralised in the bilingual brain, which is a similar proposal to one theory that stuttering is caused by incomplete or different lateralisation of speech and language in DS. In the third section of this chapter, we review the brain imaging literature on the bilingual brain and point out the similarities between stuttering and bilingualism in terms of the brain areas involved. These common neural bases for speech motor control, inhibition and language switching may explain in part the higher risk of stuttering seen in children raised in multilingual environments (e.g. Howell *et al.*, 2009).

2   Background to Brain Imaging Methods

Non-invasive imaging methods allow us to examine the structure and function of the human brain in exquisite detail across the lifespan in health and disease. Techniques such as computerised tomography (CT), single photon emission computed tomography (SPECT) and positron emission tomography (PET) involve exposure to small amounts of radiation and are expensive; their use in research is limited, therefore. The advent of magnetic resonance imaging (MRI) and, in particular, functional MRI (fMRI) in the early 1990s led to a proliferation of investigations and the blossoming of the field of cognitive neuroscience.

Functional imaging methods, such as SPECT, PET and fMRI, measure brain activity. They differ in their relative temporal and spatial resolutions.

SPECT averages brain activity over tens of minutes with a typical spatial resolution of 1 cm^3. It is typically used therefore to measure 'baseline' rates of blood flow in different brain areas. Modern PET imaging studies have spatial resolution as good as fMRI (2–3 mm^3) but, depending on the half-life of the radioisotope used, its temporal resolution is more limited. Many research studies use oxygen-15, which has a half-life of 2 minutes, and measurements are typically averaged over 60–90s during which participants perform a task. FMRI has the best spatial and temporal resolution of all the functional imaging methods in common use for research. Typically, data is acquired with a spatial resolution of 3–5 mm^3. The temporal resolution depends on the experimental design. A measurement of brain activity is typically acquired every three seconds repeatedly for several minutes. It is possible to measure activity to single brief events that occur repeatedly and frequently throughout the experiment (event-related designs). A stimulus-evoked response measured in fMRI is, however, very slow to peak; typical estimates are 4–6 seconds after the stimulus onset. If overt speech is required during the experiment, this sluggish response can be particularly advantageous, allowing the measurement to be delayed until speaking has ceased and thus avoiding artefacts due to speech-related movements (this method is often referred to as 'sparse-sampling'). In experiments not requiring overt speech, brain activity is typically measured over 20–30 second epochs, repeated several times (blocked designs).

Current structural imaging methods for research typically rely on high-resolution (1 mm^3) images that optimise the contrast between tissue types. The most common image acquired is a T1-weighted image in which cortex and subcortical structures are grey and white matter is white. Diffusion-tensor imaging (DTI) is another structural imaging technique in common usage. It has a spatial resolution of 2–5 mm^3 and measures the integrity of the white matter.

2.1 Measurements

The different techniques used to map the brain are sensitive to different signals. PET and SPECT involve injection of substances labelled with a fast-decaying radioactive chemical into the bloodstream. Depending on the compound injected, these methods reveal the brain areas in which there is increased blood flow or a change in glucose or neurotransmitter metabolism, all of which reflect increased brain activity. Using intrinsic changes in the level of oxygen in the blood, fMRI can also measure brain activity without requiring injection of any substance. The blood-oxygenation level dependant (BOLD) signal measured in fMRI arises from the different effects of oxygenated and de-oxygenated haemoglobin on the magnetic field across the head in an MRI scanner.

Structural MRI relies on measures of water content in the brain. The different tissues in the brain have different levels of water and restrict the movement of water in different ways, which results in different MR signals. On a typical structural scan (with T1-weighting), the skull and cerebro-spinal fluid (CSF) are black, the cortex and subcortical nuclei are grey (grey matter) and the fibre pathways connecting these brain areas are white (white matter). White matter structure can be examined in more detail using DTI. In diffusion images, the movement of water molecules is measured in many different directions and the relative magnitude of this movement in three orthogonal directions is represented by a ratio of values (fractional anisotropy; FA). FA is high when there is an obvious underlying structure to the tissue such as in the large fibre bundles that comprise the brain's white matter. This is because water diffuses more easily along the direction in which the fibres are running and less easily across them. FA is low in grey matter and CSF because water diffusion is not restricted in any specific direction.

2.2 Analyses

Although each of the methods mentioned above produces a different signal measurement, the data acquired are analysed using the same general statistical methods. The measurements are acquired in slices through a box of space, which contains the head. Each slice comprises many individual three-dimensional elements, known as voxels (3D pixels; Figure 4.1b, in colour section). Each voxel contains a value that represents the average signal measured at that brain location (see Figure 4.1c, in colour section). Because these voxels are fairly small (a couple of millimetres cubed) the images look quite detailed and we consider them to be high resolution; it should be noted, however, that they represent the average of signals from many thousands of neurons and glia.

In functional imaging, using PET or fMRI, the signal is acquired at each voxel during a time when the subject is either performing a task or is at rest (see Figure 4.1a, in colour section). This measurement is repeated many times under these different conditions and then averaged to show the average level of activity at that voxel during performance of a task compared to the average level of activity at that voxel during another task or during rest. The mean difference in activity levels between conditions is divided by the variance in this difference across all the time points in the scan to give a t-statistic at each voxel. To allow comparisons across studies with different degrees of freedom, t-statistics are sometimes standardised to z-statistics (unit normal distribution). For degrees of freedom greater than about 50, the values of t and z are very similar, so the conversion is not always made. The magnitude (height) of the statistic is plotted using a colour scale across each slice and in all slices in the volume (see Figure 4.1d, in colour section). The significance of the statistic, however, requires correction for the number of comparisons made (a whole brain comprises potentially more than a hundred thousand voxels) but also consideration that data from nearby voxels is likely to be similar, i.e. not independent. There are a number of methods used in brain imaging to calculate the inference of these statistics. Some take into account the extent of neighbouring voxels that have a statistic above a certain threshold, e.g. cluster statistics. Some consider the values of voxels restricted to the region of interest or predicted *a priori* and therefore apply a less strict correction. Many report uncorrected statistics at a higher than usual significance level (e.g. $p < 0.001$).

Functional imaging data can be reported for individual subjects but is more commonly presented as an average across a group. Averaging data from individuals with different sized and shaped brains requires first transforming each individual's brain images to match a template image in a standard space. Data transformed to the same standard space can then be averaged and the coordinate system for that space can then be used to report the exact location of the results. The data are usually smoothed (i.e. blurred) during this process for statistical purposes. This smoothing also compensates for the fact that even after transformation the location of the gyri and sulci in the brain are not precisely overlapping across individuals.

In structural imaging studies, a method known as voxel-based morphometry is commonly used to calculate differences or changes in brain size and shape with statistics identical to those developed for functional imaging. In this case, the voxel values reflect some measure of tissue volume (e.g. how much of the signal in a brain region comes from grey matter), or shape (e.g. how much a brain region needs to be stretched or squashed to match a brain template) or both. For DTI data, the analysed voxels have FA values or measures of diffusion in different directions. These measures of brain structure are compared on a voxel-by-voxel basis between groups of subjects or within subjects between time points related to ageing or some intervention. The statistical calculations are identical to those above, and the results are similarly problematic with respect to statistical inference. There are additional problems related to analysing diffusion data with voxel-based morphometry techniques; these relate to smoothing data and partial volume effects at the boundary between grey and white matter. One method that circumvents these problems is a conservative technique known as tract-based spatial statistics (TBSS) (Smith *et al.*, 2006), which only considers voxels in a skeleton of white matter that corresponds to the middle of fibre tracts. As above, simple statistical tests such as t-tests are used to compare values at every voxel. In this particular case, non-parametric permutation testing is typically used for inference on these statistics because the data violate conditions for the use of parametric statistics.

3   Brain Function in Developmental Stuttering

The initial studies using functional imaging to study the brain in DS used SPECT, a low resolution imaging technique, and then PET, at higher spatial resolutions, to study dopamine activity, glucose and oxygen metabolism. More recent work has resulted in larger sample sizes and the use of functional MRI. Most of these studies required subjects to read words, sentences or paragraphs during scanning rather than speak spontaneously, which might have resulted in an under representation of stuttered speech. Also, several fluency-enhancing techniques have been examined including chorus reading and delayed auditory feedback. It is worth noting that PET imaging is silent. It is therefore possible for participants to speak normally and hear themselves against a background of silence. FMRI is very noisy, requiring participants to wear ear defenders. Speech production against the background noise is problematic for two reasons: participants cannot hear themselves clearly and speech-related movements can cause artefacts in the images. Sparse-sampling designs (see above) allow participants to speak during a silent interval between measurements, which are timed to capture the delayed BOLD response to the speech produced 4–6 s earlier. This means that participants can receive normal feedback of speech and the associated movements have less effect on the images. Nevertheless, the rhythmic nature and masking effect of the scanner noise might enhance fluency. Also, participants are required to keep as themselves still as possible, which can be difficult for some individuals, in particular, for young children.

A few summaries of the functional imaging literature in developmental stuttering have reported common sites of abnormal activation. Until recently, the participants in these studies have usually been adults who stutter. In three of the five PET studies reviewed by Ingham (2001), PWS showed increased activation relative to controls in the supplementary motor area and anterior insula cortex and reduced levels of activity in auditory association cortex during speech production. These abnormal levels of activity were seen bilaterally or predominantly in the right hemisphere. A more recent meta-analysis of eight PET and functional MRI studies produced results largely in agreement with the previous summary. In the meta-analysis, three 'neural signatures' of stuttering were identified: relative to controls, PWS had increased activity in (1) the right frontal operculum or anterior insula or both and (2) the cerebellar vermis, and (3) an 'absence' of activity in auditory areas bilaterally (Brown *et al.*, 2005). Generally, during speech and irrespective of fluency, PWS showed greater levels of activity across the whole brain than fluent-speaking controls.

Our own findings in an fMRI study of sentence reading with either normal or altered feedback are in accord with this general pattern of results

(Watkins *et al.*, 2008). Adolescents and young adults who stutter (aged 14–27 years) showed more activity during speech production relative to silent baseline than did age- and sex-matched controls. When groups were compared statistically in our study, we found that during speech production, PWS compared to controls had significantly more activity in the right anterior insula and midline cerebellum consistent with two of the three 'neural signatures' revealed by the meta-analysis described above. In addition, we found that PWS had less activity (relative to controls) in the motor and premotor system bilaterally and significant overactivation in a midbrain area, close to the location of the substantia nigra and subthalamic nuclei (see Figure 4.2, in colour section). The substantia nigra and subthalamic nuclei are small structures forming part of the basal ganglia and involved in circuits between different subcortical nuclei and the cortex. Abnormal activation of the basal ganglia has been reported previously in association with both acquired and developmental stuttering (see below). It is surprising, therefore, that abnormal activation of the basal ganglia was not identified as a common abnormality in the meta-analyses described above.

The data from functional imaging studies in DS are consistent with several different theories of the underlying deficit. The right-hemisphere overactivity described in the meta-analyses is consistent with the idea that stuttering is due to atypical cerebral lateralisation or incomplete hemispheric dominance for language processing (Orton, 1928; Travis, 1978). The reduced activation of auditory cortex seen in several studies in people who stutter is consistent with abnormal interactions between motor and sensory cortices during speech production (Andrews *et al.*, 1983; Guenther, 2006). Finally, our own findings and those of others point to an abnormality in the basal ganglia or with dopamine metabolism in DS (see Alm, 2004 and references therein). We describe each of these in more detail below and evaluate the evidence for them or alternative explanations based mainly on our own findings.

3.1 Abnormal cerebral lateralisation of speech and language

The oldest explanation of stuttering that makes reference to the brain is that of Orton (1928), who suggested that stuttering is due to incomplete cerebral dominance. This appears to have been based on the increased incidence of left-handedness among stutterers and anecdotal reports of stuttering emerging following enforced use of the right hand for writing in children who earlier showed a tendency to left-handedness. Imaging findings that report increased right-hemisphere activity during speech production in PWS compared to controls appear to provide support for this idea.

One very early study to examine brain function used SPECT to scan two young adults, a female who acquired stuttering at age 13 after a head injury and a man who had stuttered since the age of four (Wood *et al.*, 1980). They were scanned while reading aloud on and off haloperidol medication, which improved fluency in both. This very preliminary study indicated right-lateralised blood flow in the posterior part of the inferior frontal gyrus (Broca's area in the left hemisphere) during stuttered speech, which reversed to be left lateralised during fluency. Blood flow in the posterior superior temporal gyrus (Wernicke's area in the left hemisphere) showed the expected left-lateralised pattern in both fluent and stuttered speech produced by these two individuals. In subsequent work on 20 PWS scanned using the same method but during rest, blood flow was found to be reduced overall relative to 78 age-matched controls and there were atypical right-greater-than-left flow asymmetries in the anterior cingulate, middle and superior temporal gyri in the PWS (Pool *et al.*, 1991).

In studies using PET or fMRI, increased right-hemisphere activity in PWS relative to controls is typically seen in the frontal opercular cortex, extending sometimes to the anterior insula and the orbito-frontal surface (Brown *et al.*, 2005; Kell *et al.*, 2009; Watkins *et al.*, 2008). Therapy that successfully improved fluency can reduce this right inferior frontal gyrus overactivity or increase left-hemisphere activity resulting in a more typical left-lateralised pattern (De Nil *et al.*, 2003; Kell *et al.*, 2009; Neumann *et al.*, 2003; Preibisch *et al.*, 2003). Rather than reflecting bilateral or right-hemisphere language dominance, some researchers speculate that this right inferior frontal activity might reflect successful compensatory activity (Preibisch *et al.*, 2003).

There is some evidence from our own unpublished studies that the overactivity of the right inferior frontal region in DS is either a reflection of speech disfluency or a cause of it. In fluent speakers given delayed auditory feedback with a long delay of 200 ms, which typically causes speech disfluencies, we saw increased activity in the right inferior frontal cortex (Watkins *et al.*, 2005). This activity was seen in the delayed feedback condition compared to another altered feedback condition, namely frequency-shifted feedback, and compared to normal feedback. Importantly, frequency-shifted feedback is not known to cause speech disfluencies in fluent speakers. We propose that the overactivity seen in the right inferior frontal region in PWS during speech production and fluent speakers while speaking during delayed auditory feedback reflects activity related to the tendency to stutter. Activity in a right-hemisphere network centred on the inferior frontal region (including the frontal operculum and anterior insula) has been described as involved in braking or stopping motor responses (Aron *et al.*, 2007). Of particular relevance is a study of response inhibition of speech in which activity in the right frontal operculum increased when participants received a signal to stop (i.e. inhibit) their planned speech response (Xue *et al.*, 2008).

In sum, although initially the reports of overactivity in the right hemisphere in DS, revealed by brain imaging, seemed consistent with Orton's proposal of incomplete cerebral dominance, further studies are needed to elaborate on the precise functional role of these regions. By combining methods such as transcranial magnetic stimulation with functional imaging it is possible to test some of the suggestions proposed above (e.g. in aphasia, Martin *et al.*, 2009).

3.2 Abnormal auditory-motor interactions during speech production

A consistently observed abnormality seen in functional imaging studies of DS is reduced activity or 'inactivity' of the auditory cortices bilaterally (Braun *et al.*, 1997; Brown *et al.*, 2005; Ingham, 2001). This has been attributed to an increased suppressive effect on auditory cortex activity from repeated overactivation of motor areas due to the excessive motor symptoms of stuttering. It has been suggested that this decrease in activity is the result of impaired efference copy; a signal from motor to sensory areas that is thought to be involved in predicting the sensory consequences of actions (see Guenther, 2006). The fact that altering auditory feedback appears to increase activity in auditory cortices and improves fluency in PWS suggests that the reduced activity seen under normal feedback is indeed detrimental to fluency.

In our own study, the activity in left auditory cortex was significantly reduced in PWS relative to controls during speech production. We also saw significantly less activity bilaterally in the ventral premotor cortex and sensorimotor cortex at the level of the representation of the face in PWS. As mentioned above, it has been suggested that the reduced activity in the auditory cortices is due to the increased suppressive effects of excessive motor cortex activity. According to our analysis, the motor cortices are significantly less active in PWS than in controls during speech production, which makes it unlikely to have increased its suppression of auditory areas. In an ongoing study, we are exploring the relationship between activity in motor and auditory areas further using functional connectivity. We looked at the correlation between fMRI activity in the left sensorimotor cortex at the level of the face representation and left auditory cortex (lateral Heschl's gyrus) during periods of silent baseline and speech production with normal, delayed or frequency-shifted feedback. During speech production, controls showed an increase in the correlation between these areas relative to the correlation during baseline and this increased correlation did not significantly change when feedback was altered from normal. In PWS, however, the correlation between activity in motor and auditory areas reduced during speech production with normal feedback from its baseline levels (i.e. during silence). When feedback was altered, especially in the delayed auditory feedback condition, the correlation increased from the silent baseline condition to the same level as that seen in controls. This decoupling of activity during normal feedback revealed by functional connectivity analysis is consistent with theories proposing abnormal interactions between sensory and motor cortex during speech production in stuttering, and is possibly due to abnormal efference copy (Andrews *et al.*, 1983). It also suggests that the mechanism underlying the known fluency-enhancing effects of altered auditory feedback could involve correction of the coordination of activity between motor and sensory cortices during speech production.

3.3   Abnormal basal ganglia function

For many years, the function of the nuclei that comprise the basal ganglia has been implicated in stuttering. Early imaging studies using PET and SPECT described overactivity and excessive dopamine metabolism in the striatum of PWS. Wu and colleagues (1995) used PET to measure glucose metabolism in four right-handed DS (three men and one woman) and four younger and fluent controls during reading aloud either alone or in unison, which enhances fluency in the DS. During stuttered speech the DS group showed decreased activity in the left hemisphere, notably in Broca's and Wernicke's areas and the right cerebellum. During fluency and in comparison with the fluent controls, these regions showed normal levels of metabolism but the left caudate nucleus showed reduced metabolism and the substantia nigra increased metabolism. In a subsequent study (Wu *et al.*, 1997), PET was used to measure dopamine activity in three male DS and six male controls, all right handed. DS showed considerably higher levels of dopamine activity in several cortical and subcortical structures though the anatomical specificity of this technique and the lack of structural images makes it difficult to be confident about the location of these differences.

Stuttering acquired due to neurological impairment can be associated with lesions of the basal ganglia and thalamus (Ludlow & Loucks, 2003). Alm (2004) reviewed the evidence for a causal role of basal ganglia impairment and dopamine in developmental stuttering and proposed a mechanism whereby dysfunction in these circuits impaired the timing of cues for initiation of segments of sequences of speech sounds. This theory is supported by reports that stuttering symptoms improve on dopamine antagonists consistent with the notion that there is an excess of dopamine in DS (Maguire *et al.*, 2000; Wu *et al.*, 1997). In Parkinson's disease, however, the relationship between dopamine activity and speech fluency is less clear; patients are reported to develop stuttering with the onset of disease (i.e. during dopamine depletion) and also to worsen on dopaminergic medication (e.g. L-Dopa) (Anderson *et al.*, 1999; Louis *et al.*, 2001). As seen in DS, patients with Parkinson's disease also benefit from external cues to initiate and perform sequences of movements fluently. For example, auditory rhythmic or visual structured cues can improve gait fluency in Parkinson's (Glickstein & Stein, 1991). It is possible, therefore, that in DS the basal ganglia dysfunction plays a role in the abnormal integration of motor and sensory information for speech production as discussed above.

Our own fMRI study revealed a large area of overactivity in the midbrain during speech produced by DS (Watkins *et al.*, 2008). This region was not active relative to baseline in the controls. Overactivation of a similar area was reported by Giraud and colleagues (2008), who also found a significant positive correlation between activation of the caudate nucleus and stuttering severity; this abnormal activity normalised after successful stuttering therapy (see also Kell *et al.*, 2009). The candidate structures that might contribute to activity in the midbrain region include the subthalamic nuclei, substantia nigra, red nucleus and pedunculopontine nucleus. With the resolution typical of whole-brain fMRI studies, it is not possible to resolve which specific nuclei were overactivated in the PWS scanned in our study. Abnormal activity in each of these different nuclei would implicate distinct cortico-subcortical loops and would therefore have significant implication for which networks are likely involved. Dysfunction in these nuclei and circuits might result in an impaired ability to produce timing cues for initiation of submovements of an overlearned motor sequence such as speech. Outputs from the basal ganglia to the medial premotor cortex are thought to be involved in the execution of self-initiated, well-learned, complex and sequential movements (see Alm, 2004 and references therein). On the other hand, Alm proposed that fluent speech in PWS is mediated by engaging the lateral premotor system and cerebellum, which might also lead to increased activity in these areas (see also Guenther, 2006; Howell & Sackin, 2002).

Another candidate nucleus for contributing to functional overactivity in the midbrain region is the pedunculopontine nucleus, which receives inputs from the cerebellum and is reciprocally connected with cerebral cortex, subthalamic nucleus and globus pallidus (Jenkinson *et al.*, 2009). This nucleus is thought to be involved in the initiation and modulation of stereotyped movements (although principally gait) and along with the subthalamic nucleus is a target for therapy in the treatment of Parkinson's disease (Jenkinson *et al.*, 2005).

Studies that have correlated stuttering severity or looked at changes due to improved fluency suggest a normalisation of patterns of activity in the right inferior frontal gyrus and basal ganglia (e.g. Giraud *et al.*, 2008; Preibisch *et al.*, 2003). This suggests that the abnormalities in these regions could be related. Furthermore, connectivity analyses have revealed a triangular network involved in inhibitory motor control comprising the right frontal operculum, subthalamic nucleus and supplementary motor area (Aron *et al.*, 2007). Further work is needed to establish if the functional abnormalities in DS seen in these regions reflect a common underlying impairment.

3.4   Summary of abnormal brain activity associated with developmental stuttering

Functional brain imaging studies in DS have revealed consistent abnormalities in function during speech tasks in terms of overactivity of right-hemisphere cortical areas, particularly in the inferior frontal gyrus (homologous with Broca's area) and underactivity of the auditory cortex bilaterally. In addition, abnormal activity in two subcortical systems involved in the control of movement, namely the cerebellum and basal ganglia, has been reported though with less consistency. Whether a common basis exists for all the abnormalities described has yet to be determined. Finally, sex differences need to be addressed. One study suggests very similar patterns of activity between males and females who stutter but also found positive correlations between stuttering and basal ganglia activity in females, whereas stuttering correlated with activity in the cerebellum in males (Ingham *et al.*, 2004). This might explain the lack of commonly observed abnormal activity associated with DS in the basal ganglia in the meta-analysis (Brown *et al.*, 2005), which described a consistent overactivation of the cerebellar vermis, as noted to correlate with stuttering in the males studied by Ingham and colleagues.

4   Brain Structure in Developmental Stuttering

Many studies of the brain anatomy in PWS focused their attention on the peri-Sylvian cortex, the location in the left hemisphere of areas that are important for expressive and receptive speech and language, namely Broca's and Wernicke's areas respectively (see Figure 4.3, in colour section). Despite the variety of methods used in these studies, some common abnormalities have emerged in association with DS. These include differences in the volume or shape of cortical areas, hemispheric volume asymmetries and white matter microstructure.

4.1   Volume and shape differences

Using volumetric measurements of structural MRI scans, Foundas and colleagues were among the first to examine the cortical areas surrounding the Sylvian fissure in PWS. They found no differences in grey matter volumes of frontal regions including the pars triangularis and pars opercularis, which together comprise Broca's area in the left hemisphere (Foundas *et al.*, 2001). In contrast, the volumes of posterior speech and language regions, typically associated with language comprehension and speech perception (i.e. Wernicke's area), were significantly increased in volume in PWS. This increase was seen in the left and right hemispheres and the normal pattern of a leftward size asymmetry in this region was reduced in DS (Cykowski *et al.*, 2007; Foundas *et al.*, 2001).

A number of unusual sulcal patterns in the peri-Sylvian region have also been described. Foundas and colleagues (2001) noted an extra diagonal sulcus (a shallow indentation on the lateral surface of the pars opercularis; see Figure 4.3, in colour section) in one or both hemispheres of 5 out of 16 people who stutter. This abnormality was only seen in 2 of the 19 right-handed male stutterers (and in at least two controls) studied by Cykowski and colleagues (2008), however. Both studies also reported extra gyri along the upper surface of the Sylvian fissure (frontal, central and parietal operculum; see Figure 4.3, in colour section). Foundas describes these in either the left or the right or in both hemispheres in nearly all the PWS she studied, but in the right-handed males who stutter studied by Cykowski this increase was seen only in the right hemisphere. The number of gyri in the left hemispheres of right-handed males who stutter did not differ from that in controls in Cykowski's study. Moreover, this group of right-handed males who stutter had the same number of sulci or gyri in the right hemisphere as they had in the left hemisphere, whereas the controls had significantly fewer sulci in the right hemisphere compared to the left. So the difference in PWS was due to an increased number of gyri in the right hemisphere that is normally decreased in number relative to the left.

A handful of studies have examined the brains of PWS using the whole-brain automated technique known as voxel-based morphometry (VBM). Despite almost identical methods, these studies report quite different results. One study found no differences in grey matter between a group of 10 stutterers and 10 controls but reported white matter increases in several regions underlying inferior frontal, precentral and superior temporal cortex in the right hemisphere (Jancke *et al.*, 2004). Another study found increased grey matter in a group of 26 right-handed male stutterers in the posterior superior temporal gyrus bilaterally, left posterior inferior frontal gyrus (pars opercularis, ventral premotor and anterior insula cortex), left anterior temporal lobe and right cerebellum (Beal *et al.*, 2007). The same study reported increased white matter in PWS underlying the right posterior inferior frontal and left middle temporal cortex. No regions of lower grey or white matter volume were found in the stuttering group compared to controls. The third study to use the VBM method (Chang *et al.*, 2008) examined grey matter volume in two groups of boys who were persistent in or recovered from DS. Compared to controls, the combined group of persistent and recovered DS had reduced grey matter volume bilaterally in the posterior inferior frontal gyrus, supplementary motor area, left supramarginal gyrus, right sensorimotor cortex and right temporal cortex. This reduction in grey matter in children who stutter relative to controls contrasts with those showing grey matter increases in adults who stutter (Beal *et al.*, 2007; Cykowski *et al.*, 2007; Foundas *et al.*, 2001); the authors suggest, therefore, that the increases seen in adults reflect reorganisational plasticity due to stuttering, rather than a causal role in stuttering.

A recent VBM study of adult males with persistent stuttering and developmental stutterers who recovered in adulthood spontaneously (i.e. without assistance) found decreased grey matter volume in a combined group of persistent and recovered stutterers in comparison with fluent-speaking controls (Kell *et al.*, 2009). Reductions were found in the left inferior frontal gyrus for both persistent and recovered groups. In the persistent group, grey matter volume in the left inferior frontal gyrus significantly correlated with stuttering severity; the more severe stutterers had lower grey matter volume in this region. The persistent group also showed reduced grey matter volume in the left middle frontal and supramarginal gyri, similar to the findings in children (Chang *et al.*, 2008). Adults who recovered showed no significant differences in grey matter volume compared to adults with persistent stuttering, however. This differs to the findings in children where in comparison to boys with persistent DS, those who recovered had significantly more grey matter in the cingulate gyrus and less grey matter in the temporal lobe, motor cortex and cerebellum bilaterally. It should be noted that comparisons between persistent and recovered stutterers are hampered by the difficulties inherent in identifying stuttering and recruiting individuals who 'recovered' from DS without detailed measurement of their stuttering severity before recovery. Also, it seems reasonable to suppose that recovery is mediated by a variety of means and that 'recovered' populations will be heterogeneous, therefore.

4.2 Hemispheric asymmetries

In the normal human brain, the study of the structural asymmetries thought to underlie lateralised brain function was stimulated by findings of a leftward asymmetry of the planum temporale, which is located on the superior surface of the temporal lobe close to Wernicke's area (Geschwind & Levitsky, 1968) (see Figure 4.3, in colour section). When abnormal functional organisation is suspected, as has commonly been the case in developmental disorders such as dyslexia, autism, schizophrenia and stuttering, researchers have examined for the presence of typical brain asymmetries. The most commonly observed structural brain asymmetries in the normal population are the left-greater-than-right planum temporale asymmetry and the brain 'torque'. The brain 'torque' involves protrusion of the right frontal and left occipital lobes creating indentations on the inner surface of the skull known as petalias. The right frontal petalia is due to a longer and wider right frontal lobe compared to the left. The left occipital petalia is due to a longer and wider left occipital lobe compared to the right.

In one of the earliest brain imaging studies of DS, Strub and colleagues used CT scans to examine the brains of a brother and sister who stuttered (Strub *et al.*, 1987). The normally observed rightward frontal lobe width and length asymmetries were found in the sister who was left-handed but were unusually leftward in the brother who was more ambidextrous. The normally observed leftward occipital width asymmetry was rightward in both siblings. Whether these asymmetries are related to the left-handedness of these siblings or their stuttering or whether both the left-handedness and atypical brain asymmetries are indicative of anomalous cerebral dominance remains an open question.

In general agreement with this early study, Foundas *et al.* (2003) also reported no difference between two groups of 14 stutterers and 14 controls in the degree of the rightward frontal asymmetry, but found reduced or absent leftward occipital asymmetry in association with DS. The volume of the planum temporale was significantly greater in stutterers (n = 16) than controls in both hemispheres and the planum temporale asymmetry was reduced (Foundas *et al.*, 2001). Stutterers with abnormal (i.e. rightward) asymmetry of the planum temporale had more severe stuttering than those with typical leftward asymmetry. Furthermore, delayed auditory feedback improved the fluency of the group of stutterers with rightward planum asymmetry (n = 5) to the same level as the group with leftward planum asymmetry (n = 9) but it had no effect on the fluency of the latter group (Foundas *et al.*, 2004). Interestingly, five controls in this study had rightward planum temporale asymmetry. This raises the question as to whether the rightward asymmetry should really be considered atypical. It is certainly not exclusively associated with stuttering but it is possible that it poses an additional risk factor for stuttering severity.

Jancke and colleagues (2004) reported a reduced leftward asymmetry of a white matter region of interest underlying the posterior part of the superior temporal cortex (i.e. the planum temporale) in a group of 10 stutterers. A whole-brain analysis of grey matter in the same group revealed no volume differences compared to controls and no altered asymmetry.

Many previous studies reported data from groups that were mixed with respect to sex and handedness. Recently, two studies have restricted their analysis to right-handed males who stutter to avoid other explanations of anomalous cerebral asymmetry in both structure and function; left-handers and females are thought to be less lateralised than males

(Watkins *et al.*, 2001). In their study of 19 right-handed adult males who stutter, Cykowski *et al.* (2007) found typical patterns of asymmetry for frontal and occipital poles and widths and for the planum temporale, with no significant differences compared to controls. Chang *et al.* (2008) studied two groups of right-handed boys aged 9–12 years with persistent DS (n = 8) or who had recovered from DS (n = 7) 2 or 3 years after onset. These two groups did not differ from each other or from controls in any measurements of asymmetry, including the planum temporale. It is possible, therefore, that the previous findings of abnormal asymmetry in people who stutter were influenced by the inclusion of females who stutter and left-handed individuals.

4.3   White matter microstructure

Using diffusion weighted imaging, three studies report reduced fractional anisotropy in the white matter underlying the central operculum in both children and adults who stutter (Chang *et al.*, 2008; Sommer *et al.*, 2002; Watkins *et al.*, 2008). Using a whole-brain voxel-wise approach, Sommer and colleagues (2002) were the first to report diffusion data in a group of 15 stutterers. Relative to controls, FA was significantly reduced in the white matter directly underneath the left ventral sensorimotor cortex, at the level of the representations of the articulators. These authors proposed that a disconnection of the white matter tracts connecting frontal and temporal language cortices underlies stuttering (Buchel & Sommer, 2004). We acquired diffusion-tensor data, using 60 diffusion directions in a group of 17 stutterers aged between 14 and 27 years. Using TBSS (Smith *et al.*, 2006), we replicated the previous finding of reduced FA in white matter close to the left ventral sensorimotor cortex (Watkins *et al.*, 2008). We also found reductions in FA in homologous right-hemisphere regions. Furthermore, the reduced FA in the left ventral premotor white matter lay directly under cortical areas that were found to be functionally abnormal in PWS. In their study of boys who persisted in or recovered from stuttering, Chang and colleagues (2008) found reduced FA for the combined persistent/recovered group relative to controls in the white matter underlying the sensorimotor cortex in the left hemisphere, in the corticospinal/bulbar tracts bilaterally and in the left posterior white matter underlying the inferior parietal cortex. In sum, three separate reports of FA measurements in stutterers describe a deficit in the white matter close to the cortical sensorimotor representations of the articulators in the left hemisphere (see Figure 4.4). White matter tracts in this region include those connecting the overlying cortical areas with subcortical structures, cortico-cortico u-fibres and possibly branches of large white matter tracts like the arcuate fasciculus and superior longitudinal fasciculus that provide connections between the posterior temporal cortex, inferior parietal areas and lateral prefrontal cortex. As these regions contain speech-related areas, a parsimonious explanation of stuttering is that it is due to disruption of the tracts connecting these regions (Buchel & Sommer, 2004).

In contrast to these three studies showing reduced FA, a recent DTI study of adults who persistently stutter revealed increased FA relative to controls in the anterior portion of the corpus callosum (forceps minor) and white matter underlying the left orbitofrontal cortex (Kell *et al.*, 2009). Areas of increased and decreased FA were seen in the left superior longitudinal fasciculus (although the decreases were only seen at an uncorrected significance level). Increased FA is slightly difficult to explain in terms of an abnormality as it could be because diffusion in the principal direction increased perhaps due to increased axon diameter or because diffusion in the two axes orthogonal to the principal one decreased, perhaps reflecting increased myelination, which means further barriers to diffusion in those directions. The authors speculate that the increased FA might reflect hyperconnectivity in DS due to a failure during development to reduce superfluous axons. The areas showing reduced FA in adults with persistent DS were close to those described in the three previous studies (see Figure 4.4, in colour section), namely the white matter underlying left sensorimotor cortex.

4.4 Summary of findings of abnormal brain structure associated with developmental stuttering

The most consistent differences in brain structure associated with DS are those in white matter microstructure described above. In the cortex, some studies report an increase in cortical volume in the posterior superior temporal gyrus and a possible reduction in the leftward asymmetry of this region. The variability in the results of the studies of cortex might be due to unusual patterns of sulci and gyri in PWS. They might also reflect variability introduced by combining data from males and females who stutter and from left- and right-handed individuals. Larger samples of each of these groups would clarify these findings. Finally, longitudinal studies are warranted given the suggestion from the study of children with persistent stuttering and recovered stutterers who showed grey matter decreases rather than the increases documented in several adult cohorts. It is important to determine whether the brain differences described reflect reorganisation of function and experience-dependent plasticity and are, therefore, a consequence of stuttering rather than a cause.

5 Brain Imaging Studies of Bilingualism

When people speak more than one language, they can differentiate and process the language of the heard or written word, they can produce words in the selected language and they can control or inhibit production of a non-selected language. These abilities raise the question as to whether the two languages of the bilingual are represented in distinct or over-lapping areas of the brain. This question was originally posed by Pitres (1895) after observing the variable recovery patterns of bilingual aphasic patients. The question about the organisation of multiple languages in the brain has been investigated by electrical stimulation of the cerebral cortex in conscious patients undergoing brain surgery, by examining bilingual aphasic patients, and with experimental studies in normal bilingual participants, but it has proven difficult to determine conclusively whether different languages share the same neural substrate. Penfield denied that separate neuronal mechanisms existed for each language (Penfield, 1953), whereas others have proposed that partially distinct cerebral areas may be involved, especially when the second language is learned after the normal period of language acquisition (Ojemann & Whitaker, 1978; Paradis, 1997). Over the decades there has also been much debate about whether bilinguals might have greater right-hemisphere involvement for language processing than monolinguals. Reports from bilingual patients with brain damage and from some experimental studies obtained with healthy bilinguals gave rise to the suggestion that there may be a greater degree of right-hemisphere involvement in language processing in bilinguals than the level typically found in monolinguals (Albert & Obler, 1978; Galloway & Scarcella, 1982). Similar proposals have been put forward about the possibility of greater right-hemisphere lateralisation in developmental stuttering (see Section 3.1).

5.1   Brain function in bilinguals

In recent times, bilingual brain organisation has started to be explored by neuroimaging methods because, unlike lesion studies, which depend on experiments of nature, a particular advantage of functional neuroimaging is that it is possible to conduct controlled experiments. It is striking how, to date, the brain imaging literature related to bilingual processing has focused exclusively on adults with a dearth of research on the cerebral organisation of two languages during the course of child development.

Despite the advantage that neuroimaging studies confer for study-ing bilingual brain organisation, the results from studies with bilingual adults remain equivocal. Some studies argue that different neural tissue is involved in first (L1) and second languages (L2) (Dehaene *et al.*, 1997; Kim *et al.*, 1997), whereas others support the claim for a similar neural repre-sentation across languages in bilingual individuals (Chee, 2006). It is now becoming increasingly clear that the degree to which brain regions are involved in bilingual language processing is modulated by factors such as age of L2 acquisition (Wartenburger *et al.*, 2003) and language proficiency (Chee *et al.*, 2004; Perani *et al.*, 1998), and that the cerebral representation of L1 and L2 might be affected by the type of language-processing skills engaged or by the particular language under investigation (Frenck-Mestre *et al.*, 2005; Tan *et al.*, 2003; Xu *et al.*, 2006). It has been argued that age of exposure might not affect all domains of language equally; while lexical and semantic aspects are relatively spared, syntax and phonology appear to be most vulnerable (Weber-Fox & Neville, 1996). Within the first year of life, speech-perception skills of infants change from language-general to language-specific as a result of their language experience (Kuhl, 1998; Sebastian-Galles, 2006; Werker & Tees, 1984). Age of first exposure is the single largest determinant of native-like speech perception and production skills in L2 learners (Flege *et al.*, 1999; Johnson & Newport, 1989).

In our early studies, we used PET to investigate whether language processing in L2 involves the same neural substrates as that of L1 in healthy bilingual adults who learned their L2 after the age of five years. We investigated the brain areas that are involved in tasks requiring semantic searches both within and across L1 and L2. English-French-proficient bilingual subjects were required to perform tasks that involved a semantic search (synonym generation) in both their L1 (e.g. *weep–cry*) and L2 (*breuvage – boisson*) and also to translate their L1 into L2 (*house – maison*) and vice-versa (*arbre – tree*). Two baseline control tasks required word repetition in each language. Sensory-input and motor-output demands were thus similar in all conditions, since they involved listening to a single word and producing a single spoken response. We observed activity in the left inferior frontal cortex in each generation task as compared to the repetition baseline (see Figure 4.5, in colour section). The pattern of activity was similar irrespective of whether the search took place in the L1 or in the L2 and irrespective of whether the search was within a language or across languages. For all the word generation conditions, a series of left-hemisphere peri-Sylvian peaks were activated and we did not find evidence that the L2 was represented differently to the L1. No right-hemisphere cortical activations were observed in any condition and our results did not support the notion of increased right-hemisphere activity for L2. This is in keeping with the view that those components of language that are represented in the left hemisphere in monolinguals are no less lateralised in bilingual speakers (Paradis, 1992).

What was striking and unpredicted in our study was that we observed increased activation in the left basal ganglia (putamen) whenever native English speakers produced an output response in their second language, French (Klein *et al.*, 1995); this was evident when subjects performed a translation into their L2, but not the inverse, when they were translating their L2 into L1 (see Figure 4.5, in colour section). Activity in the left putamen was also observed when subjects repeated words in their L2, but not in their L1. We interpreted this finding as reflecting the role of the left basal ganglia in the complex motor timing involved in speaking a language that has been acquired later in life. In a follow-up study (Klein *et al.*, 2006), we again interpreted the increased activation in the left putamen/insula for L2 production in terms of a greater role of the left basal ganglia in the coordination of speech articulation, it being further assumed that articulation of a second language is more effortful than that of a first.

Impairments in the motor control of speech have been attributed to lesions in the 'lenticular zone', which includes the insula, claustrum, white-matter fibre tracts passing through the external and internal capsule, the caudate nucleus and lentiform nucleus (putamen and pallidum) (Dronkers, 1996; Marie, 1971). Typically, patients with subcortical aphasias are non-fluent; they are reluctant to initiate speech and show voice disorders, disrupted articulation often leading to mispronunciation, and occasionally a foreign accent syndrome (FAS). The latter is a rare speech disorder characterised by an inability to make the normal phonetic and phonemic contrasts of one's native dialect, thus conferring on the patient's native language a peculiar quality that is perceived by listeners as a foreign accent (Blumstein *et al.*, 1987; Graff-Radford *et al.*, 1986; Gurd *et al.*, 1988). Present knowledge of the neural basis of FAS is limited, as only a few cases have undergone detailed lesion analyses. Most cases with published lesion information have had left-hemisphere damage. Localisation has not been uniform, but all cases have involved either primary motor cortex, inferior frontal cortex (ventral premotor or pars opercularis) or the striatum of the basal ganglia (Kurowski *et al.*, 1996). This finding of FAS may link with reports that speaking in a foreign accent can improve speech fluency in developmental stuttering (e.g. Mowrer, 1986) and also points to the striatum as playing a role in effortful coordination of speech.

Crinion and colleagues (2006) have recently focused their research on the role of the left caudate nucleus in monitoring and controlling the language in use. They used fMRI in groups of highly proficient German-English and Japanese-English bilinguals and found evidence for increased activity in the left caudate nucleus when there is change in language, suggesting a possible role for the left caudate nucleus as a regulator of language output control. Results from neuropsychological studies of bilingual patients also point to the left caudate nucleus as being involved in language control (Abutalebi *et al.*, 2000; Perani & Abutalebi, 2005). In a case study of a trilingual patient with a lesion to the white-matter surrounding the head of the left caudate nucleus, these authors have argued that patients with damage to the left caudate nucleus have difficulties characterised by a pathological mixing among languages in oral production tasks and in control of the language of output. It has been argued that anatomically the left caudate nucleus plays a critical role in control-ling and selecting automatic motor sequences such as those necessary for articulation (Crinion *et al.*, 2006; Jueptner & Weiller, 1998).

The work described above is interesting in that it highlights the increas-ing attention on the role of brain regions that are outside the traditional left peri-Sylvian areas in bilingual language processing (Perani & Abutalebi, 2005); a similar role for these subcortical brain regions has been noted with reference to stuttering.

5.2 Brain structure in Bilinguals

Although there has been increasing interest in using morphometric approaches to examine language learning-related structural brain changes (Golestani *et al.*, 2007; Lee *et al.*, 2007), surprisingly few studies have looked at anatomical correlates of bilingual processing and to our knowl-edge none have looked at structural abnormalities in bilingual stutterers. Using VBM, Mechelli and colleagues (2004) were the first to explore dif-ferences in L1 and L2 anatomy. The only difference they observed was increased grey-matter density in the left inferior parietal cortex, with the degree of structural reorganisation in this region being modulated by the proficiency attained and the age at acquisition. A more recent study (Grogan *et al.*, 2009) showed that the volume of pre-SMA and head of the caudate nucleus bilaterally are associated more with phonemic fluency than semantic fluency, and that this effect is stronger for L2 than L1 in the caudate nuclei. These authors suggest that phonemic relative to semantic fluency might rely more on internal articulatory processing. Ullman (2001) has suggested that the basal ganglia, including the caudate nucleus, form part of the procedural memory system that is involved in learning the assembly of sequences of phonemes to form words. Grogan and colleagues (2009) thus hypothesise that the left head of the caudate nucleus may be involved when the language processing system can-not rely entirely on automatic mechanisms and has to recruit controlled processes as well.

6 Concluding Remarks

We have provided an overview of some of the issues raised from the brain imaging literature in the field of bilingualism in general and in the field of stuttering research. Clearly the field of brain imaging and research on bilingual stutterers is still in its infancy. To our knowledge, the ques-tion of structure and function using modern brain imaging tools has not yet been directed towards examining bilingual stutterers. However, given that differences in stuttering severity between languages in bilinguals may be the result of a difference in language proficiency (usually more stut-tering is observed in the less proficient language; Jankelowitz & Bortz,

1996; Van Borsel *et al.*, 2009), or age of acquisition (Van Borsel *et al.*, 2009; Watt, 2000), and that these are in fact similar factors thought to have an influence on brain structure and function in the field of bilingualism in general, it seems reasonable to assume that work in the more general field of brain imaging and bilingual language processing might also be relevant for understanding the neural basis of developmental stuttering.

With tools for functional and anatomical imaging such as the ones described above, it is clear that in the future, studies of the language systems of both monolingual and bilingual individuals who stutter should shed light on the neural systems that mediate language, with possible implications long term for language intervention techniques.

References

Abutalebi, J., Miozzo, A. and Cappa, S.F. (2000) Do subcortical structures control 'langauge selection' in polyglots? Evidence from pathological language mixing. *Neurocase*, 6, 51–56.

Albert, M. and Obler, L. (1978) *The Bilingual Brain: Neuropsychological and Neurolinguistic Aspects of Bilingualism*. New York: Academic Press.

Alm, P.A. (2004) Stuttering and the basal ganglia circuits: A critical review of possible relations. *Journal of Communication Disorders*, 37(4), 325–369.

Anderson, J.M., Hughes, J.D., Rothi, L.J., Crucian, G.P. and Heilman, K.M. (1999) Developmental stuttering and Parkinson's disease: The effects of levodopa treatment. *Journal of Neurology, Neurosurgery and Psychiatry*, 66(6), 776–778.

Andrews, G., Craig, A., Feyer, A., Hoddinott, S., Howie, P. and Neilson, M. (1983) Stuttering: A review of research findings and theories circa 1982. *Journal of Speech and Hearing Disorders* 48, 226–245.

Aron, A.R., Behrens, T.E., Smith, S., Frank, M.J. and Poldrack, R.A. (2007) Triangulating a cognitive control network using diffusion-weighted magnetic resonance imaging (MRI) and functional MRI. *Journal of Neuroscience* 27(14), 3743–3752.

Beal, D.S., Gracco, V.L., Lafaille, S.J. and De Nil, L.F. (2007) Voxel-based morphometry of auditory and speech-related cortex in stutterers. *Neuroreport* 18(12), 1257–1260.

Blumstein, S.E., Alexander, M.P., Ryalls, J.H., Katz, W. and Dworetzky, B. (1987) On the nature of the foreign accent syndrome: A case study. *Brain and Language* 31(2), 215–244.

Braun, A.R., Varga, M., Stager, S., Schulz, G., Selbie, S., Maisog, J.M., *et al.* (1997) Altered patterns of cerebral activity during speech and language production in developmental stuttering. An H2(15)O positron emission tomography study. *Brain* 120 (Pt 5), 761–784.

Brown, S., Ingham, R.J., Ingham, J.C., Laird, A.R. and Fox, P.T. (2005) Stuttered and fluent speech production: An ALE meta-analysis of functional neuroimaging studies. *Human Brain Mapping* 25, 105–117.

Buchel, C. and Sommer, M. (2004) What causes stuttering? *PLoS Biology* 2(2), 0159–0163.

Chang, S.E., Erickson, K.I., Ambrose, N.G., Hasegawa-Johnson, M.A. and Ludlow, C.L. (2008) Brain anatomy differences in childhood stuttering. *Neuroimage* 39(3), 1333–1344.

Chee, M.W. (2006) Dissociating language and word meaning in the bilingual brain. *Trends in Cogitiven Sciences* 10(12), 527–529.

Chee, M.W., Soon, C.S., Lee, H.L. and Pallier, C. (2004) Left insula activation: A marker for language attainment in bilinguals. *Proceedings of the National Academy of Sciences of the United States of America* 101(42), 15265–15270.

Crinion, J., Turner, R., Grogan, A., Hanakawa, T., Noppeney, U., Devlin, J.T., *et al.* (2006) Language control in the bilingual brain. *Science* 312(5779), 1537–1540.

Cykowski, M.D., Kochunov, P.V., Ingham, R.J., Ingham, J.C., Mangin, J.F., Riviere, D., *et al.* (2007) Perisylvian sulcal morphology and cerebral asymmetry patterns in adults who stutter. *Cerebral Cortex.*

Cykowski, M.D., Kochunov, P.V., Ingham, R.J., Ingham, J.C., Mangin, J.F., Riviere, D., *et al.* (2008) Perisylvian sulcal morphology and cerebral asymmetry patterns in adults who stutter. *Cerebral Cortex* 18(3), 571–583.

De Nil, L.F., Kroll, R.M., Lafaille, S.J. and Houle, S. (2003) A positron emission tomography study of short- and long-term treatment effects on functional brain activation in adults who stutter. *Journal of Fluency Disorders* 28(4), 357–379; quiz 379–380.

Dehaene, S., Dupoux, E., Mehler, J., Cohen, L., Paulesu, E., Perani, D., *et al.* (1997) Anatomical variability in the cortical representation of first and second language. *Neuroreport* 8(17), 3809–3815.

Dronkers, N.F. (1996) A new brain region for coordinating speech articulation. *Nature* 384(6605), 159–161.

Flege, J.E., Yeni-Komshian, G.H. and Liu, S. (1999) Age constraints on second-language acquisition. *Journal of Memory and Language* 41, 78–104.

Foundas, A.L., Bollich, A.M., Corey, D.M., Hurley, M. and Heilman, K.M. (2001) Anomalous anatomy of speech-language areas in adults with persistent developmental stuttering. *Neurology* 57(2), 207–215.

Foundas, A.L., Bollich, A.M., Feldman, J., Corey, D.M., Hurley, M., Lemen, L.C., *et al.* (2004) Aberrant auditory processing and atypical planum temporale in developmental stuttering. *Neurology* 63(9), 1640–1646.

Foundas, A.L., Corey, D.M., Angeles, V., Bollich, A.M., Crabtree-Hartman, E. and Heilman, K.M. (2003) Atypical cerebral laterality in adults with persistent developmental stuttering. *Neurology* 61(10), 1378–1385.

Frenck-Mestre, C., Anton, J.L., Roth, M., Vaid, J. and Viallet, F. (2005) Articulation in early and late bilinguals' two languages: Evidence from functional magnetic resonance imaging. *Neuroreport* 16(7), 761–765.

Galloway, L.M. and Scarcella, R. (1982) Cerebral organization in adult second language acquisition: Is the right hemisphere more involved? *Brain and Language* 16(1), 56–60.

Geschwind, N. and Levitsky, W. (1968) Human brain: Left-right asymmetries in temporal speech region. *Science* 161(837), 186–187.

Giraud, A.L., Neumann, K., Bachoud-Levi, A.C., von Gudenberg, A.W., Euler, H.A., Lanfermann, H., *et al.* (2008) Severity of dysfluency correlates with basal ganglia activity in persistent developmental stuttering. *Brain and Language* 104(2), 190–199.

Glickstein, M. and Stein, J. (1991) Paradoxical movement in Parkinson's disease. *Trends in Neurosciences* 14(11), 480–482.

Golestani, N., Molko, N., Dehaene, S., LeBihan, D. and Pallier, C. (2007) Brain structure predicts the learning of foreign speech sounds. *Cerebral Cortex* 17(3), 575–582.

Graff-Radford, N.R., Cooper, W.E., Colsher, P.L. and Damasio, A.R. (1986) An unlearned foreign 'accent' in a patient with aphasia. *Brain and Language* 28, 86–94.

Grogan, A., Green, D.W., Ali, N., Crinion, J.T. and Price, C.J. (2009) Structural correlates of semantic and phonemic fluency ability in first and second languages. *Cerebral Cortex* 19(11), 2690–2698.

Guenther, F.H. (2006) Cortical interactions underlying the production of speech sounds. *Journal of Communication Disorders* 39(5), 350–365.

Gurd, J.M., Bessell, N.J., Bladon, R.A. and Bamford, J.M. (1988) A case of foreign accent syndrome, with follow-up clinical, neuropsychological and phonetic descriptions. *Neuropsychologia* 26(2), 237–251.

Howell, P., Davis, S. and Williams, R. (2009) The effects of bilingualism on stuttering during late childhood. *Archives of Disease in Childhood* 94(1), 42–46.

Howell, P. and Sackin, S. (2002) Timing interference to speech in altered listening conditions. *Journal of the Acoustical Society of America* 111(16), 2842–2852.

Ingham, R.J. (2001) Brain imaging studies of developmental stuttering. *Journal of Communication Disorders* 34(6), 493–516.

Ingham, R.J., Fox, P.T., Ingham, J.C., Xiong, J., Zamarripa, F., Hardies, L.J., *et al.* (2004) Brain correlates of stuttering and syllable production: Gender comparison and replication. *Journal of Speech, Language and Hearing Research* 47(2), 321–341.

Jancke, L., Hanggi, J. and Steinmetz, H. (2004) Morphological brain differences between adult stutterers and non-stutterers. *BioMedCentral Neurology* 4, 23.

Jankelowitz, D.L. and Bortz, M.A. (1996) The interaction of bilingualism and stuttering in an adult. *Journal of Communication Disorders* 29(3), 223–234.

Jenkinson, N., Nandi, D., Aziz, T.Z. and Stein, J.F. (2005) Pedunculopontine nucleus: A new target for deep brain stimulation for akinesia. *NeuroReport* 16(17), 1875–1876.

Jenkinson, N., Nandi, D., Muthusamy, K., Ray, N.J., Gregory, R., Stein, J. F., *et al.* (2009) Anatomy, physiology, and pathophysiology of the pedunculopontine nucleus. *Movement Disorders* 24(3), 319–328.

Johnson, J.S. and Newport, E.L. (1989) Critical period effects in second language learning: The influence of maturational state on the acquisition of English as a second language. *Cognitive Psychology* 21(1), 60–99.

Jueptner, M. and Weiller, C. (1998) A review of differences between basal ganglia and cerebellar control of movements as revealed by functional imaging studies. *Brain* 121 (Pt 8), 1437–1449.

Kell, C.A., Neumann, K., von Kriegstein, K., Posenenske, C., von Gudenberg, A.W., Euler, H., *et al.* (2009) How the brain repairs stuttering. *Brain* 132(Pt 10), 2747–2760.

Kim, K.H., Relkin, N.R., Lee, K.-M. and Hirsch, J. (1997) Distinct cortical areas associated with native and second languages. *Nature* 388, 171–174.

Klein, D., Milner, B., Zatorre, R.J., Meyer, E. and Evans, A.C. (1995) The neural substrates underlying word generation: A bilingual functional-imaging study. *Proceedings of the National Academy of Sciences of the United States of America* 92(7), 2899–2903.

Klein, D., Zatorre, R.J., Chen, J.K., Milner, B., Crane, J., Belin, P., *et al.* (2006) Bilingual brain organization: A functional magnetic resonance adaptation study. *Neuroimage* 31(1), 366–375.

Kuhl, P.K. (1998) The development of speech and language. In T.C. Carew, R. Menzel and C.J. Schatz (eds) *Mechanistic Relationships Between Development and Learning* (pp. 53–73). New York: Wiley.

Kurowski, K.M., Blumstein, S.E. and Alexander, M. (1996) The foreign accent syndrome: A reconsideration. *Brain and Language* 54(1), 1–25.

Lee, H., Devlin, J.T., Shakeshaft, C., Stewart, L.H., Brennan, A., Glensman, J., *et al.* (2007) Anatomical traces of vocabulary acquisition in the adolescent brain. *Journal of Neuroscience* 27(5), 1184–1189.

Louis, E.D., Winfield, L., Fahn, S. and Ford, B. (2001) Speech dysfluency exacerbated by levodopa in Parkinson's disease. *Movement Disorders* 16(3), 562–565.

Ludlow, C.L. and Loucks, T. (2003) Stuttering: A dynamic motor control disorder. *Journal of Fluency Disorders* 28, 273–295.

Maguire, G.A., Riley, G.D., Franklin, D.L. and Gottschalk, L.A. (2000) Risperidone for the treatment of stuttering. *Journal of Clinical Psychopharmacology* 20(4), 479–482.

Marie, P. (1971) The third left frontal convolution pays no special role in the function of language. In M.F. Cole and M. Cole (eds) *Pierre Marie's Papers on Speech Disorders* (pp. 51–71). New York: Hafner.

Martin, P.I., Naeser, M.A., Ho, M., Treglia, E., Kaplan, E., Baker, E.H., *et al.* (2009) Research with transcranial magnetic stimulation in the treatment of aphasia. *Current Neurology and Neuroscience Reports* 9(6), 451–458.

Mechelli, A., Crinion, J.T., Noppeney, U., O'Doherty, J., Ashburner, J., Frackowiak, R.S., *et al.* (2004) Neurolinguistics: Structural plasticity in the bilingual brain. *Nature* 431(7010), 757.

Mowrer, D. (1986) Reported use of a Japanese accent to promote fluency. *Journal of Fluency Disorders* 12(1), 19–39.

Neumann, K., Euler, H.A., von Gudenberg, A.W., Giraud, A.L., Lanfermann, H., Gall, V., *et al.* (2003) The nature and treatment of stuttering as revealed by fMRI A within- and between-group comparison. *Journal of Fluency Disorders* 28(4), 381–409; quiz 409–410.

Ojemann, G.A. and Whitaker, H.A. (1978) The bilingual brain. *Archives of Neurology* 35(7), 409–412.

Orton, S.T. (1928) A physiological theory of reading disability and stuttering in children. *New England Journal of Medicine* 199, 1046–1052.

Paradis, M. (1992) The Loch Ness Monster approach to bilingual language lateralization: A response to Berquier and Ashton. *Brain and Language* 43(3), 534–537.

Paradis, M. (1997) In A.M.B. de Groot and J.F.Kroll (eds) *Tutorials in Bilingualism: Psycholinguistic Perspectives* (pp. 331–354). Mahwah, NJ: Lawrence Erlbaum Associates.

Penfield, W. (1953) A consideration of the neurophysiological mechanisms of speech and some educational consequences. *Proceedings of the Academy of Arts and Science* 82, 199–214.

Perani, D. and Abutalebi, J. (2005) The neural basis of first and second language processing. *Current Opinion in Neurobiology* 15(2), 202–206.

Perani, D., Paulesu, E., Galles, N.S., Dupoux, E., Dehaene, S., Bettinardi, V., *et al.* (1998) The bilingual brain. Proficiency and age of acquisition of the second language. *Brain* 121 (Pt 10), 1841–1852.

Pitres, A. (1895) Etude sur l'aphasie chez les polyglottes. *Review of Medicine* 15, 873–899.

Pool, K.D., Devous, M.D., Sr., Freeman, F.J., Watson, B.C. and Finitzo, T. (1991) Regional cerebral blood flow in developmental stutterers. *Archives of Neurology* 48(5), 509–512.

Preibisch, C., Neumann, K., Raab, P., Euler, H.A., von Gudenberg, A.W., Lanfermann, H.,*et al.* (2003) Evidence for compensation for stuttering by the right frontal operculum. *Neuroimage* 20(2), 1356–1364.

Sebastian-Galles, N. (2006) Native-language sensitivities: Evolution in the first year of life. *Trends in Cognitive Sciences* 10(6), 239–241.

Smith, S.M., Jenkinson, M., Johansen-Berg, H., Rueckert, D., Nichols, T.E., Mackay, C.E., *et al.* (2006) Tract-based spatial statistics: Voxelwise analysis of multi-subject diffusion data. *Neuroimage* 31(4), 1487–1505.

Sommer, M., Koch, M.A., Paulus, W., Weiller, C. and Buchel, C. (2002) Disconnection of speech-relevant brain areas in persistent developmental stuttering. *Lancet* 360(9330), 380–383.

Strub, R.L., Black, F.W. and Naeser, M.A. (1987) Anomalous dominance in sibling stutterers: Evidence from CT scan asymmetries, dichotic listening, neuropsychological testing, and handedness. *Brain and Language* 30(2), 338–350.

Tan, L.H., Spinks, J.A., Feng, C.M., Siok, W.T., Perfetti, C.A., Xiong, J., *et al.* (2003) Neural systems of second language reading are shaped by native language. *Human Brain Mapping* 18(3), 158–166.

Travis, L.E. (1978) The cerebral dominance theory of stuttering: 1931–1978. *Journal of Speech and Hearing Disorders* 43, 278–281.

Ullman, M.T. (2001) The neural basis of lexicon and grammar in first and second language: The declarative/procedural model. *Bilingualism: Language and Cognition* 4(2), 105–122.

Van Borsel, J., Merlaen, A., Achten, R., Vingerhoes, G. and Santens, P. (2009) Acquired stuttering with differential manifestation in different languages: A case study. *Journal of Neurolinguistics* 22, 187–195.

Wartenburger, I., Heekeren, H.R., Abutalebi, J., Cappa, S.F., Villringer, A. and Perani, D. (2003) Early setting of grammatical processing in the bilingual brain. *Neuron* 37(1), 159–170.

Watkins, K.E., Patel, N., Davis, S. and Howell, P. (2005) *Brain Activity During Altered Auditory Feedback: An fMRI Study in Healthy Adolescents.* Paper presented at the 11th Annual conference of the Organization of Human Brain Mapping, Toronto, Canada.

Watkins, K.E., Smith, S.M., Davis, S. and Howell, P. (2008) Structural and functional abnormalities of the motor system in developmental stuttering. *Brain* 131(Pt 1), 50–59.

Watkins, K.E., Paus, T., Lerch, J.P., Zijdenbos, A., Collins, D.L., Neelin, P., *et al.* (2001) Structural asymmetries in the human brain: A voxel-based statistical analysis of 142 MRI scans. *Cerebral Cortex* 11(9), 868–877.

Watt, N. (2000) Analysis of language factors in a multilingual stutterer. *South African Journal of Communication Disorders* 47, 5–12.

Weber-Fox, C.M. and Neville, H.J. (1996) Maturational constraints on functional specializations for language processing: ERP and behavioral evidence in bilingual speakers. *Journal of Cognitive Neuroscience* 8, 231–256.

Werker, J.F. and Tees, R.C. (1984) Cross-language speech perception: Evidence for perceptual reorganization during the first year of life. *Infant Behavior and Development* 7, 49–63.

Wood, F., Stump, D., McKeehan, A., Sheldon, S. and Proctor, J. (1980) Patterns of regional cerebral blood flow during attempted reading aloud by stutterers both on and off haloperidol medication: Evidence for inadequate left frontal activation during stuttering. *Brain and Language* 9(1), 141–144.

Wu, J.C., Maguire, G., Riley, G., Fallon, J., LaCasse, L., Chin, S., *et al.* (1995) A positron emission tomography [18F]deoxyglucose study of developmental stuttering. *Neuroreport* 6(3), 501–505.

Wu, J.C., Maguire, G., Riley, G., Lee, A., Keator, D., Tang, C., *et al.* (1997) Increased dopamine activity associated with stuttering. *Neuroreport* 8(3), 767–770.

Xu, Y., Gandour, J., Talavage, T., Wong, D., Dzemidzic, M., Tong, Y., *et al.* (2006) Activation of the left planum temporale in pitch processing is shaped by language experience. *Human Brain Mapping* 27(2), 173–183.

Xue, G., Aron, A.R. and Poldrack, R.A. (2008) Common neural substrates for inhibition of spoken and manual responses. *Cerebral Cortex* 18(8), 1923–1932.

Part 2

Monolingual Language Diversity and Stuttering

Chapter 5

The Speech and Language Characteristics of Developmental Stuttering in English Speakers

PETER HOWELL AND SARAH RUSBRIDGE

Summary

Work on whether language factors lead to developmental stuttering in English is described. The impact of language factors on stuttering: (1) at the lexical level and below; and (2) at the supralexical level are critically examined. Formal language factors and usage properties (variation in performance due to variation in language use) are examined. Syntactic and prosodic units for specifying suprasegmental factors are examined. The concluding section considers two alternative approaches to unifying the findings from the review. The first links lexical and supralexical factors that affect stuttering together according to their formal properties. According to this approach, an utterance like 'it is Spring' would be analyzed at the lexical level into word types (function, function, content), phonological properties (whether or not the words start with consonant strings) and lexical usage properties (how frequently each word occurs) and so on. At the supralexical level, all words would be specified into prosodic or syntactic forms.. The second approach proposes that phonological properties can be used on regions of speech to specify linguistically and motorically difficult stretches independent of formal usage properties. The ensuing easy and hard segments can be used to specify 'suprasegmental' contexts that then allow dynamic patterns of interaction between higher cognitive planning processes and motor organizational processes to be examined. This approach has the advantage that it can be applied to languages with very dissimilar structure to English.

1 Introduction

Yairi and Ambrose (2005) give the mean age of onset of developmental stuttering as 33 months. Around 80% of children recover before teenage but recovery after teenage is rare (Andrews & Harris, 1964). It has long been suspected that language factors may account for why stuttering starts and for its early course of development (Bernstein Ratner, 1997,

2005; Bloodstein, 2006). This chapter reviews aspects of the structure of the English language that have been claimed to be associated with the onset of stuttering and how it develops over the course of a child's early development. After some essential background information about stuttering in English (its epidemiology and assessment) has been given in Section 2, Sections 3 and 4 review language factors organized under the themes lexical and superlexical properties.

Several things commend examination of English: (1) It is the international language of science, the media and commerce around the world; (2) Cross-linguistic research in stuttering usually takes findings from English and seeks to establish whether the patterns are similar in other languages (Jayaram, 1981; Preus *et al.*, 1982); (3) Comparison of stuttering between English and the other languages may identify universal features of stuttering. These points all justify a review of the work on the relationship between the structure of English and patterns of stuttering. However, focusing on English has drawbacks. For instance, aspects of language not seen in English cannot be addressed. Thus, as English is not a tone language, examination of tonal features is not possible. Some differences between English and other languages will be highlighted within this chapter. The way that stuttering is affected by language properties that do not occur in English is addressed by other chapters in this part of the book.

To conduct the examination, it is necessary to consider what stuttering is, how it develops into its persistent form and how the structure and use of the English language encountered at different points in development affects stuttering. In the work considered here, stuttering is identified and its severity is assessed based on overt symptoms in speech. Stuttering has effects on socio-emotional adjustment that would not be involved in such assessments but, as this volume is about language, we will not consider these factors. Basing assessment on overt speech makes it possible that some individuals who do not show overt symptoms will be missed. For example, some children who stutter are quiet in class and have all the symptoms of selective mutism (Howell, 2007), and some adults claim to stutter, but do not do so overtly (so-called covert stuttering).

2   Stuttering Definitions/Symptoms

Particular care needs to be taken when comparing studies within and between languages, as to whether stuttering has been assessed in the same way. If, for instance, stuttering is assessed differently in two studies that look at the same factor in different languages, then it is not possible to say whether differences are due to the forms of language or the different ways of characterizing stuttering. Unfortunately, there are many schemes for assessing stuttering and this multiplicity increases the chance that studies are not comparable. Indeed, the field of stuttering research suffers from a lack of standardization that would prevent this problem. That said, there are things that commend the different schemes that are used. The best thing that can be done (which is part of good scientific practice anyway) is to be clear about all methodological aspects of studies (symptoms, assessments etc.). Readers will then have the wherewithal to see for themselves whether different findings across studies comparing different languages can be attributed to language differences or are attributable to different ways in which stuttering was assessed. In the following, some of the important schemes that have been used for assessing the course of stuttering for English are described.

2.1 Symptom counts

Some popular assessment methods that count symptoms are considered. A well-known attempt that took the symptom approach to identify cases of stuttering was that of Johnson (1959). He specified eight types of disfluency. These were: (1) Interjections (sometimes called filled pauses); (2) Word repetitions; (3) Phrase repetitions; (4) Part-word repetitions; (5) Prolongations; (6) Broken words (or blocks); (7) Incomplete phrases (sometimes called abandonments) and (8) Revisions. The main point to note is that none of the disfluencies on this list are exclusively seen in people who stutter. Therefore, there is no single symptom that indicates whether a person is a stutterer or not. Johnson was aware of this, but he did not abandon his list. It led him to a particular view about stuttering, namely that there is continuity between speech in typically developing children and children who stutter. The continuity idea allows individuals to morph between stuttering and fluency which implies a continuous severity dimension between these types of speech. Equally importantly, it allows grades of recovery (partial through full) to occur.

2.1.1 Schemes that group disfluencies

Other authors have taken symptoms from Johnson's list and used their clinical experience to identify which of these are more, and less, typical of stuttering. These schemes were principally developed so that following the course of the disorder (into persistence or recovery) could be improved. Inevitably, since the proposals are subjective, the grouping proposals have led to disputes about what should, and should not, be included in the more, and less, typical classes. Prolongations, part-word repetitions and broken words are usually agreed to be more typical of stuttering. Phrase repetitions, revisions, incomplete phrases and interjections are usually considered less typical of stuttering. The main dispute has been whether whole word repetitions should, or should not, be considered typical of stuttering (related to this, see discussion of Riley's SSI-3 in Section 2.2. which, in the main, does not consider most whole-word repetitions as stutterings). Conversely, Yairi and Ambrose (2005) included whole-word repetitions in their class of stuttering-like disfluencies (SLD, more typical of stuttering) as well as prolongations, part-word repetitions and broken words. The remaining disfluencies appear in the list of other disfluencies (OD, less typical of stuttering) which are discarded in stuttering analyses. This scheme is almost identical to that used by Conture (2001) in his within word/between word scheme.

Howell and Au-Yeung (2002) and Howell (2004, 2010a, b) used a scheme that classified whole-word repetitions into two classes depending whether the words they occurred on were from function or content word classes. Function words are pronouns, articles, prepositions, conjunctions and auxiliary verbs, whilst content words are nouns, main verbs, adverbs and adjectives (Hartmann & Stork, 1972; Quirk *et al.*, 1985). Empirical evidence (reviewed in Section 3) suggests that, statistically speaking, whole-word repetitions on function words are less problematic (more a feature of typically developing speech) than those on content words. Furthermore, theoretical considerations suggest that whole function word repetitions have a role in maintaining fluency whereas whole content word repetitions are one indication of fluency problems (Howell, 2004, 2010a; Howell & Au-Yeung, 2002). Howell's scheme shares one feature with Johnson's in that it proposes that a speaker can morph to being fluent (recover). It also proposes that speakers who persist in stuttering have a different pattern of symptoms over development to fluent speakers (Howell, 2007; Howell *et al.*, 2010).

It is not adequate to argue that widespread use of a scheme supports its use, as do some researchers who think whole-word repetitions are characteristics of stuttering (Reilly *et al.*, 2009). Wingate (2001) had some principled reasons for opposing the view that whole-word repetitions were typical of stuttering. He argued that whole-word repetitions should be excluded from lists of SLD as they are common in typically developing children's speech. Authors who also take the position not to count whole-word repetitions as stuttering include Bernstein Ratner and Sih (1987), Kloth *et al.* (1999), Riley (1994) and Wall *et al.* (1981) as discussed in Howell (2010b). Rather, the issue whether whole-word repetitions should, or should not, be included as instances more typical of stuttering is one that should be investigated empirically (Anderson, 2007; Howell, 2010c). The Lidcombe consortium uses a perceptual method for evaluating stuttering that is only considered in passing here because of its inherent subjectivity (see Roberts, this volume for detail).

A 3% threshold has been specified as an acceptable proportion of SLD in fluent speakers for English (Yairi & Ambrose, 2005). The warning about whether SLD were assessed using the same or different procedures across the languages applies here. The 3% threshold is not equivalent when different methods are used (see discussion in Section 2.1). For English, SSI-3 based on digital recordings has been assessed as a way of separating fluent speakers from speakers who continue to stutter and, in empirical analyses, it has been shown that the SSI-3 scores of speakers who recover are not statistically distinguishable from fluent control speakers (Davis *et al.*, 2007). SSI-3 on digital recordings has also been assessed as a way of dividing persistent from recovered speakers (Howell *et al.*, 2006), and for validating questionnaires that separate persistent from recovered speakers (Howell *et al.*, 2009b).

2.2 Severity of stuttering

An initial diagnosis of stuttering is always based on the symptoms in the person's speech. The diagnosis can then be formalized by making symptom counts and applying a threshold to establish whether the person stutters or not, or by perceptual assessment. The objectivity of perceptual methods has been questioned (Kully & Boberg, 1988) which is one reason for using symptom counts. Admittedly, the focus on speech symptoms will miss some features of the disorder (e.g. the socio-emotional ones mentioned earlier) but does seem appropriate for assessing how language impacts on the disorder.

The symptoms participants show have also to be documented in all research (not just that involving language). Riley's (1994) stuttering severity instrument version three (SSI-3) is the *de facto* standard for English for characterizing the symptoms of individuals or groups of people who stutter. Version four (SSI-4) has appeared recently and is downward compatible with SSI-3 (thus assessments made with SSI-3 are not obsolete). SSI-4 may eventually supercede SSI-3. SSI-3 and SSI-4 assessments are based on frequency of symptoms, the duration of a selected set of the longest disfluenceis and records of secondary characteristics over a variety of speech contexts (e.g. spontaneous monologues, readings). Severity assessments use percentage of stuttered syllables, average duration of the set of disfluencies selected that have the longest durations, and a physical concomitants assessment (e.g. distracting sounds, facial grimaces, etc.). Stuttering behaviors are defined as 'repetitions or prolongations of sounds or syllables (including silent prolongations)' (p. 4). The SSI-3 also notes which behaviors are not included within the definition of stuttering: 'Behaviours such as rephrasing, repetition of phrases or whole-words, and pausing without tension are not counted as stuttering. Repetition of one-syllable words may be stuttering if the word sounds abnormal (shortened, prolonged, staccato, tense, etc.); however, when these single-syllable words are repeated but are otherwise spoken normally, they do not qualify as stuttering using the definition just stated' (p. 4).

The SSI-3 is widely accessible, its reliability and validity have been assessed and norms for English have been published (Riley, 1994). Using speech obtained in various contexts gives the assessments good external validity. The SSI-3 assessment instructions have been translated into other languages. Following a prescribed and standard procedure in different languages is commendable. Usually, however, the test has not been evaluated statistically and standardized after translation. It should be cautioned that the norms for English do not apply when SSI-3 is translated to other languages. Also, the manual is flexible about how stuttering is assessed and it is not certain whether the permitted alternatives produce equivalent answers.

A variety of methods of assessment are employed in research studies. This includes analyses of spontaneous speech, comparison of speech performance scores of individuals who stutter against published norms and a wide range of experimental tasks. There are advantages and disadvantages to each method. Thus, spontaneous speech has the highest external validity and experiments least. Conversely, there is the least amount of control over spontaneous speech and the most when experimental material is employed.

Symptoms are assessed (for estimating severity or as part of a study) in different ways when different methods are employed. The methods range from those: (1) made as a person speaks (Boey *et al.*, 2007); (2) using counter boards where all the syllables spoken are registered by taps with one hand and the stuttered syllables alone with taps on the other hand (a related procedure is included in SSI-4); (3) using detailed transcriptional analysis of samples of stuttered speech (Howell & Huckvale, 2004; Howell *et al.*, 2009a). The first two do not necessarily require a permanent recording of the speech. If the approach of making judgments whilst interviewing participants is adopted, no check can be made about how stuttering events are time-locked to the audio signal.

The transcription procedure is used in the University College London (UCL) speech group laboratory, among others. The transcriptions are based on recordings where sections can be selected, replayed and reviewed, and the results are permanently stored in alignment against the speech recordings. Transcriptions are time-consuming to make but clearly provide the most accurate information and are available for reanalaysis in different ways. The transcription process is being made quicker with convenient packages and software to semi-automate the process (Howell & Huckvale, 2004) and will eventually either become an essential requirement or a reference standard against which other assessment methods are evaluated. Due to the enhanced accuracy, more disfluencies are located than with the other methods where symptoms are more prone to be missed (though arguably, other assessment methods are probably satisfactory for clinical report). As mentioned, the difference in accuracy of the various methods makes comparison between reports using different assessment methods difficult. Also, only gross reliability assessments are possible when there are no permanent recordings of what was counted as a disfluency and where it occurred in the speech. Mention was made earlier about the desirability of standardizing assessment procedures across labs (as SSI-3 does for severity). Publicly available reference recordings, such as the UCLASS database, provide a means for assessing current, and developing new, standards (Howell & Huckvale, 2004; Howell *et al.*, 2009a). They allow individuals working on other languages to learn and check the ways assessments have been made in English before developing new ones (either similar ones for the investigator's own language or entirely new methods).

In summary, it is essential to check whether the same schemes have been used when examining research within one language, or comparing results from studies across languages. When grouping schemes are used, results should be assessed both for the more (e.g. SLD) and the less (e.g. OD) typical classes of disfluencies since only one of these classes might differ between languages (e.g. the less typical class might operate the same across languages whereas the more typical class might differ). We have limited our comments to symptom-based assessments. Other authors prefer to use perceptual assessments or questionnaire instruments for assessing stuttering. Many of the same issues raised here apply when these alternative methods are used. For example, if item selection has to be modified in any significant way for a questionnaire used in two languages (items dropped from one questionnaire or additional items added), comparison across languages would be precluded.

3 Lexical Factors that May Affect Stuttering

People who stutter may have a language-processing deficit relative to controls. Several such language processing deficits exist. Any problem in these processes would be revealed either as timing problems in production (i.e. preparing speech by the time it needs to be output) or a higher chance of language processing breaking down in people who stutter than controls (i.e. a greater propensity to make errors by people who stutter).

In their quest for identifying processing deficits in people who stutter, some authors have compared the receptive (perceptual) abilities for language processing of people who stutter and those who do not. The motivation for doing this is not immediately obvious given that stuttering is a problem in speech production (Wingate, 2002). The usual justification is to point out that speech production and perception are linked together so a problem in perception might affect production. In the stuttering area, generally speaking, the way production and perception are linked has not been specified in sufficient detail to motivate the view that a perceptual deficit on one or more language characteristic could lead to stuttering and there are production theories that do not require a link between production and perception (Howell, 2004, 2010a; Howell & Au-Yeung, 2002).

A further issue when investigating stuttering, as mentioned briefly in Section 2.1, concerns what methods for obtaining samples should be employed, particularly when children's speech has to be assessed. Two popular methods are to record spontaneous speech samples and to elicit material using imitation tasks where a speaker (usually a child) has to repeat sentences modeled to him or her. Speaking spontaneously has higher external validity than imitating the experimenter's speech as it is a natural reflection of the child's current language ability. The higher external validity commends assessment of spontaneous speech. Additionally, it can be argued that imitation tasks may present language that under- or over-estimates a child's current language ability, so it is not a good way of testing how language factors affect stuttering (although it may be more appropriate for older speakers). A counter to this argument is that there is less control over spontaneous utterances than there is in imitation tasks. Both these methods have a place and neither alone is ideal.

It has been argued that factors that put a child at risk of starting to stutter (precipitating, or onset factors) need to be distinguished from those that lead to a child continuing to stutter (perpetuating, or course of stuttering factors) factors (Howell, 2007; Howell *et al.*, 2008). Where possible, the evidence on how language factors put a child at risk of starting, and continuing, to stutter are mentioned for each of the language processes examined here. It should be noted that there are only a limited number of spontaneous production and imitation studies on language factors. Those studies employing children all examined them after stuttering had started so they are not optimal for identifying risk factors for onset of stuttering. However, some studies have examined children shortly after onset where language factors that put a child at risk of starting to stutter may still be operating. Stuttering that is still occurring at teenage is unlikely to resolve (Andrews & Harris, 1964) and studies up to this age may reveal what language factors put a child at risk of perpetuating in their stuttering. Other factors may begin to operate when teenagers continue stuttering into adulthood (e.g. it is possible that anxiety and low self-esteem may emerge). Another limitation is that there are few cross-sectional and longitudinal studies that examine a range of ages.

The issue about which symptoms should be used to assess stuttering, discussed in Section 2.1, raises a further consideration about comparisons across different ages. Children who stutter show a lot of whole-word repetition (Bloodstein & Gantwerk, 1967; Bloodstein & Grossman, 1981) whereas older speakers show less (Howell, 2007). Thus, if stuttering is assayed by a measure that includes whole-word repetitions, more whole-word repetitions would be expected near onset of stuttering and fewer when the children are older. The imbalance across ages in the proportion of whole-word repetitions out of all stuttering symptoms makes cross age-group comparisons similar to comparisons involving different metrics (i.e. ones that include whole-word repetitions versus those that do not). This would not be a problem if whole-word repetitions are true symptoms of stuttering, but would be if they are not. Once there is a definitive answer about whether whole-word repetitions are stuttering or not (Wingate, 2001; Yairi *et al.*, 2001), only the results with appropriate symptom counts will stand. Until then, readers need to interpret results according to which metric was employed and be attentive to this matter when comparing across studies. Data protection legislation requires long-term storage of research data, and researchers should be coding such data so that they can be easily recomputed when new recommendations about what symptoms are stuttering are adopted (Howell, 2010b).

The focus of this book is on multilingual and bilingual issues in stuttering. It is not possible to review everything that is potentially relevant from work on English participants. Only the work on language is considered and, mainly, work on stuttering in children is reviewed. This age group was focused on because there are potential parallels between what causes stuttering to begin when language is learned and how it changes during the early course of development, whether a speaker is learning their first or an additional language. There is a detailed examination of selected studies rather than a comprehensive review. The properties that are examined are divided into: (1) lexical and sub-lexical factors and (2) supralexical factors.

3.1 Formal properties of lexical and sublexical material

Lexical and sublexcical variables can be specified formally (parts of speech, word type, morphology and phonological structure of syllables) or in terms of speakers' use of the language structures (measured in terms of word frequency, neighborhood density and age-of–acquisition (AoA)). The impact that formal and usage properties have on stuttering has been examined by dividing materials into separate classes along the selected dimension for the variable (e.g. function versus content) and seeing whether different stuttering rates are associated with the resulting classes. Studies on stuttering that have examined the variables indicated are discussed.

3.1.1 *Parts of speech*

Brown (1937) examined stuttering rates on 23 'parts of speech' by 32 adults who stuttered. In a first analysis, parts of speech were ranked with respect to the percent of stuttering for each word type. Brown then collapsed the 23 categories into eight major parts of speech. The eight parts of speech are listed in Table 5.1 with auxiliaries (which are function words) listed separated from main verbs (which are content words). The entries are ranked from easiest (least stuttering) to most difficult (most stuttering).

Table 5.1 Order of difficulty of nine parts of speech for by 32 adult speakers who stutter. The table is adapted from Brown (1937) (here auxiliary verbs are separated from other verbs). Assignment of each part of speech into function (F) and content (C) word classes who stuttered is indicated at the right

Adapted from Brown (1937)	
Easy (least stuttering)	
Articles	F
Auxillary verbs	F
Prepositions	F
Conjunctions	F
Pronouns	F
Main verbs	C
Adverbs	C
Nouns	C
Adjectives	C
Hard (most stuttering)	

3.1.2 Function and content words

Brown's data shows that most stuttering in adults occurs on content words. Thus, in Table 5.1, the parts of speech that are function (F) or content (C), using the definition given earlier, are indicated at the right. The content words all appear at the bottom of the list, which shows content words are stuttered more than function words by adults. The difficulty experienced on content words could be because of many inherent differences between the two word forms. For example, the differences could have arisen because content words are produced by different brain mechanisms, or because they have a statistical tendency to carry complex phonological properties such as lexical stress, strings of consonants or because they occur less frequently than function words.

Bloodstein and Gantwerk (1967) found that the opposite tendency occurs in children who stutter who had higher rates of stuttering on function words. This study did not specify what symptoms were considered as stutters (they were simply referred to as 'stutterings'). However, Bloodstein and Grossman (1981) recorded the spontaneous speech (elicited picture descriptions) of five children who stuttered aged between 3;10 and 5;7 years where the symptoms considered to be stutters were specified. The symptoms were sound or syllable repetition, word repetition, phrase repetition, prolongation of a sound, hard attack on a sound, inappropriate pause, and audible secondary characteristics such as gasping. Note that whole-word repetitions were considered as stutters. They reported that for most of their participants, proportionately more function words than content words were stuttered.

As discussed in Section 2.1, there is dispute about whether whole-word repetitions should be considered as stutters or not and this affects interpretation of this study. The main reason for excluding whole-word repetitions as stutters is that they are regularly observed in the speech of typically developing children as well as children who stutter (Howell *et al.*, 1999). Consequently, they would not distinguish children who stutter from typically developing children. Inclusion of whole-word repetitions could have led to the Bloodstein and Grossman result as they occur frequently in children's speech and tend to happen on function word classes unlike other types of stutter. If Wingate (2001) is correct that whole-word repetitions should not be considered as symptoms of stuttering, children showing high rates of these symptoms should be excluded from samples who stutter. Stuttering rate on function words would then reduce because whole-word repetitions occur mostly on that type of word. Thus the high rate of stuttering on function words in children who stutter may be an artifact due to misdiagnosis of some children as stutterers. Wingate's argument would be less applicable to adults who stutter, who have lower rates of whole-word repetition but have high rates of symptoms that occur on content words. The appropriate way to settle the debate about whether whole-word repetitions are stutterings is empirically. One way this could be done would be to see whether the imbalance in the type of words that are disfluent still occurs when whole-word repetitions are excluded from analyses. Until such analyses have been conducted, the best thing that can be done is to document what symptoms were considered as stutters in the studies that are considered.

Howell *et al.* (1999) reported stuttering rates on function and content words on cross-sectional data of 51 stuttering and 68 non-stuttering English-speaking individuals of five different age groups (2–6 years; 7–9 years, 10–12 years, teenagers and adults). Analysis was based on conversations involving a fluent interviewer. The stuttering symptoms that were marked included word and part-word repetition and segmental or syllabic prolongations. Again it is of note that whole-word repetitions were counted.

Function words that appeared before content words were almost the only function words that were stuttered and these alone were examined. As shown in Figure 5.1, fluent speakers had a higher percentage of disfluency on these function words compared to content words. The rates of disfluency on function words and on content words changed over age groups for the speakers who stutter: For the 2–6-year-old speakers who stuttered, there was a higher percentage of disfluencies on function words than content words. In subsequent age groups, disfluency decreased on function words and increased on content words.

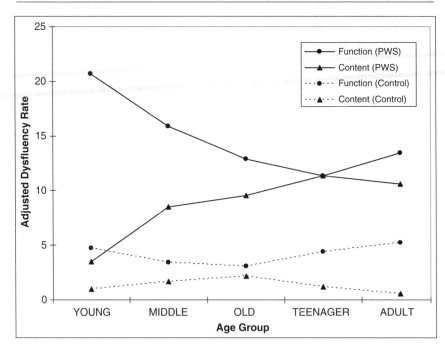

Figure 5.1 Stuttering rate on function and content words for speakers in different age groups. Stuttering rate was adjusted so that differences in absolute stuttering rates between age groups did not influence the results

Although the Howell *et al.* (1999) data showed a change from stuttering on function words to content words as age increased, a limitation is that the data are cross-sectional. Consequently, some of the children who stuttered at younger ages would have recovered by the time they reached the ages of the older groups as described earlier. The possibility that this affected the pattern of results was ruled out in longitudinal work by Howell (2007). Seventy-six children between the ages 8 and 12 years plus were followed up. All the children were diagnosed as stuttering at the outset of the study (around age 8). The children were assessed by instruments completed by the parents, by the children themselves and by a researcher at 12 plus to establish whether they were still stuttering or not. Recall 12 plus is the age at which stuttering should have recovered if it was going to (Andrews & Harris, 1964). Forty-one children recovered and 35 persisted.

Spontaneous speech samples at age 8 and 12 years plus were transcribed and marked for disfluencies. Whole-word and phrase repetitions were grouped together into one category (these were expected to occur predominantly on function words). Part-word repetitions, prolongations and broken words were grouped together (these were expected to occur predominantly on content words).

The balance between these disfluency-groupings changed in different ways over the test ages depending on whether the children persisted or recovered at 12 plus. The data for the recovered speakers showed that the average number of whole-word and phrase repetitions on function words went down as well as the number of part-word repetitions, prolongations and broken-word disfluencies on content words. The reduction of the number of disfluencies of word and phrase repetitions and of part-word repetitions, prolongations and broken disfluencies represented a proportional reduction of both disfluency groupings to levels shown by fluent speakers (recovered speakers converged on what fluent speakers did).

The data for the persistent speakers showed that the average number of whole-word and phrase repetitions per two-minute period on function words went down but the number of part-word repetitions, prolongations and broken disfluencies on content words went up. The latter showed that these speakers diverged from the speakers who recovered and that there was a shift from disfluency on function to content words.

It is not immediately obvious why more stuttering on function words than content words should occur based on lexicality per se. All children make a transition from producing one-word utterances (at around 1 year of age) to producing multiword utterances occurs at around 2 years of age (Labelle, 2005). Different types of words are spoken at these stages. Content words are the main types produced at the one-word stage (Bloom, 1970; Brown, 1973; Radford, 1990). Function words are introduced into utterances when they start to produce multi-word utterances at around age 2 (Labelle, 2005). It seems unlikely that use of the more difficult, content word forms accounts for why some children start to stutter as they have been using: (1) content words before stuttering started (at the one-word stage); (2) function words before stuttering started (using function words from age 2 which is almost a year before the average child starts to stutter). As discussed in Section 4, some authors have sought to explain the different rates of stuttering on function and content words in terms of the role they have in supralexical language processes (prosody and syntax). These accounts also need to explain why stuttering symptoms migrate across word types (from function to content) as age increases.

Returning to the issue about whether there are inherent differences between function and content words, it appears that the two word types are processed in different parts of the brain and that the parts of the brain involved differs between typically developing and stuttering individuals. If content and function words classes are processed in different parts of the brain by all speakers, this would, in principle, allow individuals to have selective problems on the different word types. Pulvermüller (1999) argued that processing of function words depends on structures in the left hemisphere of the brain whilst content words seem to be processed in both hemispheres. This conclusion was based primarily on work with aphasic patients, although the findings have been generalized to typical cases as well as to patients suffering from a range of language disorders (Caramazza & Berndt, 1985; Chiarello & Nuding, 1987; Gevins *et al.*, 1995). Pulvermüller pointed out that there is a sparsity of data from cases that have controlled for word frequency and word length of the stimuli used in tests and that there are few studies that have used direct measure of brain activity such as Electroencephalography or fMRI. Though processing of word classes in different brain regions could account for problems in one word form or the other, it could not immediately account for the change in stuttering from occurring on function to content words with age.

Neuroimaging studies have shown that the processing of function and content words is different in people who stutter. Speakers who stutter show a distortion of the normal pattern of left hemispheric dominance (Kroll *et al.*, 1997). The different pattern could reflect different functional problems experienced with the two word classes because processing them relies on the two hemispheres to different extents. Alternatively, people who stutter may have structural abnormalities in the left cerebral hemisphere that then lead to the problems with both word classes (which both depend on left hemisphere processing according to Pulvermüller, 1999). There is no clear-cut answer as to whether the structural or functional account applies at present. Also, no account has been offered about why developmental changes in stutter types occurs across ages.

The argument that young children have problems on function words (Howell, 2007) is questioned by statements made by Yairi and Ambrose (2005: 68). They state that they have observed blocks and prolongations in children around the period where stuttering starts. The symptoms Yairi and Ambrose mention tend to occur on content words (Howell, 2007). This suggests that stuttering may be more like adult forms (i.e. appear on content words) in some cases. At present, Yairi and Ambrose's data are not available for public scrutiny and no case reports have appeared, so these claims cannot be verified.

It is important to note that Howell *et al.* (1999) in the original and subsequent work selected utterances with function words before content words for analysis. If an utterance like 'I trampled on it' (FCFF) is examined, there are three function words in this utterance, but only the one before the content word would be repeated or have pauses around it. Thus, word class per se cannot be the determinant of stuttering; otherwise all function words would have a similar chance of being stuttered. Function words that appear before content words have two properties: (1) The function words appear prior to difficult words; (2) the disfluencies themselves occur on easy words (from the function word class). (The work on phonological word (PW) in Section 4.1 offers one account of a process that might explain these.) Function and content words dissociate in three ways (symptom type, whether they are contextually dependent and whether or not they are a response to difficulty of the word type): The symptoms that occur on function words are whole-word repetitions and pauses that depend on them being positioned before the content word they are associated with and they are not due to difficulty of the word class (statistically, function words are simple compared to content words). In contrast, symptoms on content words involve parts of the word (part-word repetition, prolongation and breaks within the word), they are independent of position but are due to difficulty of these words. Properties of different languages offer a rich potential source for testing these observations.

3.1.3 Morphology

There is surprisingly little work on word morphology and stuttering. One study in Marshal (2005) looked at whether nouns and verbs with inflectional endings attracted more stuttering than non-inflected words in spontaneous speech, based on the reasoning that the addition of inflectional affixes altered the phonology of the word. The inflections investigated were those which added an additional consonant at the end of the word (and so may result in a word-final consonant cluster, e.g. 'hope' to 'hoped'). Specifically, these were: (1) plural marking on nouns (the cat, the cats); (2) tense on verbs (I lie, you lie, I lied, you lied); (3) third-person singular agreement on verbs (I lie, he lies, I want, he wants). In 16 stuttering male adults aged between 16 and 47 years (all male) no effect of inflectional ending on stuttering rate was observed. Given that English has a simple inflectional system relative to many of the other languages of the world and that inflections in English happen on the final parts of words, more cross linguistic work on this feature is vital.

3.1.4 Syllable constituency

Syllable constituency refers to how syllables are composed. Differences in syllable constituency can be used as an alternative method for quantifying differences in complexity between function and content word classes, variation in the complexity within each of these word classes and differences in complexity across languages.

3.1.4.1 Phonological measures of difficulty

In addition to parts of speech, Brown (1945) examined other factors that could affect stuttering in adults, two of which occurred within words. The first was word length. Words that had five or more letters were designated as difficult relative to words with four or less letters. The second was the phone that words *started* with. Words that started with any consonant other than /ð, t, h, w and ɥ/ were designated difficult and words starting with consonants outside this set, or vowels were designated easy.

Brown's factors are simplistic in some ways according to present stan-dards. For example, it would be better to specify word length in terms of number of phonemes rather than number of letters. Also, examination of other aspects of onsets (such as whether onset consonants are part of a string or not) would be recommended.

Since this pioneering work, several other phonological factors have been examined to establish what properties make some words more dif-ficult than others. There is general agreement about the importance of consonant strings at syllable (or more specifically word) onsets (Wingate, 2002). Thus, prolongations, part-word repetitions and word breaks tend to occur around syllable onsets. This suggests that syllable onsets may have an important role in determining stuttering.

3.1.4.2 Consonant strings, consonant manner (late emerging consonants) and length in syllables (Throneburg et al.'s 1994 scheme)

Throneburg *et al.* (1994) examined whether words that contained dif-ferent phonological factors influenced stuttering rate in the spontaneous speech of 24 children who stuttered (9 girls, 15 boys; age 29–59 months, mean 40.5 months). SLD, including whole-word repetitions, were counted as stuttering (Section 2.1.2) and the children were close in age to when the disorder started.

The phonological properties of words that contained SLD were exam-ined as well as the word immediately following them (as controls). Throneburg *et al.* (1994) considered that the word following a disfluency was a suitable control because: (1) Preschool-age children have difficulty distinguishing word boundaries (Kamhi *et al.*, 1985); (2) Stuttering has been considered to be a response that occurs in anticipation of word diffi-culty (Bloodstein, 1972). This may apply to word repetitions (whole-word or phrases with whole words), but would not apply to part-word repeti-tions, prolongations and word breaks. Authors who exclude whole-word repetitions as symptoms of stuttering would question whether the second justification about the control material was appropriate.

Each word was examined to see if it contained: (1) Developmentally late emerging consonants (LEC, composed of fricatives, affricates and liquids (Sander, 1972)); (2) Consonant strings (CS); (3) Multiple sylla-bles (MS). CS and LEC were not restricted to onset, they could appear in any syllable position. All possible combinations of the three factors were examined. Thus words could have none of these factors (e.g. *bat*), just one of these factors (CS, MS or LEC with respective examples *bent*, which has CS in final position, *potatoe* which is multisyllabic and *chair* which has LEC), and combination of two of the factors (CS and MS, CS and LEC, LEC and MS with examples *bunting, scream, bathing*) and words that contained all three factors (e.g. *Christmas*). A fact to note is that words with initial CS that do not have an LEC are rare. Thus, some of the phonological features are more likely to appear in initial than other positions.

The proportion of SLD and control words for each of the eight categories ((2 × MS) × (2 × CS) × (2 × LEC)) of phonological difficulty was calculated and the proportion of these that were stuttered was estimated. None of the three factors (LEC, CS and MS) occurred significantly more often in words with SLDs than in the overall sample. The proportion of disfluent and immediately following words in each of the eight phonological difficulty categories closely resembled the expected values based on chance. Further analyses were conducted based on stuttering severity and after categories were collapsed into single, double or all three features, but no differences were found between words with SLD and controls. They concluded that the phonological difficulty of the disfluent word, and the fluent word following it, did not contribute to stuttering.

Howell and Au-Yeung (1995a) replicated the Throneburg *et al.* (1994) study using three age groups (2;7–6; 6;0–9;0 and 9;4–12;7) and included a fluent control group matched in age to the stuttering groups. The same transcription and disfluency assessment procedures were used as in Kadi-Hanifi and Howell (1992), using a broad phonetic transcription in fluent regions and a narrow phonetic transcription in disfluent regions. The disfluency assessments included whole-word repetitions which Throneburg *et al.* also included. No main effect of phonological category was found.

Both these studies suffer from a number of problems. Additional analyses ought to be done to examine different symptom types since whole-word repetitions may occur prior to difficult words whereas disfluencies like part-word repetition and prolongation have no relationship with the following word as argued earlier. Also, function and content words ought to be examined separately since they attract different types of stuttering (Howell, 2010b). Finally, as stuttering occurs in initial syllable and word position (Brown, 1945; Wingate, 2002), the effect CS and LEC factors have when they appear in these positions ought to be examined. There may also be some interaction between CS and LEC such that when they occur in the same word position, this enhances their difficulty. Thus, a word like 'school' that has a CS and LEC that occur in word-initial position would be expected to cause more difficulty than 'quiz' where the CS occurs before the vocalic segment and the LEC after it.

To start to address these issues, Howell *et al.* (2000) examined CS and LEC dependent on word position separately on function and content words. Spontaneous speech samples were obtained in 51 participants who stuttered from three age groups: 3–11 years, $N = 21$; 11–18 years, $N = 18$, > 18 years, $N = 12$.

No effects of phonological difficulty were reported for function words. For content words, analyses showed that the CS and LEC factors occurred at different rates across the age groups used. A more detailed breakdown of LEC and CS in content words was also reported; all nine combinations of three LEC by three CS positions were examined (no LEC, word-initial LEC, non-initial LEC combined with no CS, word-initial CS and non-initial CS). Usage of certain of these nine categories varied over age groups showed that in general, simple forms (LEC and/or CS absent) occurred less often as age increased whereas forms with these features were used more often. The ratio of stuttering (proportion of stuttered words in a particular word class divided by the proportion of all words in that word class) showed that the frequency of stuttering on content words remained high for adult speakers when CS and LEC both occurred in a content word and when they appeared in word-initial position. As the effect was specific to the adults, the effects of phonological difficulty may have more to say about the course of stuttering well after onset and may be linked to the predominant type of symptom that occur on content words (prolongations etc.). In sum, CS and LEC affected the chance of stuttering of content words being stuttered when these factors occurred at the start of these words.

3.1.4.3 *Index of phonetic complexity, Weiss and Jakielski (2001)*

Macneillage and Davis (1990) suggested that motor constraints affect early speech development in predictable ways. Jakielski (1998) used this and developed an Index of Phonetic Complexity (IPC) based on her observations of babbled speech. Eight factors occurred early in speech development namely:

(1) Non-rhotacized vowels occurred most frequently.
(2) Final syllables tended to be open.
(3) Words were comparatively short.
(4) Young children used dorsal place of articulation less frequently than older children.
(5) Nasals, stops and glides were most common in cluster-token segments.
(6) Singleton consonants were reduplicated in the younger age group, whereas variegated consonants emerged increasingly often as children got older.
(7) There was a tendency for children to move from producing singleton consonants to clusters as they got older.
(8) Clusters progressed from homorganic to heterorganic place of articulation with age.

Words that did not have these properties were considered hard. For example, words with open final syllables were marked easy (factor 2) and words with closed final syllables as hard. Jakielski used these properties to obtain IPC scores of words by counting how many hard factors a word had.

Weiss and Jakielski (2001) determined whether the IPC score indicated which speech sounds children who stutter found difficult. They analyzed speech samples from structured and unstructured conversations, in 13 children who stuttered aged between 6 and 11 years.

IPC values were obtained for all words in 25 sentences and for words with a within-word disfluency (part- and whole-word repetitions and prolongations) separately. IPC values for the stuttered words would be expected to be higher than the IPC values of all words. Weiss and Jakielski correlated this difference with age of the 13 children. Sentence-based IPC scores were also obtained and analyzed in a similar way. None of a number of analyses conducted showed any relation between the difference in IPC values between all words and stuttered words and age. As with Throneburg *et al.* (1994), function and content words were not analyzed separately and no distinction was made between initial and final positions.

Howell *et al.* (2006) replicated the Weiss and Jakielski (2001) study distinguishing between function and content words and looked at a range of age groups of English children (42 speakers in the age ranges 6–11 (16), 11 plus–18 (16) and 18 plus (10)). The stuttering symptoms included were part-word and whole-word repetitions and segmental prolongations.

Stuttering rate on the content words of teenagers and adults, but not younger speakers, correlated with the IPC score suggesting that at least some of the factors may have an acquired influence on stuttering (rather than an innate universal basis, as the theory behind Jakielski's work suggests). Disfluency on function words in early childhood appears to be responsive to factors other than phonetic complexity.

The fact that significant effects were only found for the older age groups and that the effect was specific to content words suggest that phonological difficulty is associated with the later course of stuttering rather than its onset for English speakers at least. This may be because older speakers show proportionately more disfluency on content words that are associated with specific types of disfluency.

Dworzynski and Howell (2004) have applied the IPC procedure to German and Howell, and Au-Yeung (2007) applied it to Spanish. With both these languages, as with English, no relationship occurred between IPC score and stuttering rate for function words, but did for content words. Howell *et al.* (2006) also established which IPC factors showed the best relationship with stuttering for the three languages (English, German and Spanish). IPC factors 3, 5 and 7 (multi-syllable, manner and contiguous consonants) were significant for all languages and for the majority of age groups. As noted earlier, these factors correspond approximately with Throneburg *et al.*'s MS, LEC and CS, respectively.

Altogether four studies have shown a relationship between phonological complexity of content words and stuttering rate for content words particularly for older speakers who stutter (Dworzynski & Howell, 2004; Howell & Au-Yeung, 1995a; Howell & Au-Yeung, 2007; Howell *et al.*, 2006) and the main factors involved correspond approximately with those used by Throneburg *et al.* (1994). This suggests different role for stuttering on function words that may be linked with symptom type (whole-word repetition predominates on this word type). Moreover, the findings apply across languages.

3.2 Usage metrics on lexical material

All parts of speech are not used with the same frequency and the structural properties of speech causes some words to have many related words (their neighbors) whereas others do not. These (and other) factors derive from the particular experience a speaker has, rather than the formal properties of language just discussed, and they are referred to collectively as usage properties.

Usage properties are starting to be examined in stuttering (although word frequency has been examined for many years). The ones currently receiving attention are word frequency (the number of times a given word occurs in a language, Kucera & Francis, 1967); neighborhood density and associated statistics (neighborhood density refers to the number of words that differ in phonetic structure from another word based on a single phoneme that is either substituted, deleted or added, Luce & Pisoni, 1998), AoA (words acquired early may be better learned and less prone to error or disfluency than words acquired late Gilhooly & Logie, 1980).

Many usage properties differ across function and content word categories. For example, function words appear more frequently than content words, words with more neighbors may be more difficult to retrieve than words with few neighbors and words acquired early may be easier to access than those acquired later. All of these properties indicate differential access for words that differ on these aspects and the ease with which a word is accessed may have an impact on whether that word is stuttered or not. It may be the case that one or more of these properties has precedence over the other usage and formal properties as the factor that determines whether words are likely to be stuttered. After presenting evidence about links between word frequency, neighborhood density and AoA, a proposal about how these might be used to develop a unified measure of factors affecting word difficulty is presented.

3.2.1 Word frequency

Word frequency is often talked about as if it is a fixed property associated with a word but it is not. Words are added (e.g. in recent years, many terms associated with computing) and others are dropped from contemporary use (e.g. gas mantle, antimacassar, velocipede). As well, global changes occur in word frequency over the course of development. For instance, Wingate (2002: 253) stated that 70% of words produced are content in type in early childhood but this goes down in later childhood to 50%. There are also idiosyncratic influences on word frequency: Different words may be frequently used by children who have particular hobbies, a favorite football team or TV program. Before a child starts to use language, they have no use of any particular words and, throughout development, novel words do not match any language representations (Storkel, 2009: 292). These observations indicate limitations about how word frequency, in particular, affects children.

Nevertheless, some authors argue that the different access to content and function words is largely related to the differences in word frequencies between these two classes; i.e. words with higher frequencies (function words) are accessed and produced faster than words with low frequencies (content words). Based on this, some researchers believe that word frequency is a more important factor in lexical access than the distinction between the lexical classes (Gordon & Caramazza, 1985).

Early work on stuttering showed that older children and adults who stutter tended to stutter more on words that occurred less frequently in language (Danzger & Halpern, 1973; Hubbard & Prins, 1994; Schlesinger *et al.*, 1965; Soderberg, 1966). However, work that would allow a more definitive conclusion would also have controlled for the impact that word type may exert over lexical access. Also, the only study we have located that looked at word frequency and stuttering in children is Anderson (2007). This is discussed in the next section as neighborhood density was also examined.

3.2.2 Neighborhood density and associated measures

Neighborhood density has been used to examine speed of lexical access in people who stutter. Arnold *et al.* (2005) tested nine 3–5-year-old children who stuttered in a priming experiment. The technique involves an auditory sentence or syllable being presented (the prime). Participants then describe a picture (the probe) and speech initiation time (SIT) is measured. When the auditory prime matches some aspect of the probe, the planning time needed for the production of different elements in the phrase is reduced. For the Arnold *et al.* (2005) material, neighborhood density was confounded with some syllable constituent properties. Thus, the dense set has no consonants strings (gun, key, hat, pig, sock) whereas all the members of the sparse set have consonant strings (heart, tree, start, fork, spoon). It is of note that the material was just content in type and no examination of individual symptom types was performed.

Frequency measures associated with neighborhood density are used as well as scores of number of neighbors. Thus, phonological neighborhood frequency is the mean frequency of occurrence of a target word's neighbors. Anderson (2007) illustrated the latter by noting that the phonological neighbors of the word dog (e.g. bog, hog, dig, log, etc.) tended to occur less frequently in language (mean frequency of 11.0 per million) than the phonological neighbors of the word cat (e.g. cattle, that, etc.). Anderson (2007) looked at the effects of neighborhood density and word frequency on stuttering in children. Fifteen children who stuttered (10 males, 5 females) aged between 3;0 and 5;2 years were recorded in a play task in conversation with a parent. Yairi and Ambrose's (2005) SLD were located in initial analyses (in later analyses individual symptoms were examined as described below). Though Anderson did not select either function or content words for examination, she carefully matched each stimulus and its control for word class. Words containing SLD were randomly paired with the first subsequently produced fluent word that matched it on a predetermined set of dimensions.

An important feature of Anderson's study was that she looked at the impact of these variables on individual symptom types. In particular, she looked at whole-word repetitions, part-word repetitions and prolongations. Neighborhood density failed to influence the susceptibility of words to be stuttered for any of the types of disfluency. Anderson (2007) reported that words that had a part-word repetition or a sound prolongation disfluency were lower in word frequency and neighborhood frequency than fluent control words, but these frequency variables did not have an effect on single syllable word repetitions (Howell, 2010c).

One other density measure that ought to be examined is onset density (Vitevitch, 2002). Since most stuttering occurs on the first parts of syllables and words, Vitevitch's (2002) work has shown the importance of onset neighbors. His work is on perception and uses fluent participants, but the procedure could be adapted for analysis of productions to examine stuttered speech.

3.2.3 Age-of-acquisition

It has been proposed that for children, lexical access of a word may be more dependent on the age at which a word is acquired rather than how frequently they have experienced the word (De Moor *et al.*, 2001). Research arguing for the importance of AoA considers that children generally learn a small set of content words before they employ function words and this results in faster lexical access for the content words that have been learned early. De Moor *et al.* (2001) reported that lexical access in children is not predicted better by word frequency than the age at which a word is acquired. De Moor *et al.* went on to argue that word frequency has less impact on lexical access in children, than in adults, because young speakers have not yet been exposed to frequency effects.

Gilhooly and Logie (1980) have demonstrated that AoA effects continue to occur into adulthood (early acquired words are more easily accessed than later acquired words). However, no studies have compared the size of such effects across the lifespan. An interesting finding on the topic was reported by Newman and German (2002). They showed that AoA effects decreased as children mature. Newman and German's findings suggest that any effect may be decreased or eliminated with maturation so this could be a factor that has more influence at stuttering onset than in its later course.

AoA may be a factor which is of importance in determining which sounds children who stutter find difficult. Anderson (2008) reported the effects of priming on materials with different AoA in groups of children who stuttered and controls (22 children in each group aged between 3;1 and 5;7 years). All children's picture naming latencies and errors were reduced following repetition priming and in response to early AoA words relative to late AoA words. AoA and repetition priming effects were similar for children in both fluency groups, except that children who stuttered benefited significantly more, in terms of error reduction, than controls from repetition priming for late AoA words.

The words used were content in type and separate symptoms were not examined. Although AoA has received much less attention than word frequency in the literature, it would seem to merit further work. Function words are acquired later than some content words. It is possible to match function words to selected content words and establish whether there are lexical effects (or effects associated with the different lexical types).

3.3 Summary, conclusions, future directions and cross-linguistic work with respect to lexical factors

To summarize the situation so far, parts of speech have been abandoned as an area of study, probably because this level of detail is considered unnecessary when looking at the relationship with stuttering. There is some evidence that function and content words are linked to different stuttering symptoms (different symptoms occur on each word class and variables that affect content words do not affect function words). Although this suggests that lexical class is an important determinant of stuttering, it is cautioned that knowing whether a word is function in type does not allow the likelihood of stuttering to be predicted. In particular, function words that precede content words are often repeated, whereas function words that follow content words are not. Thus, the likelihood of stuttering cannot be predicted from word class alone. The phonological properties at the onset of content words (CS and LEC) are related to the likelihood of the word being stuttered. The impact usage factors have on stuttering has not been examined for separate word types. However, they have been examined on separate symptom types which are linked to different word types. Whole-word repetitions that usually occur on function words show no effect of usage variables whereas part-word repetitions and prolongations that usually occur on content words do show effects of word frequency and neighborhood frequency. AoA has been shown to have an effect on stuttering in a priming experiment (Anderson, 2008) but its effects on spontaneous speech remain to be investigated.

All these factors may contribute towards understanding whether a particular utterance is difficult for a person who stutters. Some of the usage variables may be superfluous insofar as they are subsumed by other variables (those considered and others still to be investigated). The operative variables can be identified by various statistical techniques and the residual variables can be combined to produce a combined metric of word difficulty. Two approaches as to how such a metric could be developed are described.

Method one – Metric independent of lexical class: It was mentioned that lexical class (of function words in particular) does not always relate to word difficulty. The first metric would drop lexical class for this reason and produce a lexical-class free measure. An implementation of this approach would be to assess all words for CS/LEC and MS, obtain their age-normed word frequency and neigborhood frequency scores and AoA. This list of variable is likely to be incomplete and will need extending as knowledge increases (this is a reason why data should be archived so new computations can be made as additional information becomes available). With sufficient data, statistical approaches like discriminant function analysis and logistic regression could be used to obtain an equation that weights each of these components. Archived data should be pooled where possible (sharing data has obvious advantages). As mentioned, some data for English are already publicly available (Howell & Huckvale, 2004; Howell *et al.*, 2009a). More properties would need to be included to specify the properties of language other than English (e.g. mora for Japanese and tone for Mandarin).

Method two – Metrics that use lexical class to define contextual units: The shift of stuttering from function to content words may be explained on the assumption that there is a contextual unit that can include both lexical types and entire such units are involved when language is produced (see Section 4). Unlike the previous method, this approach retains lexical status and the main reason for this is that the different word types are associated with different disfluency types (function words are often repeated as wholes whereas content words involve disfluency on their onsets). Also, the likelihood of stuttering on function words is contextually dependent and this may pose a problem for lexical-free difficulty metrics too (although this needs to be established). Whereas position in a contextual unit can be ascertained for function and content words as described in the next section, it is less obvious how lexical-free metrics could distinguish the two types of easy words (corresponding to function words that precede or follow a content word) that are stuttered at

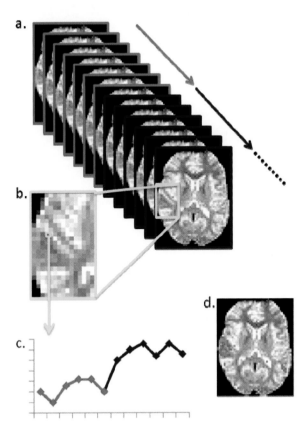

Figure 4.1 Analysis of brain imaging data. Functional imaging data are shown in this figure but the same approach can be used to analyse images of brain structure (e.g. grey matter maps). (a) Multiple images are acquired under different conditions over time in one individual (e.g. task – blue or rest – red) or in different groups of individuals (e.g. patients – red and controls – blue). (b) Enlarged view of part of a brain image to show the individual elements, known as voxels. (c) The signals are measured in each voxel across time in different conditions or for each individual in a group and statistically compared between conditions or groups. (d) A colour map of the thresholded statistic is overlaid on a brain image to show the voxels that are significantly different in terms of activation during task vs. rest or structure in patients vs. controls

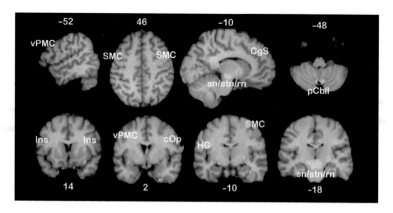

Figure 4.2 Summary of abnormal brain activity during speech in DS (Watkins *et al.*, 2008). Coloured areas overlaid on a structural brain image show the location of significant increases (yellow) or decreases (blue) in activation in a group of young people who stutter compared to controls (figure data taken from Watkins *et al.*, 2008, permission pending). Numbers next to the images indicate the location of the slice in standard space. vPMC – ventral premotor cortex, SMC – sensorimotor cortex, CgS – cingulate sulcus, sn/stn/rn – substania nigra/subthalamic nucleus/red nucleus, pCbll – posterior cerebellum, Ins – insula, cOp – central operculum, HG – Heschl's gyrus

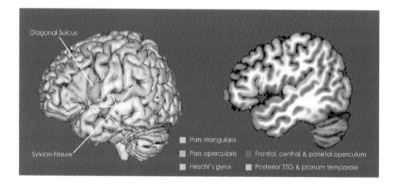

Figure 4.3 Peri-Sylvian language areas that have received a great deal of attention from studies of brain structure in developmental stuttering. Left, a three-dimensional lateral surface rendering of an MRI brain scan. The Sylvian Fissure is the largest fissure visible on the lateral surface. Broca's area comprising the pars triangularis and pars opercularis are cortical regions in the frontal lobe. Wernicke's area is located at the posterior end of the Sylvian fissure on the superior temporal gyrus (STG). Right, a sagittal slice through the left hemisphere showing the operculum (lip) of the Sylvian fissure and structures not visible on the surface. Heschl's gyrus runs transversely across the top of the temporal lobe inside the Sylvian fissure. Primary auditory cortex is located on Heschl's gyrus. The planum temporale is a triangular surface of cortex lying behind Heschl's gyrus extending to the end of the Sylvian fissure

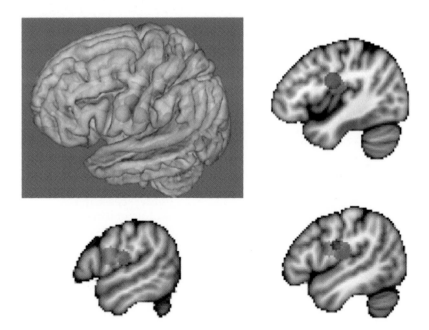

Figure 4.4 Abnormal white matter microstructure in developmental stuttering: replication across three studies. Top left panel shows a semi-opaque three-dimensional surface rendering of an average of 152 brains. The internal spheres show the location of significant differences between stutterers and controls from three separate studies (purple/pink – Watkins *et al.*, 2008; blue – Chang *et al.*, 2008; green – Sommer *et al.*, 2002). Top right panel shows a sagittal slice through the left hemisphere located 42 mm from the midline. Bottom right and bottom left panels show sagittal slices 6 mm and 12 mm more lateral than that shown in the top right panel

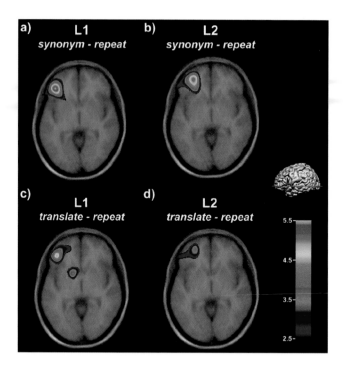

Figure 4.5 Brain activations in bilinguals processing L1 and L2. Positron emission tomography (PET) subtraction images showing mean average cerebral blood flow (CBF) increases in the group of English-French bilinguals superimposed on the average MRI brain scan: (a) subtraction of word repetition from synonym generation in L1; (b) subtraction of word repetition from synonym generation in L2; (c) subtraction of word repetition from translation from L1 English into L2 French; (d) subtraction of word repetition from translation from L2 French into L1 English. The range of t-values for the PET data is coded by the colour scale, and the left hemisphere is on the left side in all horizontal sections. Visible in Figure 4.5 is the idea that all generation tasks activate the left frontal region but that additional activity is observed in the left basal ganglia (putamen) when speaking in the L2 (Figure 4.5c)

different rates. A further argument for using a contextual unit is that this allows the process as speakers morph over ages from stutters occurring on one type of word to another with associated changes in symptom type to be investigated (Howell, 2004; Howell, 2010a, b). A lexical-class-based method would include word characterization as function or content and, for the function words, whether these precede or follow their content word. This would not preclude use of the same usage and formal factors as established with the lexical-class free method). Method two will probably produce quick and appropriate results for English whereas method one (that needs more information before it can be implemented) would seem to have more potential as a universal scheme. The next section considers two contextual units that conceivably could serve the role of specifying which function words are and are not likely to be stuttered. Once again, cross-language work should play an important role in testing the adequacy of the different contextual units for predicting stuttering.

4 Supralexical Factors that Affect Stuttering

Word-based accounts were considered in the previous section. A limitation pointed out was that in order to account for shifts from stuttering on function to content words as age increases, a contextual unit is required that includes both these word types on at least a proportion of such units. Two possible contextual units that meet the requirement that they should include both lexical types are considered in this section (phonological words and syntactic units). Both have addressed (to different extents) the issue of metrics for variation in difficulty and whether stuttering is more likely at the boundaries of their respective units. The phonological word (PW) is a contextual unit that groups words together based on phonological properties. They contrast with syntactic units which group words together with respect to their particular grammatical role that are considered as an alternative subsequently in this section.

4.1 Phonological or prosodic words support for use in disfluency analysis

Function and content words can be used to specify phonological or prosodic words (PW) in English both of which refer to the same segment.

4.1.1 The structure of PW

Selkirk (1984) used the term 'prosodic word' that groups together function and content word classes. Content words are, according to Selkirk, the core of a PW. One content word occurs in a PW and the function words are optional and play a subsidiary role. Function words only have weak unstressed forms, not the strong stressed forms that content words can take. For English, grouping elements in terms of function and content word classes is of interest because of the link between these word classes and different stuttering symptom types.

The way function and content words link together in English was described by Selkirk (1984) as follows: 'It is also characteristic of function words that they may exhibit an extremely close phonological connection, or juncture, with an adjacent word – usually to the word that follows but sometimes to one that precedes' p. 336, Later in the same text, Selkirk developed the argument with regard to the role of function words further:

> We claim that these and other ways in which function words are not treated like 'real' words in the grammar are to be attributed to a single principle, the *Principle of the Categorical Invisibility of Function Words* (PCI), which says (essentially) that rules making crucial appeal to the syntactic category of the constituent to which they apply are blind to the presence of function word constituents. (p. 337)

Terminologically, a content word is a *host* (also called *head*). Function words belong to the class of *clitics*. A function word preceding the host is a *proclitic*, and a function word positioned after the host is an *enclitic*. Examples of proclitic plus host for English are 'a fence' and 'can pile' and an example of host and enclitic is 'give it'.

4.1.2 Link between PW and stuttering

The significance of the concept of PW for stuttering arises from that fact that a single phonological constituent can extend beyond one lexical item. Extending beyond a single lexical item provides the context to understand fluency breakdown and the different classes of fluency symptoms that ensue. The UCL speech team adopted the interpretation of the PW based on the notion that isolated function words are not PWs (as pointed out by Levelt, 1989; Selkirk, 1984 and others). Instead, function words are viewed as prefixes or suffixes to a neighboring content word (Au-Yeung *et al.*, 1998; Howell *et al.*, 1999). Following Selkirk, the UCL group defined a PW on lexical criteria as consisting of a single content word (C) plus adjacent function words (F) leading to the general form $[F_nCF_m]$, where n and m are integers greater than or equal to zero. Consider for instance the utterance 'I look after her cats'. There are two function words between the two content words 'look' and 'cats'. Au-Yeung *et al.* (1998) and Howell *et al.* (1999) developed Selkirk's (1984) semantic sense unit rules to establish which function words are associated with each content word.

Selkirk's sense unit rules maintained that two constituents C_i, C_j form a sense unit if (a) or (b) is true of the semantic interpretation of the sentence:

(a) C_i modifies C_j (a head)
(b) C_i is an argument of C_j (a head).

The extensions to the rules made by Au-Yeung *et al.* (1998) were:

(c)   both C_i and C_j modify C_k (a head)
(d)   both C_i and C_j are arguments of C_k (a head).

Applying these rules to the 'I look after her cats' example, it is necessary to determine whether one or both of the function words that appear after 'look' are prefixes to the content word 'cats', or suffixes of 'look'. Applying the rules to this example, 'after' is part of the same PW that includes 'look' (it is a phrasal verb and forms a special meaning with 'after'). The function word 'her' is a prefix of 'cats'. Thus, the sentence has the following PW form: [I look after]$_{PW}$ [her cats]$_{PW}$.

PW have been interpreted as showing the important roles that different classes of disfluency have on stuttering (Howell, 2004, 2010a, b). According to Howell's account, the core problem that leads to disfluent symptoms is that a speech sound is not ready for motor output (which arises from word difficulty, identified using properties reviewed in the section on lexical factors). Certain disfluencies from Johnson's list (Section 2.1.1) can be regarded as ways of delaying the forthcoming speech that is not ready. The particular symptoms that have this role are pauses, whole-word repetition and phrase repetition. Stalling allows the speaker more time to prepare the difficult material and avoid disfluencies on this material. By implication, if the speaker does not stall, they advance to the problematic unit and this results in part-word repetitions, prolongations and broken words which are all signs that the speech sound was not fully prepared for motor output. Several authors working on fluent speech have also proposed that whole-word repetition serves the role of delaying the time at which the following word is produced (for example, Blackmer & Mitton, 1991; Clark & Clark, 1977; Maclay & Osgood, 1959; MacWhinney & Osser, 1977). It is of note, however, that these accounts have not linked whole-word repetition to function words nor have they indicated that whole-word repetitions occur at the start of PW, nor have they pointed out what type of disfluency ensues if stalling does not happen (advancing occurs).

Next it is necessary to consider the evidence for these observations. The interest in PW is that they are structural units built around a single word on which difficulty is focused. There is always one and only one content word which is statistically more likely to have higher difficulty than the function words that can also occur in these units. Ways of estimating the difficulty of function and content word classes and variation of difficulty of words within these classes were considered in detail in the syllable constituency and usage sections above. PW are specifically used to group together words around a content word. The reasons why PW are necessary is that they offer a principled account of the role of different symptom types, explain why different symptom type groupings are associated with different word types (function and content) and offer an explanation of stuttering development into persistent and recovered forms.

4.1.3 Evidence about PW contexts and stuttering

To summarize the arguments in the previous section, PW are important because they: (1) have a single difficult nucleus; and (2) represent a contextual unit that allows the process by which words of different lexical types with different levels of difficulty lead to different symptoms. This section examines the evidence for the second of these issues. Three aspects of PW that have relevance to stuttering are discussed: (1) The symptoms that occur on or around any function words prior to a content word stall the attempt at a content word that is not fully prepared; (2) The symptoms that occur on content words indicate a premature advance to the content word that is not fully prepared; (3) There is a reciprocal relation between the symptom classes indicated in the previous two points.

(1) *The symptoms that occur on or around any function words prior to a content word stall the attempt at a content word that is not fully prepared.* Stallings occur on (or before) function words that precede the content word in a PW. Thus, for instance, a speaker may say 'I I dropped it' (repetition of the function word 'I'), but not 'I dropped it it' (the function word after the content word is not repeated. The UCL team's account is that whole-word repetition (single, or more than one, word) is used to delay the attempt at production of the content word (which is why this class of symptoms is called stallings). To play this role, stallings have to occur on simple words (i.e. function words) that precede the content word (pausing on, and repeating enclitics would not be able to serve this role). Stallings are common in early childhood stuttering. As noted, the class of stallings includes the whole-word repetitions that are excluded as symptoms of stuttering by some authors (Section 2.1.2). The prediction that whole-word repetition occurs predominantly on function words that precede a content word, but not on function words that follow the content word has been supported for selected constructs for fluent English speakers (Strenstrom and Svartvik, 1994). The authors reported that subject personal pronouns (which appear before verbs in English, i.e. proclitic in PW) have a greater tendency to be produced disfluently than object personal pronouns (which appear after verbs in English and are enclitic in PW).

(2) *The symptoms that occur on content words indicate a premature advance to the content word that is not fully prepared.* If the speaker does not stall when the next word is not fully prepared, the content word will be attempted based on an incomplete plan. This results in the fragmentary types of disfluency that characterize the advancing class.

An operational definition is needed to test the prediction that words are not fully prepared. Difficulty is taken as an indication of how well prepared words are. Hence, the prediction requires that: (1) word type (content words); (2) symptom type (advancings); and (3) difficulty will have a joint impact on stuttering rate. Pairwise links between all three elements have been documented.

As mentioned in Section 3.1.4.3, four studies have shown a relationship between phonological complexity and stuttering rate for content words which supports the link between (1) and (3) (Dworzynski & Howell, 2004; Howell & Au-Yeung, 1995a, 2007; Howell *et al.*, 2006). All these studies also showed no effects of phonological difficulty for function words (as required for the prediction about stallings above).

A link between advancing symptoms and difficulty (2) and (3) was supported by Anderson (2007). She examined separate symptom types and whether they were affected by variables that related to difficulty (Anderson, 2007). Symptoms from the advancing class (part-word repetition and prolongation) were affected by difficulty variables (word, and neighborhood, frequency). This study also showed that a symptom from the stalling class (whole-word repetition) was not affected by difficulty variables.

A link between word types and symptom type (1) and (2) was established by Howell (2007). He showed that advancings (part-word repetitions, prolongations and word breaks) occur on content words and stallings (pauses and whole-word repetitions) occur on function words. Taken together, the Anderson (2007), Howell (2007), Dworzynski and Howell (2004), Howell and Au-Yeung (1995a), Howell and Au-Yeung (2007) and Howell *et al.* (2006) studies offer support for the views that: (1) advancings happen on content words and they are affected by variables that reflect difficulty; (2) stallings happen on function words and they are not affected by the difficulty of these words. The first view supports the prediction that the symptoms that occur on content words indicate a premature advance to the content word that is not fully prepared.

The stalling/advancing interpretation represents an alternative perspective to the discussion about selecting disfluency types for inclusion or exclusion based on whether they are more or less typical of stuttering (Section 2.1.2). In the current account all the events mentioned from Johnson's list are disfluencies though each event represents one of two different processes (delaying or tackling problems on content words that are not ready for output).

(3) *Evidence for a reciprocal relation between different symptom types*

(a) The account of stalling and advancing implies that if speakers stall, they will avoid advancings and if speakers advance, they have not stalled. Data have been reported that support the prediction that both disfluency groupings rarely happen together within a PW. Thus, column 4 of Table 5.1 in Howell *et al.* (1999) showed that the percentage of words with disfluency on both the precontent function word and the content word itself was always less than 5% for all the different fluency and age groups used in that study. Similar results were obtained for Spanish (Au-Yeung *et al.*, 2003) where the percentage of words with disfluency on both the precontent function word and the content word itself was always less than 3% for all the different fluency and age.

(b) As stallings happen on or around initial function words and advancings occur on the content word, reciprocity between stallings and advancings predicts that when disfluency rates on function words are high, the rate on content words should be low and vice versa. Bloodstein's work suggests that children show high rates on function words whereas Brown's work shows that adults will show high rates on content words so age groups can be used to examine this prediction. A change in the reciprocal relationship between word types that are stuttered on across ages was shown in Figure 5.1 (Section 3.2.3.2) for English data (Howell *et al.*, 1999). Similar results have been reported for Spanish (Au-Yeung *et al.*, 2003) and German (Dworzynski *et al.*, 2004).

(c) Priming function and content words. There is experimental support for the view that function and content words in a PW require different amounts of planning time because of their relative difficulties and that manipulating the timing of each of these using a priming technique aids or hinders fluency in a way that is consistent with word types having reciprocal effects on processing time and fluency.

Savage and Howell (2008) looked at priming in PW such as 'He is swimming' and 'She is running' (both have function-function-content word, FFC, form). On a trial, a child was primed either with function words (e.g. they heard, and repeated, 'he is') or a content word (e.g. they heard, and repeated, 'swimming'). A cartoon (the probe) was then displayed depicting an action that had to be described, and speech initiation time and disfluency rate were measured. When the auditory prime matched an aspect of the probe (e.g. 'he is' was primed and the picture was of a boy, or 'swimming' was primed and this was the action), the planning time needed for the production of the primed elements in the phrase was reduced.

The account that function words delay attempts at the content word and if this is not done, the content word plan will not be complete and, hence, be prone to error predicts that priming either the function or the content word (the elements in PW) will have opposite (i.e. reciprocal) effects on fluency. Priming a function word should reduce its planning time, allowing it to be produced more rapidly. When rate of production of a function word is increased, pressure is placed on having the content word plan ready earlier. The reduction of planning time for the function word would enhance the time pressure for preparing the content word, and increase the chance that it is produced disfluently (of either the stalling or advancing type). Priming the content word reduces its planning time (as with function words). But this time priming should reduce the disfluency rate on function and content words (priming the content word accelerates planning and decreases the chances of plan-unavailability, which should be reflected in a reduction of disfluency on the function or content word). Savage and Howell (2008) confirmed these predictions in children who stuttered and controls (mean age 6 years). Priming function words increased disfluencies on function and content words whereas priming content words reduced disfluencies on function and content words.

4.1.4 Summary about the link between prosodic structure and stuttering

There is substantial evidence for English and a limited number of other languages that the complexity of content word nuclei is related to stuttering in PW (Anderson, 2007; Dworzynski & Howell, 2004; Howell, 2007; Howell & Au-Yeung, 1995a, 2007; Howell *et al.*, 2006). This aspect is not explained well by syntactic accounts. Like the syntactic accounts, PW offers an account of location of symptoms. The PW account seems more complete than the syntactic account in at least two respects: (1) It offers an explanation of the positioning of different forms of stuttering symptoms and how they change developmentally that syntactic accounts do not; (2) PW pass the test of predicting empirical observations about the distribution of symptom counts that syntactic accounts fail (Pinker, 1995), see p. 137, and specific analyses have favored PW accounts of stuttering location over utterance and syntactic accounts (Au-Yeung *et al.*, 1998).

4.2 Syntactic structure, boundaries and stuttering

Two issues about the relationship between syntax and stuttering are examined: (1) whether some syntactic structures attract more stuttering than others; and (2) whether stuttering is more likely to occur ay syntactic boundaries than at other positions in utterances.

4.2.1 Syntactic structure and stuttering

This section examines studies that looked at specific types of syntactic construction and whether they affected stuttering in speakers of various ages (Bernstein Ratner & Sih, 1987; Palen & Peterson, 1982; Ronson, 1976; Wells, 1979).

Bernstein Ratner and Sih (1987)

Bernstein Ratner and Sih (1987) looked at a variety of sentence types that varied in syntactic complexity and length. The length variable was based on the addition of embedded phrases and clauses. It did not have any relationship with stuttering and is not discussed here. Eight children who stuttered and eight typically developing children, aged between 3.11–6.4, served as participants. They performed an elicited imitation task in which the syntactic complexity of the imitated sentences was manipulated, and the effects of these variables on fluency and accuracy of sentence reproduction were investigated.

The disfluencies that are specific to stuttering were differentiated from those disfluencies that are present in the speech of all children. The following categories of disfluency were tallied for both groups of children: Full- and part-word repetition, phrase repetition and false start, filled pause (*urr, well,* etc.), unfilled pause, prolongation and dysrhythmic phonation. Separate tallies were made for the children who stuttered of the incidence of disfluency behaviors that 'primarily defined stuttering'. These were multiple sound and syllable repetitions, extended prolongations and dysrhythmic phonation. A fact of note is that whole-word repetitions were *not* included as symptoms of stuttering. They do not appear in the percentage of *stuttered* syllables but they are listed in the counts of disfluent syllables used for assessing the fluent children.

They ranked their 10 syntactic categories in order of increased complexity using other literature as a guidance. Bernstein Ratner and Sih state that 'Generally speaking, the developmental literature suggests that children first master simple S-V-O (subject-verb-object) structures that they then are able to negate and invert to form interrogatives' (Klima and Bellugi, 1966; Menyuk, 1969; Wells, 1985). The predicted order of syntactic complexity (PRED) based on others' findings and the 'authors' intuitions' was as follows:

(1) Simple active affirmative declarative: The boy found the lady.
(2) Negative: The boy didn't find the lady.
(3) Question: Did the boy find the lady?
(4) Passive: The boy was found by the lady.
(5) Dative: The boy found the lady a chair.
(6) Prepositional Phrase: The boy is finding the lady with the red hair.
(7) Coordinate with forward reduction: The boy is finding the lady or the man.
(8) Right-embedded relative clause: We had thought that the boy found the lady.
(9) Left-embedded complement clause: That the boy found the lady was a lie.
(10) Center-embedded relative clause: The chair that the boy found the lady was broken.

Scores were obtained for both groups of children (control and stuttering) for the percentage of sentences containing at least one typical disfluency

(SDYS), the percentage of typical disfluent syllables (SYLLDYS) and the percentage of sentences changed during imitation (CHANGED). PRED correlated with SDYS, SYLLDYS and CHANGED for the typically developing children. Similar analyses for the children who stuttered only led to a significant correlation between PRED and SDYS and CHANGED. Based on these results, there is some indication of a relationship between syntactic complexity and typical disfluencies for both groups of speakers.

The analyses of percent syllables stuttered (SYLLSTUTT) in each sentence type and percentage of sentences containing at least one stutter (SSTUT) can only be done for the children who stutter. The correlations of SYLLSTUTT with PRED was not significant. The correlation of SSTUT with PRED was significant which suggested an effect of syntactic complexity on stuttering.

Bernstein Ratner and Sih (1987) concluded that their investigation supported the notion that syntactic complexity, as defined by progressive addition of late acquired sentence constructions in child language, was correlated with children's abilities to fluently imitate sentences. This is the case whether normal or stuttering children's performances was examined; the effect was not unique to children who stutter. A major question raised about this study is why an independent measure of complexity was not used. Whilst the authors noted that there was some correspondence between their ordering and those used by others (see earlier discussion), they also pointed out that the ordering in these studies differs from their own in several ways, though they did not expand on this. It is reasonable to specify which individual syntactic constructions are considered simple and which are considered complex (Bernstein, 1981). However, putting material in rank order that: (1) ignores available schemes (i.e. those from the fluent literature); (2) bases the selected ordering on unspecified and subjective criteria; is problematic. The obvious questions are whether orderings based on other authors' work would have resulted in a correlation with syntactic complexity and, if not, whether this ordering was selected by Bernstein Ratner and Sih because it led to a significant correlation.

Ronson (1976)

Ronson (1976) tested 16 adult males who stuttered who were aged between 19 and 29 years. The participants were divided into three severity groups. Symptoms of stuttering were part-word repetitions, word repetitions, phrase repetitions, interjections of sounds and syllables, revisions, tense pauses and disrhythmic phonations. Each participant read aloud 36 test sentences which were either SAAD (simple, active, affirmative, declarative) (e.g. 'The kind gentle teacher helped the seven new children'), negative (e.g. 'The kind gentle teacher didn't help the seven new children') or passive sentence types (e.g. 'The seven new children were helped by the kind gentle teacher'). All sentences were constructed with words of three frequency types; however, no interaction was reported between disfluency on passive sentences and word frequency for any of the three severity groups. An interaction was found for simple active affirmative declaratives and negatives for the severest group only; that is, disfluency increased as word-frequency level decreased within SAAD and negative sentences. The more severe adult stutterers were found to have problems with certain syntactic constructions.

Palen and Peterson (1982)

Palen and Peterson (1982) tested 15 children aged 8–12 using the same procedures as Ronson. Similar to Ronson (1976), no relationship between disfluency and passive sentences was found. An interaction was found for negatives (for the severest group only), but not for simple active affirmative declaratives. Passives are rarely produced at all ages and it is probable that children do not understand them until they are beyond age three; however, these structures do not appear to be problematic for stutterers in their later life. Negatives, however, do apparently cause problems, indicating that more complex structures attract stuttering in the age range 8–12 years.

Wells (1979)

Wells (1979) compared stuttering rates (which included whole-word repetitions) of 20 male adults (aged 18–45 years) who stuttered on sentences extracted from spontaneous speech samples that had a single embedded clause with sentences that had multiple embedded clauses. She reported significantly more disfluencies in sentences with multiple embedded clauses than those with a single embedded clause, and this effect also depended on severity of stuttering. Although no statistical analyses are reported, Wells noted that there was a trend towards more frequent stuttering in utterances which contained a postverbal, as opposed to preverbal, relative clause. Within postverbal relative clauses, the NP is functioning as both the object of the main clause and the subject of the relative clause. Within preverbal relative clauses, the NP functions as the subject of both the main and relative clause. Here, unlike in Hannah and Gardner's study reviewed below, there was an effect of syntactic complexity for embedded structures even though both studies examined similar (adult) populations. However, both studies seem to indicate that embedded clauses are problematic for stuttering.

4.2.2 Syntactic boundaries and stuttering

Four studies that have examined stuttering at syntactic boundaries are reviewed in this section (Hannah & Gardner, 1968; Bernstein, 1981; Wall *et al.*, 1981, Howell & Au-Yeung, 1995a).

Hannah and Gardner (1968)

Hannah and Gardner (1968) examined the location of stuttering within spontaneous speech samples from eight participants. Participants ages were not given, though it is clear they were adult (as indicated by the abstract and reference was made to the group comprising seven men and one woman). The disfluencies examined were sound, word and phrase repetitions, any prolongations, blocks and other filled and unfilled pauses unrelated to the normal juncture phenomena. They reported that stuttering was more often associated with syntactic position than syntactic complexity. That is, stuttering occurred more often in postverbal than in preverbal or verbal units within the sentence (no correlation was found between disfluency and subject, verb and object/complement/optional adjunct). The postverbal unit might contain a noun phrase or an expansion such as a relative clause. Not all expansions of the postverbal unit correlated significantly with disfluency rate; however, when the expansion was a coordinate or embedded clause, a positive and significant relationship was noted.

Bernstein (1981)

Bernstein (1981) examined whether stuttering occurred at boundary or non-boundary positions in eight children who stuttered (mean age 6;3) and eight control children (mean age 6;4) and whether particular syntactic structures attracted more stuttering. Both participant groups had six males and two females. In this paper, boundary refers to the boundary of constituent structures generally at the level of the phrase but once (potentially) referring to an embedded clause (complement). Spontaneous speech samples were obtained and complete sentences of type noun phrase-auxiliary-verb phrase were selected for analysis.

Bernstein stated that the symptoms 'hesitations, repetitions, prolongations, and filled pauses' were noted. The subsequent analysis of where stuttering was located, clarify that whole-word repetitions were considered as stuttered disfluencies. The word that followed the stuttering incident was taken as the locus in the case of hesitations and filled pauses.

Bernstein (1981) reported two main findings: First, it was reported that although both groups had more disfluencies at constituent boundary than non-boundary (constituent internal) positions, children who stuttered had more disfluencies at constituent boundaries (disfluency rates at non-boundary positions did not differ between the groups). Second, stuttering was associated with verb phrases (VP): 'VP attracted a significantly high degree of disfluency for the young stutterers. Disfluency on this particular constituent was not significantly represented in the speech of the normal children.' The study does not provide descriptive statistics and lacks detail on what statistical tests were performed. The literature on fluent speech suggests that whole-word repetitions and filled pauses are more likely to occur at syntactic boundaries. Analysis of these symptoms comparing them with the remaining symptoms would clarify whether the former are dominating the pattern of results. This is important given the debate about whether or not whole-word repetitions should be considered symptoms of stuttering.

Wall *et al.* (1981)

Wall *et al.* (1981) examined disfluencies that occurred at clause boundary and non-clause-boundary (henceforth referred to as non-boundary) locations within simple and complex sentences in the spontaneous speech of nine male children who stuttered, aged 4–6;6 years. Criteria outlined in Van Riper (1971) were used 'as a guide' to identify the following symptoms of stuttering: sound and syllable repetitions, prolonged sounds, prolonged articulatory postures with or without tension and broken words. Although they do not mention whether whole-word repetitions were considered as stuttering, a companion paper using the same data for analyzing whether the voicing feature affected stuttering (Wall *et al.*, 1981) excluded them. It is assumed that they were omitted from the syntax study too.

The study investigated whether the frequency of stuttering was influenced by clause boundaries, clause type, sentence complexity and the hierarchical structure of the clause. The speech samples were first broken down into sentences (incomplete sentences were excluded from analyses). The constituent structure of each sentence was analyzed, which broke the sentence down into clauses and phrases. The complexity of each sentence, the individual clause types and a hierarchy of clause-internal constituents (which were based on Johnson, 1965) were coded. The key aspects for analysis were boundary and non-boundary locations. Boundary location was regarded as the word occurring at clause onset; the boundary essentially delineated the clause.

This is a complicated study that makes it not possible to do justice to in the space allowed (even Wall *et al.*'s original report is exacting to follow given the brevity that is necessary when publishing in journals). A full description can be found in Howell (2010b). Here only the main results are given.

Wall *et al.*'s (1981) comprehensive set of analyses showed that the clause boundary influenced stuttering in young children. The authors highlighted that this may be related to sentential planning in clausal units. No indication was found that clause-internal constituents affected stuttering and interactions between stuttering and complexity were not clear cut (VP in particular).

Howell and Au-Yeung (1995)

Howell and Au-Yeung (1995) reported a replication and extension of Wall *et al.*'s (1981) analysis procedure that extended testing to children in three age groups 2;7–6 (six children who stutter and five controls); 6–9;7 (15 children who stutter and 31 controls); 9;4–12;7 (10 children who stutter and 12 controls). Symptoms counted were segment, part-word, word or phrase repetitions, segmental or syllabic prolongations and repetitions of sequences of such prolongations (this differs from that in Wall *et al.* as they excluded whole-word repetitions from their symptom list).

Howell and Au-Yeung (1995) examined usage of the various syntactic categories across age groups, a difference was found between fluent speakers and speakers who stutter, where the children who stuttered initially used more simple structures and fewer complex ones. This difference decreased over age groups (this finding is consistent with Wall, 1980) and reflects changes in syntactic ability with age.

Percentage of stutterings (actual stutter/opportunity to stutter for that category × 100) collapsed over syntactic categories at boundary and non-boundary locations were in close agreement with those of Wall *et al.* for the youngest age group (i.e. Wall *et al.*'s results were replicated). However, significantly more stuttering occurred at non-boundary positions as age increased for the children who stuttered (supported by an interaction between boundary/non-boundary stuttering position and age group in an ANOVA).

Overall, Howell and Au-Yeung found that syntactic complexity affected fluency in older speakers more so than in younger speakers, which suggested an effect of syntax in the later course of stuttering. Across age groups, stuttering was more likely at clause boundary than non-clause boundary positions, although the effect was dependent upon age.

4.2.3   Summary about syntactic structure, boundaries and stuttering

There are many questions about Bernsten Ratner and Sih's (1987) study that make it difficult to determine whether syntactic structure affects children who stutter in a different way to control children. The main one concerns how the rank order of difficulty was determined. There are several inconsistencies between the other studies (significant in one study, but not another). Although the different findings may depend on age-group tested, there is insufficient data to properly determine this at present. Examples of inconsistencies reported are that negatives were found to be problematic for older severe stutterers (Ronson, 1976) but there was no effect in children (Palen & Peterson, 1982). Embedded clauses were not problematic for adult stutterers (Wells, 1979), although a study detailed in the section on syntactic boundaries did find effects (Hannah & Gardner, 1968). Overall, there were few effects of complexity and problems were identified in studies that reported significance. Thus, the relationship between syntactic structure and stuttering is equivocal.

The results of the part of Hannah and Gardner's (1968) study that examined the location of stuttering within spontaneous speech samples reported that stuttering was more often associated with syntactic position than syntactic complexity; that is, stuttering occurred more often in postverbal than in preverbal or verbal units within the sentence (no correlation was found between disfluency and subject, verb and object/complement/optional adjunct). This was different to what Bernstein (1981) found (more stuttering at VP onsets). Wall *et al.* (1981) also found different findings to Bernstein (1981) insofar as they did not report any effect of stuttering at VP boundaries (this is partly in line with Hannah & Gardner, 1968). It was pointed out that the inconsistent findings about what boundaries attract more stuttering may be due to the fact that different studies included different symptom types. Some of the symptoms are known from work on fluent children to appear at syntactic boundaries. These are the same symptoms that have a debatable status as signs of stuttering. If it is correct to dismiss them when examining stuttering, studies that do this and find no effect of VP boundaries would provide the appropriate findings (Wall *et al.*, 1981). Until issues like whether whole-word repetitions are a distinctive sign of stuttering are resolved, it is not possible to definitely conclude whether or not more stuttering occurs at syntactic boundaries.

4.3   Summary, conclusions, future directions and cross-linguistic work with respect to supralexical contexts

Our reading of the literature suggests that prosodic units are more promising than syntactic units for determining the pattern of stuttering and how it changes over age. Here some remarks are made about comparisons between syntactic and prosodic units as predictors of disfluency followed by suggestions how lexical and supralexical influences could be integrated in an account of stuttering.

The boundaries of many types of segmental unit often coincide. Thus, the start of an utterance is also the start of a syntactic structure and of a PW. Analyses can be performed to dissociate the onset of these units to see whether each of the units is important in determining fluency. Au-Yeung *et al.* (1998) performed such an analysis to determine whether PW onsets attracted more stuttering and dissociated this from effects at the starts of utterances. Au-Yeung *et al.* showed that function words at phonological word-initial position were stuttered more than function words at other positions. However, this did not conclusively demonstrate whether this was due to the effect of a word's position in a PW or utterance. To check this, Au-Yeung *et al.* compared stuttering rate of the function words at the phonological word final position of utterance-initial phonological words and the stuttering rate of the function words at first position of the non-utterance-initial phonological words. The result showed that stuttering rate of the function words that appeared late in utterance-initial phonological words had a lower stuttering rate than function words that appeared in initial position in utterance non-initial phonological words for the five age groups used in Howell *et al.* (1999). That is, given an utterance containing two function words F1 (final in utterance-initial phonological word) and F2 (initial in utterance non-initial phonological word), [....F1]....[F2....]..., F2 is stuttered more than F1 in spite of F1's earlier position in an utterance. This analysis shows that a pure utterance position effect cannot account for the effects of phonological word position.

Similar analyses could be conducted to dissociate position effects in syntactic and PW units based on an example Pinker (1995) discussed. Pinker (1995) used the examples '[The baby]$_{np}$ [ate [the slug]$_{np}$]$_{vp}$' and '[He]$_{np}$ [ate [the slug]$_{np}$]$_{vp}$' to show pauses do not always occur at syntactic boundaries but, as we will argue, they do occur at PW boundaries. He stated that pausing is allowed after the subject NP *'the baby'*, but not after the subject NP, in the pronominal *'he'*. Note that both these positions involve the same major syntactic boundary, a subject NP, so syntactic factors alone cannot account for this difference in pause occurrence. Analysis of this example into PW suggests that these units are preferred predictors of pause location. Thus, the PW boundaries in the examples are [The baby]$_{PW}$ [ate]$_{PW}$ [the slug]$_{PW}$ and [He ate]$_{PW}$ [the slug]$_{PW}$ respectively. Pausing between *'baby'* and *'ate'* is allowed in the first sentence (as Pinker observed), as they are in two separate PW. Pausing should not occur in the second sentence (again as Pinker observed) because there is no PW boundary at the corresponding point. Thus it seems that PW are preferred units for specifying boundaries where pauses occur for this example unless the syntactic boundaries happen to correspond with PW boundaries.

The final remarks in this chapter look at how complexity on lexical items and observations about distribution of stuttering symptoms could be combined in a PW account. Specification of complexity in PW is based on the properties of the nucleus (a content word for English). Recall that the section on lexical factors advocated that formal and usage factors might both determine difficulty that is subsequently manifest as stuttering. The first method suggested to achieve this was that the difficult nucleus should be specified in terms of a range of lexical variables irrespective of word type. There would be no prespecification of what type of word served as the nucleus in a PW, and the nucleus and supralexical content would be emergent properties based on the structural and usage properties of the language elements (areas where there are consonant clusters of consonants with manners that are difficult to produce etc. would specify the nucleus, and constraints that occur on stuttering on the elements that surround them would specify the supralexical context). The second method suggested that function and content words should also be used to specify the difficult nucleus. If this is done, then PW could be deduced directly from Selkirk's definition and the distribution of symptoms examined in these pre-defined supralexical contexts.

The methods are considered here in reverse order. Method two is immediately applicable to English. This derives primarily from the fact that Selkirk's account of PW was based on this language. Consequently PW reflect many of English's structural features, though the same is not necessarily true for other languages. For English, much of the groundwork has been done for examination of symptom types within these units and work on improved measures for complexity of nuclei will undoubtedly continue. Also, there are some advantages to using pre-defined units for analysis: (1) Comparison can be made of the adequacy of PW and other units (e.g. syntactic units) in terms of how well they predict aspects of speech performance. For example, direct comparison can be made between PW and syntactic units, which are also formally defined, with respect to how well the respective measures of complexity predict stuttering rate and how well they predict the location of symptom types; (2) Restrictions about which word types are stuttered, what symptom types they involve and the location of the symptom can also be tested. For example, the positional effect where stuttering occurs on proclitics, but not enclitics can be tested.

The principle advantage of the first method is that it is not tied to any particular language. Tying PW to English is an advantage for understanding stuttering mainly for this language. Though comparisons have been made between English and other languages using PW, they are constrained by Selkirk's framework. It is unlikely that phonological systems that relate to stuttering will be developed very rapidly for other languages to offer similar advantages for those languages. Method one provides an alternative approach (language-independent perspective) that bases analyses on phonological properties that are widespread across languages.

In conclusion, it is our view that PW should be used to account for the effects of complexity and distribution of symptom types in stuttering. Method two for assessing complexity can be implemented for English at present. Method one needs more work, but it may have the additional advantage that it can be extended to languages with structures that are different to English.

References

Anderson, J.D. (2007) Phonological neighborhood and word frequency effects in the stuttered disfluencies of children who stutter. *Journal of Speech, Language, and Hearing Research* 50, 229–247.

Anderson, J.D. (2008). Age of acquisition and repetition priming effects on picture naming of children who do and do not stutter. *Journal of Fluency Disorders* 33, 135–155.

Andrews, G. and Harris, M. (1964) *The Syndrome of Stuttering. Clinics in Developmental Medicine (No 17)*. London: William Heineman Medical Books Ltd.

Arnold, H.S., Conture, E.G. and Ohde, R.N. (2005) Phonological neighborhood density in the picture naming of young children who stutter: Preliminary study. *Journal of Fluency Disorders* 30, 125–148.

Au-Yeung, J., Howell, P. and Pilgrim, L. (1998) Phonological words and stuttering on function words. *Journal of Speech, Language, and Hearing Research* 41, 1019–1030.

Au-Yeung, J., Gomez, I.V. and Howell, P. (2003) Exchange of disfluency with age from function words to content words in Spanish speakers who stutter. *Journal of Speech, Language, and Hearing Research* 46, 754–765.

Bard, E.G. and Shillcock, R.C. (1993) Competitor effects during lexical access: Chasing Zipf's tail. In G.T.M. Altmann and R.C. Shillcock (eds) *Cognitive Models of Speech Processing: The Second Sperlonga Meeting* (pp. 235–275). Hillside: Erlbaum.

Bernstein, N.E. (1981) Are there constraints on childhood disfluency. *Journal of Fluency Disorders* 6, 341–350.

Bernstein Ratner, N. and Sih, C.C. (1987) Effects of gradual increases in sentence length and complexity on children's dysfluency. *Journal of Speech and Hearing Disorders* 52, 278–287.

Bernstein Ratner, N. (1997) Stuttering: A psycholinguistic perspective. In R.F. Curlee and G. Siegel (eds) *Nature and Treatment of Stuttering: New Directions* (2nd edn) (pp. 99–127). Needham, MA: Allyn & Bacon.

Bernstein Ratner, N. (2005) Evidence-based practice in stuttering: Some questions to consider. *Journal of Fluency Disorders* 30, 163–188.

Blackmer, E.R. and Mitton, J.L. (1991) Theories of monitoring and timing of repairs in spontaneous speech. *Cognition* 39, 173–194.

Bloodstein, O. (1972) The anticipatory struggle hypothesis: Implications of research on the variability of stuttering. *Journal of Speech and Hearing Research* 15, 487–499.

Bloodstein, O. and Gantwerk, B.F. (1967) Grammatical function in relation to stuttering in young children. *Journal of Speech and Hearing Research* 10, 786–789.

Bloodstein, O. (1974) Rules of early stuttering. *Journal of Speech and Hearing Disorders* 39, 379–394.

Bloodstein, O. and Grossman, M. (1981) Early stutterings: Some aspects of their form and distribution. *Journal of Speech and Hearing Research* 24, 298–302.

Bloodstein, O. (2006) Some empirical observations about early stuttering: A possible link to language development. *Journal of Communication Disorders* 39, 185–191.

Bloodstein, O. and Berstein-Ratner, N. (2007) *A Handbook on Stuttering* (6th edn) Clifton Park, NY: Thomson Delmar.

Bloom, L. (1970) *Language Development: Form and Function in Emerging Grammars*. Cambridge, MA: MIT press.

Boey, R.A., Wuyts, F.L., Van de Heyning, P.H., De Bodt, M.S. and Heylen, L. (2007) Characteristics of stuttering-like disfluencies in Dutch-speaking children. *Journal of Fluency Disorders* 32, 310–329.

Brown, R. (1973). *A First Language: The Early Stages*. Cambridge, MA: Harvard University Press.

Brown, S.F. (1937) The influence of grammatical function on the incidence of stuttering. *Journal of Speech Disorders* 2, 207–215.

Brown, S.F. (1945) The loci of stutterings in the speech sequence. *Journal of Speech Disorders* 10, 181–192.

Caramazza, A. and Berndt, R. (1985) A multicomponent deficit view of agrammatic Broca's aphasia. In M.L. Kean (ed.) *Agrammatism* (pp. 27–63). Orlando: Academic Press.

Chiarello, C. and Nuding, S. (1987) Visual field effects for processing content and function words. *Neuropsychologia* 25, 539–548.

Clark, H. and Clark, E. (1977) *Psychology and Language: An Introduction to Psycholinguistics*. New York: Harcourt Brace.

Coady, J.A. and Aslin, R.N. (2003) Phonological neighbourhoods in the developing lexicon. *Journal of Child Language* 30, 441–469.

Conture, E.G. (2001) *Stuttering: Its Nature, Diagnosis and Treatment*. Boston, MA: Allyn & Bacon.

Danzger, M. and Halpern, H. (1973) Relation of stuttering to word abstraction, part of speech, word length, and word frequency. *Perceptual and Motor Skills* 37, 959–962.

Davis, S., Shisca, D. and Howell, P. (2007) Anxiety in speakers who persist and recover from stuttering. *Journal of Communication Disorders* 40, 398–417.

De Moor, W., Ghyselinck, M. and Brysbaert, M. (2001) The effects of frequency-of-occurrence and age-of-acquisition in word processing. In F. Columbus (ed.) *Advances in Psychology Research* (pp. 71–84). Huntington, NY: Nova Science Publishers.

Dixon, R.M.W. (1977) Some phonological rules of Yidiny. *Linguistic Inquiry* 8, 1–34.

Dixon, R.M.W. and Aikhenvald, A.Y. (2007) *Word: A Cross-linguistic Typology*. Cambridge: Cambridge University Press.

Dworzynski, K., Howell, P., Au-Yeung, J. and Rommel, D. (2004) Stuttering on function and content words across age groups of German speakers who stutter. *Journal of Multilingual Communication Disorders* 2, 81–101.

Dworzynski, K. and Howell, P. (2004) Cross-linguistic factors in the prediction of stuttering across age groups – The case of German. In A. Packman, A. Meltzer and H.F.M. Peters (eds) *Theory, Research and Therapy in Fluency Disorders* (pp. 382–388). Montreal: International Fluency Association.

German, D.J. and Newman, R.S. (2004) The impact of lexical factors on children's word-finding errors. *Journal of Speech, Language, and Hearing Research* 47, 624–636.

Gevins, A., Leong, H., Smith, M.E., Le, J. and Du, R. (1995) Mapping cognitive brain function with modern high-resolution electroencephalography. *Trends in Neurosciences* 18, 429–436.

Gilhooly, K.J. and Logie, R.H. (1980) Age of acquisition, imagery, concreteness, familiarity and ambiguity measures for 1944 words. *Behaviour Research Methods & Instrumentation* 12, 395–427.

Gordon, B. and Caramazza, A. (1985) Lexical access and frequency sensitivity: Frequency saturation and open/closed class equivalence. *Cognition* 21, 95–115.

Gordon, P.A., Luper, H.L. and Peterson, H.A. (1986) The effects of syntactic complexity on the occurrence of disfluencies in 5-year-old nonstutterers. *Journal of Fluency Disorders* 11, 151–164.

Hannah, E.P. and Gardner, J.G. (1968) A note on syntactic relationships in nonfluency. *Journal of Speech and Hearing Research* 11, 853–860.

Hartmann, R.R.K. and Stork, F.C. (1972) *Dictionary of Language and Linguistics*. London: Applied Science.

Hood, L., Lahey, M., Lifter, K. and Bloom, J. (1978) Observational descriptive methodology in studying child language; preliminary results on the development of complex sentences. In G.P. Sackett (ed.) *Observing Behavior: Vol. 1: Theory and Application in Mental Retardation* (pp. 239–263). Baltimore, MD: University Park Press.

Howell, P. (2004) Assessment of some contemporary theories of stuttering that apply to spontaneous speech. *Contemporary Issues in Communication Science and Disorders* 31, 122–139.

Howell, P. (2007) Signs of developmental stuttering up to age 8 and at 12 plus. *Clinical Psychology Review* 27, 287–306.

Howell, P. (2010a) Language processing in fluency disorders. In J. Guendouzi, F. Loncke and M. Williams (eds) *The Handbook on Psycholinguistics and Cognitive Processes: Perspectives on Communication Disorders* (pp. 437–464). London: Taylor & Francis.

Howell, P. (2010b) *Recovery from Stuttering*. New York: Psychology Press.

Howell, P. (2010c) Phonological neighborhood and word frequency effects in the stuttered disfluencies of children who stutter. Comments on Anderson (2007). *Journal of Speech, Language and Hearing Research* 53, 1256–1259.

Howell, P. and Au-Yeung, J. (1995) Syntactic determinants of stuttering in the spontaneous speech of normally fluent and stuttering children. *Journal of Fluency Disorders* 20, 317–330.

Howell, P. and Au-Yeung, J. (2002) The EXPLAN theory of fluency control and the diagnosis of stuttering. In E. Fava (ed.) *Pathology and Therapy of Speech Disorders* (pp. 75–94). Amsterdam: John Benjamins.

Howell, P. and Au-Yeung, J. (2007) Phonetic complexity and stuttering in Spanish. *Clinical Linguistics Phonetics* 21, 111–127.

Howell, P. and Huckvale, M. (2004) Facilities to assist people to research into stammered speech. *Stammering Research* 1, 130–242.

Howell, P., Au-Yeung, J. and Sackin, S. (1999) Exchange of stuttering from function words to content words with age. *Journal of Speech, Language, and Hearing Research* 42, 345–354.

Howell, P., Au-Yeung, J. and Sackin, S. (2000) Internal structure of content words leading to lifespan differences in phonological difficulty in stuttering. *Journal of Fluency Disorders* 25, 1–20.

Howell, P., Bailey, E. and Kothari, N. (2010) Changes in the pattern of stuttering over development for children who recover or persist. *Clinical Linguistics and Phonetics* 24, 556–575.

Howell, P., Davis, S. and Bartrip, J. (2009a) The UCLASS archive of stuttered speech. *Journal of Speech, Language, and Hearing Research* 52, 1092–4388.

Howell, P., Davis, S. and Williams, S.M. (2006) Auditory abilities of speakers who persisted, or recovered, from stuttering. *Journal of Fluency Disorders* 31, 257–270.

Howell, P., Davis, S. and Williams, S.M. (2008) Late childhood stuttering. *Journal of Speech, Language, and Hearing Research* 51, 669–687.

Howell, P., Davis, S. and Williams, R. (2009b) The effects of bilingualism on stuttering during late childhood. *Archives of Disease in Childhood* 94, 42–46.

Howell, P., Au-Yeung, J., Yaruss, S. and Eldridge, K. (2006) Phonetic difficulty and stuttering in English. *Clinical Linguistics and Phonetics* 20, 703–716.

Hubbard, C.P. and Prins, D. (1994) Word familiarity, syllabic stress pattern, and stuttering. *Journal of Speech and Hearing Research* 37, 564–571.

Jakielski, K.J. (1998) *Motor Organization in the Acquisition of Consonant Clusters*. University of Texas at Austin, Ann Arbor Michigan, UMI Dissertation services.

Jayaram, M. (1981) Grammatical factors in stuttering. *Journal of the Indian Institute of Science* 63, 141–147.

Johnson, N.F. (1965) The psychological reality of phrase-structure rules. *Journal of Verbal Learning and Verbal Behavior* 4, 469–475.

Johnson, W. & Associates (1959). *The onset of stuttering*. Minneapolis: University of Minnesota Press.

Kadi-Hanifi, K. and Howell, P. (1992) Syntactic analysis of the spontaneous speech of normally fluent and stuttering children. *Journal of Fluency Disorders* 17, 151–170.

Kamhi, A., Lee, R. and Nelson, L. (1985) Word, syllable, and sound awareness in language-disordered children. *Journal of Speech and Hearing Disorders* 50, 207–212.

Klima, E.S. and Bellugi, U. (1966) Syntactic regularities in children's speech. In J. Lyons and R. Wales (eds) *Psycholinguistic Papers* (pp. 183–208). Edinburgh, Scotland: Edinburgh University Press.

Kloth, S.A.M., Kraimaat, F.W., Janssen, P. and Brutten, G. (1999) Persistence and remission of incipient stuttering among high risk children. *Journal of Fluency Disorders* 24, 253–265.

Kroll, R.M., De Nil, L.F., Kapur, S. and Houle, S. (1997) A positron emission tomography investigation of post treatment brain activation in stutterers. In H.F.M. Peters, W. Hulstijn and P.H.H.M. Van Lieshout (eds) *Speech Production: Motor Control, Brain Research and Fluency Disorders* (pp. 307–319). Amsterdam: Elsevier.

Kucera, H. and Francis, W.M. (1967) *Computational Analysis of Present-day American English*. Providence, RI: Brown University.

Kully, D. and Boberg, E. (1988) An investigation of interclinic agreement in the identification of fluent and stuttered syllables. *Journal of Fluency Disorders* 13, 309–318.

Labelle, M. (2005) The acquisition of grammatical categories: A state of the art. In H. Cohen and C. Lefebvre (eds) *Handbook of Categorization in Cognitive Science* (pp. 433–457). New York: Elsevier.

Levelt, W.J. (1989) *Speaking: From Intention to Articulation*. Cambridge, MA: MIT Press.

Limber, J. (1973) The genesis of complex sentences. In T. Moore (ed.) *Cognitive Development and Acquisition of Language* (pp. 169–185). New York: Academic Press.

Luce, P.A. and Pisoni, D.B. (1998) Recognizing spoken words: The neighborhood activation model. *Ear and Hearing* 19, 1–36.

Maclay, H. and Osgood, C.E. (1959) Hesitation phenomena in spontaneous English speech. *Word* 15, 19–44.

MacNeillage, P. and Davis, B. (1990) Acquisition of speech production: Frames, then content. In M. Jeannerod (ed.) *Attention and Performance XIII: Motor Representation and Control*, Hillsdale, NJ: Lawrence Erlbaum.

MacWhinney, B. and Osser, H. (1977) Verbal planning functions in children's speech. *Child Development* 48, 978–985.

Maddieson, I. (1984) *Patterns of Sounds. Cambridge Studies in Speech Science and Communication*. Cambridge: Cambridge University Press.

Marshall, C. (2005) The impact of word-end phonology and morphology on stuttering. *Stammering Research* 1, 375–391.

Menyuk, P. and Anderson, S. (1969) Children's identification and reproduction of /w/, /r/ and /l/. *Journal of Speech and Hearing Research* 12, 39–52.

Newman, R.S. and German, D.J. (2002) Effects of lexical factors on lexical access among typical language-learning children and children with word-finding difficulties. *Language and Speech* 45, 285–317.

Nusbaum, H.C., Pisoni, D.B. and Davis, C.K. (1984) *Sizing up the Hoosier Mental Lexicon: Measuring the Familiarity of 20,000 Words (Research on Speech Perception, Progress Report No. 10)*. Bloomington: Indiana University, Psychology Department, Speech Research Laboratory.

Palen, C. and Peterson, J.M. (1982) Word frequency and children's stuttering: The relationship to sentence structure. *Journal of Fluency Disorders* 7, 55–62.

Pearl, S.Z. and Bernthal, J.E. (1980) Effect of grammatical complexity upon disfluency behavior of non-stuttering preschool-children. *Journal of Fluency Disorders* 5, 55–68.

Pinker, S. (1995) Language acquisition. In L.R. Gleitman, M. Liberman and D.N. Osherson (eds) *An Invitation to Cognitive Science* (2nd edn). Cambridge, MA: MIT Press.

Pisoni, D.B., Nusbaum, H.C., Luce, P.A. and Slowiaczek, L.M. (1985) Speech perception, word recognition, and the structure of the lexicon. *Speech Communication* 4, 75–95.

Preus, A., Gullikstad, L., Grotterod, H., Erlandsan, O. and Halland, J. (1982) En undersolkese over forekomst av stamming i en lest tekst. *Norsk tidsskrift for logopdei* 16, 11–18.

Pulvermüller, F. (1999) Words in the brain's language. *Behavioural and Brain Sciences* 22, 253–336.

Quirk, R., Greenbaum, S., Leech, G. and Svartvik, J. (1985) *A Comprehensive Grammar of the English Language* (2nd edn). London and New York: Longman.

Radford, A. (1990) *Syntactic Theory and the Acquisition of English Syntax: The Nature of Early Child Grammars of English*. Oxford: Blackwell.

Reilly, S., Packman, A., Onslow, M., Wake, M., Bavin, E., Prior, M., Eadie, P., Cini, E., Bolzonello, C. and Ukoumunne, O. (26 January 2009) Response to Howell – Onset of stuttering unpredicatable. / [E-letter], Pediatrics (17 January 2009), http://pediatrics.aappublications.org/cgi/eletters/ (accessed 17, 27 February 2010).

Riley, G.D. (1994) *Stuttering Severity Instrument for Children and Adults (SSI-3)* (3rd edn). Austin, TX: Pro Ed.

Rispoli, M. and Hadley, M. (2001) The leading edge: The significance of sentence disruptions in the development of grammar. *Journal of Speech, Language, and Hearing Research* 44, 1131–1143.

Rispoli, M. (2003) Changes in the nature of sentence production during the period of grammatical development. *Journal of Speech, Language, and Hearing Research* 46, 818–830.

Ronson, I. (1976) Word frequency and stuttering: The relationship to sentence structure. *Journal of Speech and Hearing Research* 19, 813–819.

Rowland, C. and Theakston, A.L. (2009) The acquisition of auxiliary syntax: A longitudinal elicitation study. Part 2: The modals and DO. *Journal of Speech Language and Hearing Research* 52, 1471–1492.

Sander, E.K. (1972) When are speech sounds learned? *Journal of Speech and Hearing Disorders* 37, 55–63.

Savage, C. and Lieven, E. (2004) Can the usage-based approach to language development be applied to analysis of developmental stuttering? *Stammering Research* 1, 83–100.

Savage, C. and Howell, P. (2008) Lexical priming of function words and content words with children who do, and do not, stutter. *Journal of Communication Disorders* 41, 459–484.

Schlesinger, I., Forte, M., Fried, B. and Melkman, R. (1965) Stuttering information load and response strength. *Journal of Speech and Hearing Disorders* 30, 32–36.

Selkirk, E. (1984) *Phonology and Syntax: The Relation between Sound and Structure.* Cambridge, MA: MIT Press.

Silverman, S. and Bernstein Ratner, N. (1997) Stuttering and syntactic complexity in adolescence. *Journal of Speech and Hearing Research* 40, 95–106.

Soderberg, G.A. (1966) Relations of stuttering to word length and word frequency. *Journal of Speech and Hearing Research* 9, 584–589.

Storkel, H.L. (2009) Developmental differences in the effects of phonological, lexical and semantic variables on word learning by infants. *Journal of Child Language* 36, 291–321.

Strenstrom, A.-B. and Svartvik, J. (1994) Imparsable speech: Repeats and other nonfluencies in spoken English. In N. Oostdijk and P. de Hann (eds) *Corpus-based Research into Language*, Atlanta, GA: Rodopi Amsterdam.

Theakston, A.L. and Rowland, C. (2009) The acquisition of auxiliary syntax: A longitudinal elicitation study. Part 1: Auxiliary BE. *Journal of Speech Language and Hearing Research* 52, 1449–1470.

Throneburg, R.N., Yairi, E. and Paden, E.P. (1994) Relation between phonologic difficulty and the occurrence of disfluencies in the early stage of stuttering. *Journal of Speech and Hearing Research* 37, 504–509.

Van Riper, C. (1971) *The Nature of Stuttering.* Englewood Cliffs, NJ: Prentice-Hall.

Vitevitch, M.S. (2002) The influence of onset-density on spoken word recognition. *Journal of Experimental Psychology: Human Perception and Performance* 28, 270–278.

Wall, M.J., Starkweather, C.W. and Cairns, H.S. (1981) Syntactic influences on stuttering in young child stutterers. *Journal of Fluency Disorders* 6, 283–298.

Weiss, A.L. and Jakielski, K.J. (2001) Phonetic complexity measurement and prediction of children's disfluencies: A preliminary study. In B. Maassen, W. Hulstijn, R. Kent, H.F.M. Peters and P.H.H.M. Van Lieshout (eds) *Proceedings of the 4th Conference on Speech Motor Control and Stuttering*, Nijmegen: Uitgeverij Vantilt.

Wells, G. (1985) *Language Development in the Pre-school Years.* New York: Cambridge University Press.

Wells, G. B. (1979) Effect of sentence structure on stuttering. *Journal of Fluency Disorders* 4, 123–129.

Wingate, M. (2001) SLD is not stuttering. *Journal of Speech, Language, and Hearing Research* 44, 381–383.

Wingate, M. (2002) *Foundations of Stuttering.* San Diego: Academic Press.

Yairi, E., Watkins, R., Ambrose, N. and Paden, E. (2001) What is stuttering? *Journal of Speech, Language and Hearing Research* 44, 585–592.

Yairi, E. and Ambrose, N.G. (2005) *Early Childhood Stuttering.* Austin, TX: Pro-Ed.

Chapter 6
Stuttering in Japanese

AKIRA UJIHIRA

Summary

Some important issues that are discussed concerning stuttering are whether and how language factors lead to stuttering and what symptoms should be used to diagnose stuttering. To date, these have been mainly debated using work from English. This chapter describes features of the Japanese language that require theories to be revised (the function/content word distinction and morae). Japanese provides fewer opportunities for whole-word repetition than languages like English. The implication this for diagnosis of stuttering are discussed. One prediction is that recovery rate should be lower in Japanese than English and some evidence that supports this prediction is reported.

1 Introduction

The way that the structure of English affects the patterns of stuttering in that language has been studied extensively. Stuttering has been examined to a lesser extent in other languages. Even when investigations have been conducted, the languages that have been examined tend to have a similar structure to English and, not surprisingly, the patterns of stuttering tend to be similar to those in English. Japanese, in contrast, is a language that differs in several major ways from English. Structural differences between two languages alone would not necessarily support cross-linguistic comparison of stuttering patterns. However, some of the contrasts between Japanese and English occur on language properties that have been widely implicated as determinants of stuttering in empirical research (again mainly on English). These determinants have featured in theoretical accounts of stuttering (Howell, 2004). Theories about language determinants of stuttering, which are principally based on findings from English, give a limited perspective (e.g. they may not apply to Japanese and many other Asian languages). One example of a theory which may not apply or would need major modification directly to Japanese is Bloodstein's (1995) suggestion that function words are stuttered around the time the disorder starts because there are few function words in Japanese. The second is Bernstein Ratner and Wijnen's (2007) account that stuttering begins when children start to acquire syntax because Japanese has a totally different syntax to English. These two examples suggest that empirical research on stuttering in Japanese may provide challenging ways to assess such theories that may provide indications of the directions in which they need modifying.

The principal ways in which Japanese and languages like English differ that could affect stuttering are: (1) function words are rare in Japanese (Section 5) and, consequently, there is greater reliance on particles on content words (Noda, 1989; Suzuki, 1989). In turn, the syntax of Japanese differs in several respects to English (Japanese is an agglutinative and accusative language – mentioned in Sections 3.2.1 and 3.4). Japanese has a simple phonological structure. Together with the low incidence of function words, the simple phonological structure suggests that there may be less word-to-word variation in difficulty in Japanese compared to English; (2) whereas prosodic structure is traditionally described at the level of the syllable in English, Japanese describes syllable weight in terms of the number of morae (Allen, 1973; Hayes, 1989; Hyman, 1984; Zec, 1995 and Section 4.1 below).

Theories have been proposed that identify points within syllables where speakers have problems moving forward in an utterance. For instance, early theorists had suggested that initial consonants were problematic for people who stutter (Brown, 1945). Wingate maintained that this was a simplification and that people who stutter have problems moving from the onset consonant to the following vowel (termed the rhyme, see Section 3.3). He put this as follows: 'In the case of syllables, the latent division is at the juncture of initial consonant(s) and the following vowel, the syllable nucleus' (Wingate, 2002: 328). The division of the syllable into onset and nucleus is an incomplete characterization for Japanese, which requires mora structure. As mentioned, Section 4 has details about mora structure where it is also explained how it applies to English as well as Japanese, while Section 6 shows that there are patterns of stuttering in Japanese and English associated with morae that are not apparent if syllable constituent analysis alone is performed. To summarize, one goal of this chapter is to document similarities and differences between Japanese and English and to see in what way the differences have ramifications for theories of stuttering and how Japanese could be used as an exacting way of testing such accounts.

In the domain of stuttering, theory and applied work are closely related and, metaphorically, they handshake (information is exchanged between theory so that predictions are updated by empirical findings). For instance, many theory-based ideas have been put forward about how language structure is associated with the type and frequency of different stuttering symptoms and these ideas have been applied in the diagnosis of stuttering and assessing the efficacy of treatment protocols. Some theoretical statements assume that whole-word repetitions are an important symptom of stuttering that can be used in various applications. However, the incidence of symptoms is different in Japanese and English, for example, whole-word repetitions are rarer in Japanese than English. This makes the use of whole-word repetitions in diagnosing stuttering less applicable to Japanese. Rules of thumb about diagnosis of stuttering can be used to illustrate how whole-word repetitions and other language factors would have less scope for operating in Japanese than English: One of these rules is by Conture (1990), who suggested that whole-word repetitions are symptoms in his within-word class that are a tell-tale sign that stuttering will persist. The lower incidence of whole-word repetitions in Japanese might make this rule less applicable; A second rule is that a threshold of 3% stuttering-like disfluencies (SLD) has been proposed as a criterion as to whether a child is stuttering or not (Yairi & Ambrose, 2005). SLD include whole-word repetitions but it is not clear whether this threshold is appropriate for use in Japanese because that language has fewer opportunities for speakers to produce whole-word repetitions because short words, particularly function words, are rare.

Next, a brief indication about what predictions are made about applied aspects of stuttering (diagnosis, recovery rates and treatment) and how these can be tested by comparing Japanese and English is presented (i.e. whether they confirm the assumptions or require modifications). Some theories maintain that stuttering symptoms are associated with certain language properties (Howell, 2007, 2010a; Kolk & Postma, 1997). The association between symptoms and language structure pointed out by Howell (2007) was that whole-word repetitions occur predominantly on the function word class for English. A language in which function words are less frequent than in English, such as Japanese, would be expected to have fewer whole-word repetitions. Predictions can then be made and tested about how the low frequency of whole-word repetitions affects applied aspects such as diagnosis and recovery rate between Japanese and English. In terms of diagnosis, Wingate (2002) stated that including whole-word repetitions when diagnosing stuttering leads to labeling people who do not stutter as stutterers. Therefore, misdiagnosis should be less likely to happen in Japanese speakers because whole-word repetitions are less frequent, so this problem is avoided. Another prediction follows from Wingate's view concerning recovery rate differences between Japanese and English: When the children misdiagnosed as stutterers report that they are not stuttering as they get older, they would be designated as 'recovered' and this would make recovery rate seem high. If this account is correct, elevated recovery rates (due to whole-word repetitions being used to diagnose stuttering) would be less likely in speakers of Japanese (i.e. recovery rates would appear to be lower in Japanese than English). In this chapter, epidemiological characteristics are compared between Japanese and English to establish whether the rarity of these symptoms leads to differences in patterns of stuttering between the two languages.

In terms of treatment, it has been argued that whole-word repetition has a role in facilitating the fluency of children who stutter because this symptom helps prevent them from developing more problematic symptoms like part-word repetitions, prolongations and blocks (Howell, 2010a). There is empirical support for this. For example, children who recover show high rates of whole-word repetitions relative to children who persist (Howell *et al.*, 2010). Another illustration consistent with this view is from work on operant procedures in which speakers conditioned to produce more whole-word repetitions show a reduced incidence of the more problematic symptoms (Howell *et al.*, 2001; Reed *et al.*, 2007). The implications of lower occurrence of whole-word repetitions in Japanese compared with other languages, and other differences in language factors between Japanese and English, for treatment protocols are considered (Ujihira, 2008). Other language-based theories have not usually been applied to treatment. For example, Bernstein Ratner and Wijnen's (2007 theory that syntax precipitates stuttering and determines how it subsequently develops has not influenced treatment in Japan.

2 Definition of Stuttering in Japan

Social and psychological factors are included in some definitions of stuttering (Uchisugawa, 1990) and are used by therapists in Japan because of the continuing popularity of Van Riper's and Johnson's views. The social and psychological factors are not of primary concern here where the focus is on language behavior. It has been noted that Wingate (1988) excluded word repetition as a symptom of stuttering; his approach has had some influence on Japanese research and practice (Nagafuchi, 1985). Wingate (1964) stated that 'the speech characteristics of stuttering include involuntary, audible and silent repetitions or prolongation in the utterance of short speech elements, namely: sound, syllables and words of one syllable', but there are very few one-syllable words in Japanese. This corresponds approximately with the definition of many authorities in the US, who also exclude whole-word repetitions as symptoms of stuttering (Bernstein Ratner & Sih, 1987; Dejoy & Gregory, 1985; Gaines *et al.*, 1991; Kloth *et al.*, 1999; Riley, 1994; Wall *et al.*, 1981; Wingate, 1988, 2002).

3 Language Properties that Contrast between Japanese and English that May Affect Stuttering (non-prosodic)

3.1 Function words

Other chapters in this volume have specified the type of symptoms in different languages and how they are associated with language structures.

In some cases, certain stuttering symptoms have been linked to word classes (function and content). The distinction between function and content words is less appropriate for Japanese where the role of function words is usually carried by particle endings. Put another way, interstitial function words (function words situated in the spaces between content words) that appear in English are infrequent in Japanese. There are no articles in Japanese. Most of the subject pronouns are omitted in speech. The particles tend to occur on content word endings. Also, the function words that do exist tend not to occur at the beginning of an utterance. For instance, many conjunctions are found at the end of clauses or phrases. So the function words have little influence on stuttering in Japanese. Nevertheless, as with English, a large percentage of stuttering occurs at the beginning of sentences or phrases. This suggests that some other property than function/content mediates difficulty.

3.2   Content words and particle endings (regular and irregular)

Japanese is a heavily agglutinative language (i.e. one that joins morphemes together), not an inflectional one (i.e. one that uses extra, in particular function, words to signify morphological properties). In agglutinative languages, affixes are added to the base of a word. Some agglutination occurs in other languages and examples from English illustrate what these are. Agglutination occurs in the most frequently used constructs in English, such as the plural marker -(e)s, and also in derived words such as shame·less·ness. Japanese uses agglutination to a much greater degree than does English. Agglutination occurs when functional properties appear as particles at the end of content words, especially verbs, adjectives and nouns (as mentioned in Section 3.1). The particles add to the grammatical interpretation of an utterance. For example, consider the sentence 'kusuri-o-nom-a-s-a-re-tei-mas-i-ta' (I was forced to drink/take medicine.) There are verb-conjugation and noun-particles in this sentence; the 11 hyphens (-) indicate the component divisions: word(noun)-particle(case)-stem of verb-ending of conjugation-affix(voice)-ending of conjugation-affix(voice)-affix(aspect)-affix (politeness)-ending of conjugation-suffix(tense). There are many competing options for word classifications for this and all utterances. Consequently there is no established theory of parts of speech for Japanese. In modern grammar, nouns and pronouns are considered to combine with a given case particle to form a discrete lexical unit, as in the following examples; 'watasiga' (I) 'watasio' (me) (Suzuki, 1972). There are few analyses that contrast content and function words. Morphemes stipulate the lexical or grammatical relationships.

Particles and particle endings can occur in complex and simple (regular) ways. With stative verbs (one which asserts that one of its arguments has a particular property, possibly in relation to its other arguments), the particles give specific meaning. For example, particle 'ga' linked with action verbs represents an agent situated just before 'ga', whereas, with other verbs 'ga' operates as an object as in 'ringo-ga suki' ((I) like an apple.) In this example, the pronoun is omitted which is often done in conversations.

Verbs have four kinds of conjugation (two regular and two irregular). In the regular verbs, V-stem verbs are simpler than C-stem verbs, because the latter has inflectional endings, but the former does not. Instead, V-stem verbs cling to an affix directly, 'tabe-nai, tabe-masu, tabe-te, tabe-ru, tabe-reba, tabe-yoo' (eat). C-stem verbs have conjugations such as 'nom-a-nai, nom-i-masu, nom-de, nom-u, nom-e-ba, nom-o-o' (drink). Some C-stem conjugations can include euphonic changes (phonic changes that make the sound pleasant), like non-de to non-da. Irregular verbs are 'kuru' (come) and 'suru' (do). The patterns of their conjugations are mixed with two kinds of regular patterns and some isolated form exceptions which bear little relation to the conjugation in irregular English forms like 'went', 'sought' etc. The hierarchy of complexity of verbs in Japanese is that irregulars are most complex, C-stem verbs are next and V-stem verbs are the simplest.

There are two kinds of adjectives, i-adjectives and na-adjectives. They have regular conjugations and are regarded as simple components of language.

To summarize, word forms are very different in Japanese to English, there is heavy reliance on particle endings and there is a mix of regular (simple) and irregular (complex) particle endings on the word forms that exist. These features challenge the conventional Western way of determining how language structure is linked with stuttering.

3.3 Phonology – syllable constituency

The two main constituents of a syllable are the onset consonant/s and the rhyme. The rhyme is further subdivided into the nucleus and coda. The nucleus is a sound peak (usually on a vowel). The coda is the sequence of one or more final consonants.

According to the Maximal Onset Principle (Kubozono & Honma, 2002; Prince & Smolensky, 1993), unmarked syllables are usually CV (consonant-vowel). In ancient Japanese, the syllable structure was almost exclusively CV. For historical reasons, many Chinese words entered the Japanese language. This introduced CVC and CVV structures, and sequences of VV and CC arose in compound words. In order to cope with VV and CC sequences, delete, insert and fusion processes evolved, for instance, V- insert : 'gak-u- mon' (scholarship), /s/-insert 'haru-s-ame' (spring rain), V-delete 'ar (a) iso' (rough coast), VV fusion 'nag($a^{\rightarrow}$)

e($^{\frown}i$)ki' (grief) (Kindaichi, 1976; Kubozono, 1999a). The same processes are used today for borrowed foreign words, e.g. the Japanese word for Christmas 'k-u-r-i-s-u-m-a-s-u'. The coda and the second vowel of the rhyme are extra segments for a syllable, so their status is phonologically lower than CV sequences or a nucleus. The coda in Japanese is a position for a limited number of segments, such as voiceless obstruent for the first half of geminates (e.g. ga-k-koo [gak˺koː] which has a duplication of the consonant represented in Roman script) and nasals (nasals that occupy the coda position are unstable phonetically). The second vowel of a syl-lable has the same status as the coda, however any vowel permitted in Japanese can appear there (that is the last part of a long vowel and the second vowel of diphthong can appear at the position). The pitch accent system (mora unit) that relates to the second vowel of the rhyme is vital in Japanese (Section 4.1).

3.4 Syntax

With respect to syntax, Japanese is not an ergative (treats the subject of an intransitive verb like an object) language but an accusative one (treats the subject of a verb differently to an object) as is English. The crucial property of an accusative language can be seen in English where subject pronouns (e.g. 'he') have different forms from object pronouns (e.g. 'him'). In English, verbs precede accusatives. Nominatives, whose deep structures function as agents, are often omitted in colloquial expressions in Japanese whereas they are never omitted in English. Word orders and sentence structures differ between Japanese and English. For instance, 'zoo-wa hana-ga nagai' (As for an elephant, the nose is long) is called a theme (topic) present sentence, whose structure is a theme (zoo-wa:as for an elephant) and an explanation (hana-ga nagai: the nose is long) (Mikami, 1960). The particles 'wa' and 'ga' play important roles in a sentence. The role of 'wa' in this sentence is the topic marker. Zoo is the topic of the sentence with 'wa'. Hana with 'ga' is the nominative of the predicate, nagai. So what is long? It is the nose. What is the topic? It is an elephant. In Japanese, these appear in one short sentence.

A few examples on passive expressions illustrate some of the many syntactic differences between Japanese and English. Many Japanese intransitive verbs can take a form of passive, '-a-re- or -rare-'. 'Taro-wa (ga) titi-ni sin-a-re-ta' ('Taro was affected by his father's death'). This sentence illustrates an example of the so-called 'adversative' passive, whose direct translation into English would be meaningless: 'As for Taro, his father to, was died'. However, in Japanese, the use of the passive on an intransitive verb, together with the use of the particle 'ni', shows the reader to understand the agent of the verb (die).

'*Tanakasan-ga watasi-no-musuko-ni omotya-o ageta' (Mr Tanaka gave my son a toy.) is syntactically incorrect. When the nominative of the sentence is close to the speaker, i.e. 'I give ...', ager-u is used. In this agrammatical sentence, ageta (gave) is used, but here the subject is a third person – Mr Tanaka. In these situations, when describing the 'giving' by a third party, kurer-u should be used. 'Tanaka-san ga watasi-no-musuko-ni omotya-o kureta' (Mr. Tanaka gave my son a toy.) is a correct sentence (so the kure-ta verb uses the dative case that gives the correct speaker familiarity) (Iori, 2001).

The positions of the inflection, the object and the verb in Japanese are different from those in English. From a generative grammar framework, the branches in the syntactic tree are different. Japanese branches to the left whereas English is bound on the right (Mihara, 1994).

4 Mora Structure

A mora is the minimal unit used in phonology that determines stress and timing. In all the examples of mora that follow, /-/ stands for a mora boundary and /./ for a syllable boundary which is also a mora boundary. A syllable that contains one mora is monomoraic; one with two morae is bimoraic and so on. Monomoraic syllables are also called light syllables, bimoraic syllables are referred to as heavy syllables, and trimoraic syllables are termed superheavy syllables. In general, morae are formed as follows:

(1) The syllable onset (the first consonant(s) of the syllable) does not represent any mora. For example, in the word 'jump' 'j' does not count towards a mora – the entire word has two morae.
(2) The syllable nucleus constitutes one mora in the case of a short vowel, and two morae in the case of a long vowel or diphthong. For example, in the word 'cake' the 'a' is long (/ei/), so it is two morae. The entire word contains three morae (/keik/). Consonants serving as syllable nuclei also represent one mora if short and two if long.
(3) In Japanese the coda represents one mora. In English, the codas of stressed syllables represent a mora (thus, the word 'cat' is bimoraic).

4.1 Mora in Japanese

Some examples of morae in Japanese that show the distinction between syllables and morae are given here: Nippon (ni-p.-po-n), Tokyo (To-o.-kyo-o), Osaka (o-o.-sa.-ka) and Nagasaki (na.-ga.-sa.-ki). All four of these Japanese words have four morae, even though they have two, three, three and four syllables, respectively.

4.1.1   Independent and special morae

Morae that form syllables are referred to as 'independent morae'. The independent morae that form syllables can be mono-, bi- or tri-moraic. There are also special morae that rely on preceding independent morae in words. Special morae, like independent morae, are units of temporal regulation. Several properties show that the special morae serve as an independent unit, although they do not form a syllable on their own. Special morae link between preceding and current syllables to form short syllables, CV or V, where V is a short vowel. Syllable and mora boundaries do not coincide when a syllable includes a special mora. The example 'ki-t.te' in 1(b) below illustrates this. An English native speaker listening to this word would only identify two syllables, ki and te. As another example, /na.-ra./ (the name of the old capital) is two syllables and two morae. Here the syllable boundaries coincide with the morae boundaries because /na.-ra/ does not include a special mora. In contrast /na-n.-to/ (southern capital) is constructed of two syllables and has three morae. Here the syllable and morae boundaries are not coincident as one mora boundary breaks a syllable into CV and C. /ka-n.-sa-i/ (the name of a regional area) consists of two syllables and four morae. The two morae break the syllables into CV and C and CV and V respectively. Japanese native speakers regard /na-ra/ as half the length of /ka-n-sa-i/ and 2/3 that of /na-n-to/. In other words, /na-ra/ is duple, /na-n-to/ is triple and /ka-n-sa-i/ is quadruple.

The special morae fall into four types: (a) a moraic nasal, which occupies the coda position of the syllable; (b) a moraic obstruent, or the first half of a geminate consonant; (c) the second half of long vowels; and (d) the second half of diphthongal vowel sequences. The four types are illustrated in (1) below.

(1)   (a)   ta-n. go (word), ro-n.do-n (London)
      (b)   ki-t. te (stamp), ho-s.sa (fit)
      (c)   ko-o.be (kobe), su.mo-o (wrestling)
      (d)   ka-i.si (start), ko-i.bi.to (sweatheart).

4.1.2   The roles of morae in production of Japanese

Kubozono (1999a) identified four roles of morae: (a) as a basic unit of temporal regulation (seen in music); (b) as a segmentation unit in speech perception; (c) as a unit by which phonological distance is defined; (d) as a segmentation unit whereby words or speech are broken into discrete chunks in speech production. Only the last two are relevant here.

A typical case where phonological distance is measured in morae is seen in the rules for assigning accent to loan words. The loanword accent rule is: place an accent on the syllable containing the antepenultimate mora. (shown by the diacritic/´/) as in these examples:

'o-o.-su.-to'.-ri.-a (Austria)' and 'o-o.-su.-to.-ra'.-ri.-a (Australia)'. 'ro'-n.-do-n (London)' and 'wa.-si'-n.-to.-n (Washington)'. These all obey the rule.

Another phonological process operating at the mora level is compensatory lengthening. Diphthongs are frequently monophthongized in casual speech, for example, from 'da-i.-ko-n' (radish) to 'de-e. ko-n' in Tokyo dialect. In this example, the diphthongal vowel sequence of the first syllable /dai/ is changed into a monophthong but retains bimoraic length of the entire syllable by lengthening the nuclear vowel. Both 'daikon' and 'deekon' have four morae. Vowel lengthening occurs so as to retain the length in morae. There are some syllable-based dialects in Japan that break this rule. In the Kagoshima syllable-based dialect, vowel monophthongization is not accompanied with vowel lengthening. Thus 'dai.kon.' is changed into 'de.kon'. Both 'daikon' and 'dekon' are two syllables. 'daikon' is four morae but 'dekon' is three. Here length is retained based on the number of syllables rather than morae.

The role of special morae in speech production (d) is supported by evidence from speech errors (later some support from stuttering will be considered). Examples involving metathesis, blends, substitution and repetitions are given in a-d below (taken from Kubozono, 1985; Ujihira, 2000).

(2) (a) te-k.ki-n. ko-n.-ku.-ri-i.-to → ko-k.ki-n.-te-n.-ku.-ri-i.-to (ferroconcrete)

(b) to.-ma.- re (stop) + su.-to-p.-pu (stop) → su-to.-ma-p.-pu

(c) ku.-da-n.-ka-i.-ka-n. → ku.da-i. -ka-i.-ka-n. (Kudan Hall)

(d) ta-ta-n.-go. (tango: word) a-a –i.-sa.-tu (aisatu:greeting).

In 2(a), /te/ and /ko/ are metathesized, they are independent morae in heavy syllables. In 2(b), /ma/ inserts at the place where /to/ should appear in the heavy syllable /top/. In 2(c), /n/ is replaced by /i/ to make a special mora that combines with the preceding vowel to make a heavy syllable. In 2(d), the stuttered repetition unit breaks a heavy syllable into two morae. The fragments cut off from the words (italicized) are morae.

Examples of similar error patterns for the first three types in English are as follows (taken from Fromkin, 1973):

(3) (a) Metathesis: Ch/om.sky and H/al.le → H/om.sky and Ch/al.le,

(b) Blend: Ch/om.sky + H/al.le → Ch/al.le

(c) Substitution: Ch/om.sky and H/al.le → H/om.sky and H/alle.

4.2 Mora in production of English

Morae have been used to account for the length of syllables in English and to mark the stressed syllable as the heaviest one in a word or a phrase

(Allen, 1973). As in Japanese, the light syllable is mono-moraic. The heavy syllable is bi-moraic, and the superheavy syllable is tri-moraic. Although there are schemes for specifying morae for English in terms of morphological properties, this results in a more complex system than that in Japanese. The Japanese system described above is used in the later analyses of stuttering. The following are examples of English utterances segmented into morae in the Japanese way:

(4) (a) a-sur-pri-se: /ə-ː.-sə.- pra-ɪ-z/ 3 syllables 6 morae
     (b) a-u-tu-mn-wi-n-d bri-ng-s: /ɔ́-ː.-tə-m.-wɪ-n-d.-brɪ-ŋ-z./ 4 syllables 10 morae
     (c) the-fir-s-t-sno-w: /ðə.-fə-ː-s-t.sno-ʊ./ 3 syllables 7 morae.

5 Evidence from Japanese and English Where the Two Contrast on Factors that May Affect Stuttering

5.1 Overview of methods employed in the data for report

The data reported in this chapter have appeared in several publications in Japanese (Ujihira, 1999, 2000, 2004, 2008; Ujihira & Kubozono, 1994).

5.1.1 Participants

The participants were: (1) speakers of Japanese or English; (2) speakers who stuttered or were fluent (there were four groups altogether). The Japanese stuttering group consisted of 41 adults (38 males and 3 females) whose ages ranged form 15 to 50 years. They were recruited from self-help groups in Osaka, Kyoto and Tokyo. They had undergone speech therapy where diagnosis of stuttering was made (described in Section 5.1.2). All speakers were mild cases based on Uchisugawa (1990). Spontaneous discussions that lasted between one and two hours (average one hour 15 minutes) were recorded on DAT tape.

The English stuttering group consisted of 66 adults (53 males and 13 females) who spanned the same age range as the Japanese stutterers. They were recruited from self-help groups in Los Angeles, San Francisco and Vancouver. They had all undergone speech therapy. Severity (estimated by percentage of syllables stuttered) was similar to the Japanese speakers who stuttered. The recordings were made in a similar way to those of the Japanese stutterers and were of similar duration.

The Japanese fluent group comprised 294 fluent adult Japanese speakers (237 males and 57 females) whose age ranged from 15 to 60 years. They reported no history of speech problems. The speech consisted of discussions of about 30 to 90 minutes' duration about TV programs in Japan (NHK, ABC, MBS etc.). They were recorded on DAT tape as with the previous groups.

The English fluent group consisted of 34 fluent adult English speakers (27 males and 7 females) whose age-range was the same as the Japanese controls. No history of speech problems was reported. Like the Japanese fluent control speakers, the speech consisted of discussions about TV programs (in this case CNN). Both the Japanese fluent group and the English fluent group produced some disfluencies in their spontaneous speech.

Rate of occurrence of stutters on words with selected language properties has to be estimated relative to how often words with that property occur in spontaneous speech samples in normal speech (i.e. stuttering rate has to be normalized relative to occurrence rate). Occurrence rate was estimated from all of the speech of five or six members of the corresponding group each of whom produced 2500–3000 words in total. Occurrence rate for words with each selected language property was based on all words with that property for the corresponding speakers group (e.g. Japanese stutterers).

5.2 Diagnosis

Criteria for the diagnosis of stuttering were proposed by a committee of the Japanese Society for Logopedics and Phoniatrics (Moriyama *et al.*, 1981) which used information from research into stuttering available from the West. The Japanese assessment instrument is comprehensive and speech therapists in Japan follow its criteria.

The instrument checks eight types of characteristics (symptoms as well as other features): A is stuttering symptoms which include sound and syllable repetition, repetition of small parts of words, consonant prolongation, vowel prolongation, 'stress or burst, distortion or tense, break' and block. B assesses what occurs before an utterance starts, such as preparation, and abnormal respiration; C is stuttering-like disfluencies which are specified as words and phrase repetition, speech errors, revisions, interjections, incomplete words and pauses; D concerns prosodic factors such as change of loudness, pitch and quality, and speaking on residual air; E includes symptoms outside the classifications for A–D; F assesses associated symptoms; G is about how the speaker handles situations (release mechanisms, starter, postponement and avoidance strategies); H estimates emotionality.

The instrument has four steps that check the stutterer's progress: estimation of speech rate; calculation of consistency and adaptability; severity profiling; assessment of associated symptoms (tics, head and body movements etc.). The procedures how to administer the text are given in detail and a judgment about whether a person stutters or not is based on a syntheses of all of this information (based on an item list for evaluation and summary). The summary includes information about the client's circumstances. The participants who stuttered were assessed as stuttering according to this instrument.

5.3 Severity assessment

The symptoms in Van Riper's (1992) profile of stuttering severity were assessed. Disfluent symptoms were examined separately (for example, a sound or a syllable repetition, C or V prolongation, or blocking). The speaker was considered a stutterer when stuttering rate of any of these symptoms occurred on more than 1% of all words. Uchisugawa's (1990) classification of severity by stuttering symptoms was also used. Stutters were divided into blocks, prolongations and repetitions that were then used as an indication of the severity of stuttering (the higher the number of blocks, the more serious the stuttering).

5.4 Data analysis

Whole-word repetitions were not included as instances of stuttering. As mentioned earlier when stuttering was defined, Wingate (1988) omits whole-word repetitions as a symptom. Next, in accordance with Moriyama *et al.* (1981), stuttering data were selected as follows. The symptoms of stuttering, repetitions, prolongations and blockings were identified by a phonetician or a linguist. Blocking was based on appearance of abnormal respiration before sound onset. Prolongations had to be more than one mora duration for a vowel or a consonant except for a long vowel or geminate where prolongation was estimated from the context. Repetition was easier to identify than blockings and prolongations (the main analyses are on repetition).

Repetitions appeared in all speakers' utterances and involved a constituent of a word that was repeated one or more times. The locus of repetition was on the initial syllable of the word (further breakdown is given in Section 6.2). The samples were transcribed in phonemic form and decisions regarding repetitions or units of the repetition were made by two or three specialists, agreement between them being required. The specialists majored in linguistics or applied linguistics. Decisions on the number of iterations in repetition units were based on spectrographic analysis using standard broad-band spectrograms, and linear predictive coding (LPC) spectra with equipment ws-5170 ver.2.03 made by Ono Techno system.

6 Comparison of Symptoms of Stuttering in Japanese and English

This section mainly looks at symptoms of stuttering and examines whether they are related to mora structure and phonetic transitions.

6.1 General classes of disfluency

The 1333 disfluencies from the Japanese adults who belonged to the stutterers' self-help groups were categorized as blocks, prolongations and repetitions, a block followed by a repetition, a prolongation followed by a repetition, a repetition followed by a block or a repetition followed by a prolongation. The counts of instances of these disfluencies in each category and the percentage they represent out of all disfluencies are given in Table 6.1 (Ujihira, 2000). It is apparent from this table that pure repetitions are the dominant stuttering symptom in Japanese (no equivalent data are available for English at present). It is also of note that the mixed stuttering classes (e.g. block followed by a repetition) were infrequent (each of these categories comprised less than 2% of the entire sample of stuttered disfluencies). For English, it has been reported that repetitions (whole-word repetition in particular) play a different role from prolongations and blocks (Howell, 2010a) and that these two symptom-groups occur on different word classes. The two symptom-classes (repetition versus prolongations and blocks) cannot be linked to word class in Japanese because the function/content word class distinction is not applicable, at least not in the way it operates in English. However, the fact that the symptom types do not co-occur on the same language element is consistent with the proposal that the symptom types play a different role, as was argued based on evidence from English. Although it seems unlikely that this role is mediated by different word classes, it is still possible that other language factors may be responsible.

Speakers of Japanese who stutter repeat the CV unit most often. In addition, prolongations occurred predominantly on V not C. The latter

Table 6.1 Type of symptoms of stuttering in Japanese (far left), examples (middle) where (⋆ means a locus of blocking, and :::: means prolongation of the segment) and number of occurrences and percentage of that symptom class out of all disfluencies (far right)

Symptom	Examples	Number (%)
Blocking	⋆ dʒib ɯŋ (myself)	85 (6.4)
Blocking + repetition	⋆ a a akira (Akira:man's name)	19 (1.4)
Prolongation	ʃi::::gats (April)	20 (1.5)
Prolongation + repetition	ко:::ко ko koto (koto:matter)	5 (0.4)
Repetition	ta ta ta taŋgo (word)	1189 (89.2)
Repetition + Blocking	se se se ⋆ ekakɯ (character)	9 (0.6)
Repetition + Prolongation	ɲi ɲi::::teirɯ̈ (resemble)	6 (0.5)
Total		1333 (100)

is different from English where Cs are prolonged rather than Vs (Howell *et al.*, 1986; Ujihira & Kubozono, 1994; Ujihira, 1999, 2000).

6.2 Comparison of stuttered repetitions across Japanese and English

Repetitions alone were examined next since they are the dominant symptom class in Japanese. Comparison was made for the groups of Japanese and English stutterers. For the Japanese speakers, repetitions constituted 89.2% (1189) of the disfluencies in Table 6.1. The locus of disfluency in a word should be controlled when comparisons are made across Japanese and English. The majority of stuttering in the Japanese sample was on the first syllable of the words (1119). Selection of similar material for English resulted in 566 repetitions at the beginning of the words. The relative incidences of different types of repetition (involving different parts of words) in these samples are given in Table 6.2 for Japanese and English. For both languages, repetitions were separated into the same classes based on what part of the word was repeated (the repetition unit), which may indicate the break point where stutterers have problems moving on in an utterance (Wingate, 2002, as discussed at the end of Section 1).

Repetitions occurred on words that started with consonants or vowels. Row a of Table 6.2 shows the data for repetitions on a consonant segment. Rows b, c, and d of Table 6.2 give data for CV (could be mora or syllable) repetition, repetition of a short vowel, repetition of the short vowel of a mora that has a long vowel and V repetitions, respectively. Japanese does not have consonant clusters, but English does. For English, class a1 is where the word started with a consonant string and the initial consonant was repeated and class a2 is equivalent to class a in Japanese (Table 6.2).

The label others (class g) in Table 6.2 is a category that includes multiple repetition units, for instance, two morae of repetition (çira çiraɡana/), and mixed repetition units (/ʃʃʃʃæ ʃæks/or /tttatataŋ taŋɡo/). There were few of these (less than 2% for either speaker group).

For English, 566 examples of repetition in word-initial position were available and their distribution is summarized in an equivalent way to the Japanese data in the bottom half of Table 6.2. Comparison of the percentage of words in different repetition classes shows that the two languages operate differently. In terms of elements repeated, Japanese is dominated by CV repetition (90.0% when b, c and d are summed) whereas English has most repetitions on C (50% when a.1 and a.2 are summed). In Japanese, the rate involving a mora or a mora/syllable repetition is 90% and that for English is 43.1% (summing over b, c and d for each language). Although mora exert a massive influence in Japanese, mora repetition in English stuttering is also common.

Table 6.2 Type of repetitions in Japanese (indicated in the first column), syllable type they occur on (second column), examples (third column) where (⋆ means a locus of blocking) and number of occurrences and percentage of that symptom class out of all disfluencies (fourth column). Data for Japanese stutterers are given at the top and for English stutterers at the bottom

Repetition Type	Syllable structure	Examples	Number (%)
(1) Japanese			
a. segment	CV	k k k k kega (injury)	70 (6.3)
b. mora/syllable	CV	sa sa sa sakana (fish)	746 (66.6)
c. mora	CVC	sa sa sa sampo (stroll)	151 (13.5)
d. mora	CVV	kakakaiʃa (company)	111 (9.9)
e. syllable	CVC	mon mon mondai (question)	7 (0.6)
f. syllable	CVV	kaː kaː kaː saɴ (mom)	22 (2.0)
g. others			12 (1.1)
			Total : 1119 (100)
(2) English			
a1. segment	(C)CCV…	g g greɪt (great)	45 (8.0)
a2. segment	CVC	ttteləfoʊ (telephone)	238 (42.0)
b. mora/syllable	CV	næ næ næ ʃənl (national)	74 (13.1)
c. mora	CVC	kɪkɪkɪŋ (king)	114 (20.1)
d. mora	CVV…	mamamaɪld (mild)	56 (9.9)
e. CVC in a syllable	CVCC	dʒʌs dʒʌs dʒʌst (just)	9 (1.6)
f. syllable	CVC	nʌm nʌm nʌmbər (number)	22 (3.9)
g. others			8 (1.4)
			Total: 566 (100)

The main finding in this section is that the mora is the dominant repetition unit in Japanese whereas the C-segment (onset consonants) is most frequent in English. The question naturally arises as to why Japanese stutterers repeat CV predominantly whilst English stutterers repeat C. Two factors that are known to affect stuttering in English speakers who stutter are whether words start with consonant strings or not (having strings makes the word more prone to stuttering) and whether words contain consonants acquired in early or late development. It has been shown that later acquired consonants cause words to be more difficult than those acquired early for English (Howell *et al.*, 2006), German (Dworzynski & Howell, 2004) and Spanish (Howell & Au-Yeung, 2007). All of these three languages have consonant strings (although there are fewer in Spanish than in the other two) whereas Japanese does not. All three languages make the /r-l/ distinction and these phonemes are acquired late in development (Sander, 1972). Japanese does not make the /r-l/ distinction so these phonemes would not occur and make Japanese words difficult. It is possible that problems extend beyond the onset consonants because two of the factors that operate on onsets would not operate fully in Japanese, so speakers of this language would experience a problem on later parts of words (on the V of CV rather than the onset C).

6.3 Comparison of selected types of repetition between Japanese and English stutterers and non-stutterers

An analysis across languages (Japanese and English) and fluency group (stutterers versus fluent speakers) was made to establish whether these four groups have problems at different break-points. For the stutterers, the three commonest types of repetition have breaks at different points. These are after the consonant (C); consonant-vowel (CV) or the CVC portion up to the start of the second syllable (break after CVC). These three types of repetition are illustrated in the examples in (5) (sango, Japanese for coral) and (6) (candle, the English word).

(5) (a) /s s s s saŋgo/   (b)/sa sa saŋgo/   (c)/saŋ saŋgo/
(6) (a)/k k k k kændl/   (b)/kæ kæ kændl/   (c)/kæn kændl/

There were 243 examples from Japanese stutterers and 201 examples from English stutterers. The Japanese fluent speakers had 522 examples and the English fluent speakers had 106 examples. All these subset samples are words whose head syllable was CVC or CVV because the intention was to examine the dominant break-point in a syllable; C-repetition, CV-repetition or CVC/V repetition. Table 6.3 gives the percentage for each of the three types out of repetitions in all three classes. Data for Japanese speakers are given in the top part (with stutterers in the first row and fluent speakers in the second row) and for English speakers in the bottom part (again with speakers who stutter in the first row and fluent speakers in the second row).

Table 6.3 shows that the rate of CV repetition relative to other types of repetition was significantly higher in Japanese non-stutterers' samples than stutterers' samples ($\chi^2 = 75.45$, df $= 2$, p < 0.005). There was a lower rate of C repetitions in the non-stutterers', compared to the stutterers' samples (although it should be noted that Ns are low). The stutterer/non-stutterer differences suggest that Japanese speakers who stutter have a

Table 6.3 Repetition at C, CV and CVC/V break points for Japanese (top section) and English (bottom section) speakers. Within each section there are examples of words that have the different break points followed by data for stutterers and controls (next two rows). The numbers in the total column are sample counts (these are represented as a % of all three types of repetition inside the bracket

Type	C	CV	CVC/V	Total
Japanese	/s s s saŋgo/	/sa sa saŋgo/	/saŋ saŋgo/	
Stutterer	14 (5.8)	205 (84.3)	24 (9.9)	243 (100)
Non-stutterer	5 (0.9)	479 (91.8)	38 (7.3)	522 (100)
English	/k k k k kændl/	/kæ kæ kændl/	/kæn kændl/	
Stutterer	118 (58.7)	65 (32.3)	18 (9.0)	201 (100)
Non-stutterer	66 (62.3)	32 (30.2)	8 (7.5)	106 (100)

slight tendency to have problems at onset shown by the higher rate for stuttering speakers than controls. The relatively lower rate of repetition by stutterers on CVs suggests a form of trading relationship (i.e. the more problems experienced on consonants, the fewer repetitions there are on CV).

The differences between stutterers and non-stutterers is greater in Japanese than in English. Prosodic or phonological structures may potentially lead to the differences (prosodic features like morae are used more in Japanese than English and these may pose particular problems for people who stutter). Although the association of morae with Japanese has just been emphasized, it is of note that most of the English speakers, both stutterers and non-stutterers, also broke the syllable into CV and C or V as did the Japanese speakers.

7 Language Factors: Comparison of Language Determinants in Japanese and English

7.1 Position effect

Stuttering occurs predominately at the beginning of a word or a phrase, and to about the same degree in Japanese as English. Thus, according to previous studies, the rates of stuttering occurrence at word-initial positions are 92.5%–99.5% in English (Wingate, 1979), and 94.9% in Japanese (Ujihira, 2000). Bloodstein and Bernstein Ratner (2007) argued that high rates of stuttering on function words arose because these words start utterances. This argument is questioned by the Japanese data because function words are rare and those that do exist tend to occur less frequently at the onset, than at the offset, of an utterance.

7.2 Phonetic transition

The problem point in repetitions like /ta ta takai/ ('high') and /sa sa ŋka/ ('join') may arise because of difficulty in making the transition between the vowel and the following consonant (/k/, a plosive, and /ŋ/, a nasal, respectively). Repetitions were located and the transition between the vowel and following segment were examined and the last segment was classified by its manner. The data for Japanese stutterers and controls are shown in Table 6.4 and similar data for English stutterers and controls are shown in Table 6.5. The percentage of stuttering on the different transitions is shown and the occurrence rate of these transitions is also indicated in the tables. Percentage of stuttering was compared against occurrence rate across stutterers and controls for each language.

There were significant differences between repetition rate and occurrence rate on the different transitions between stutterers and non-stutterers. Both Japanese and English showed the same tendency. The first involved transition from a vowel to a plosive in the stutterers' samples (Japanese: $\chi^2 = 174.7$, df $= 1$, p < 0.005, English: $\chi^2 = 7.80$, df $= 1$, p < 0.01). There were no corresponding differences for the non-stutterers. The second involved the phonetic transition from a vowel to nasal. Here the rate of disfluency in transitions from vowel to nasal was significantly higher than occurrence rate in non-stutterers (Japanese: $\chi^2 = 46.4$, df $= 1$, p < 0.005, English: $\chi^2 = 11.32$, df $= 1$, p < 0.005). See Tables 6.4 and 6.5 for details.

To summarize, there were high rates of repetitions for stutterers when the segment required a transition from a vowel to a plosive. In contrast for non-stutterers, repetitions occurred mainly in transition from vowels

Table 6.4 Rates of all types of repetition on transitions from a vowel to the consonants manner shown in the left-hand column. The data are from Japanese speakers and results for stutterers are at the left and non-stutterers at the right. Under each speaker group, percentage of repetitions on the transition category indicated is given on the left and occurrence rate of those transitions is given at right

From V to	*Stutterer*		*Non-stutterer*	
	Repetition	*Occurrence*	*Repetition*	*Occurrence*
Plosive	474 (47.1)	695 (28.3)	334 (27.2)	809 (33.0)
Fricative	91 (9.0)	170 (6.9)	86 (7.0)	175 (7.1)
Tap or Flap	102 (10.1)	183 (7.4)	119 (9.7)	299 (12.2)
Nasal	214 (21.2)	661 (26.9)	368 (29.9)	537 (21.9)
Approximant	16 (1.6)	34 (1.4)	23 (1.9)	69 (2.8)
Vowel	111 (11.0)	715 (29.1)	299 (24.3)	564 (23.0)
Total	1008 (100)	2458 (100)	1229 (100)	2453 (100)

Table 6.5 Rates of all types of repetition on transitions from a vowel to the consonants manner shown in the left-hand column. The data are from English speakers and results for stutterers are at the left and non-stutterers at the right. Under each speaker group, percentage of repetitions on the transition category indicated is given on the left and occurrence rate of those transitions is given at right

From V to	Stutterer		Non-stutterer	
	Repetition	*Occurrence*	*Repetition*	*Occurrence*
Plosive	81 (33.2)	717 (25.5)	41 (25.9)	533 (20.2)
Fricative	37 (15.2)	426 (15.2)	21 (13.3)	460 (17.4)
Trill	36 (14.8)	340 (12.1)	11 (7.0)	176 (6.6)
Nasal	36 (14.8)	625 (22.2)	49 (31.0)	540 (20.4)
Approximant or Vowel	54 (22.0)	703 (25.0)	36 (22.8)	938 (35.4)
Total	244 (100)	2811 (100)	158 (100)	2647 (100)

to nasals. The sonority values are maximally different for vowels and plosives (Selkirk, 1984). According to Selkirk's sonority index, vowels are most sonorant and have values of 8–10, and plosives are least sonorant at 1–2. Concatenating a vowel and plosive juxtaposes sounds with the most difference in sonority. This large difference aids perception but works against the principle of least effort that has been proposed for production (Martinet, 1960; Takebayashi, 1996; Trask, 1996). The transition from a vowel to a nasal, that attracted most disfluency for the non-stutterers, involved a shorter distance in the sonority hierarchy (nasals have a sonority value of 5 on the sonority index). The transitions from a vowel to a nasal fit closer to the principle of least effort than transitions from a vowel to a plosive and so they should be easier to produce. The transitions that the stutterers showed highest rate of disfluency were the most difficult to pronounce, as expected, but the one that the non-stutterers experienced most difficulty were ones that should have been easy to produce these. In brief, stutterers' CV repetitions occur on hard transitions whereas non-stutterers' CV repetitions occur on easy ones.

For English, repetitions also commonly involved the C. Thus it is necessary to examine the transitions from Cs to phones with other manners for this language. Incidence of repetition of C units is low in Japanese irrespective of speaker group (Table 6.2) and is not performed for them (either stutterers or controls). C repetitions in English were analyzed in the same way as with CV-unit repetitions (Table 6.6). For the stutterers, there were 238 repetitions and the number of words in the base rate condition was 192. The corresponding numbers for the non-stutterers were 85 repetitions out of 2037 words. The result of the analysis showed the same tendency as

Table 6.6 Rates of all types of repetition on transitions from a consonant to the phoneme manners shown in the left-hand column. The data are from English speakers and results for stutterers are at the left and non-stutterers at the right. Under each speaker group, percentage of repetitions on the transition category indicated is given on the left and occurrence rate of those transitions is given at right

English phonetic transition, C-unit repetition (%)

From V to	Stutterer		Non-stutterer	
	Repetition	*Occurrence*	*Repetition*	*Occurrence*
Plosive	95 (40.0)	632 (32.9)	16 (18.8)	768 (37.7)
Fricative	55 (23.1)	680 (35.4)	25 (29.4)	560 (27.5)
Nasal	29 (12.2)	244 (12.7)	4 (4.7)	155 (7.6)
Trill	26 (10.9)	109 (5.7)	2 (2.4)	130 (6.4)
Approximant or Vowel	33 (13.8)	256 (13.3)	38 (44.7)	424 (20.8)
Total	238 (100)	1921 (100)	85 (100)	2037 (100)

in the case of vowel transitions out of CV-unit repetitions described above (Tables 6.4 and 6.5). The dominant phonetic transitions of stutterers were from plosive to vowel (here for the C repetitions, the transition from a trill to the vowel was also significant). The effects of both of these were significant (for the former, $x^2 = 5.51$, df $= 1$, p < 0.05 and for the latter: $x^2 = 10.92$, df $= 1$, p < 0.005). On the other hand, the highest rate of phonetic transition for non-stutterers was from an approximant to a vowel which was significant, too ($x^2 = 28.1$, df $= 1$, p < 0.005). The full results are given in Table 6.6.

This result also showed that the type of phonetic transition that leads to C repetitions differed between stutterers and non-stutterers. As in the case of CV-unit repetitions, an easy phonetic transition from one articulation to another tended to produce repetitions in non-stutterers' samples. On the other hand, in stutterers' samples, again it is the difficult phonetic transition from one articulation to another (plosive-vowel) that tended to produce repetitions. Also of interest is the fact that the type of transition where stutterers' repetitions occurred most frequently was the one that produced the least repetitions for the non-stutterers.

The final types of transition examined were just looked at for Japanese speakers who stutter (there were insufficient data for the other groups). For this group, the transitions from voiceless C to V, and from voiced C to V, were examined (Table 6.7). A transition from voiced C to V should be easier than one from a voiceless C to V. The transitions from voiceless C or voiced C to subsequent V were both significantly higher for the stuttered repetitions than occurrence rate ($x^2 = 14.73$, df $= 1$, p < 0.005)

Table 6.7 Rates of all types of repetition on transitions from a consonant to a vowel in Japanese speakers who stutter. The voicing on the consonant from which the transition started is indicated in the left column (onset). Percentage of repetitions on the transition category indicated is given in the central column and occurrence rate of those transitions is given in the right column

Onset	Repetition	Occurrence rate
[+voiced]	16 (22.9)	882 (45.8)
[−voiced]	54 (77.1)	1045 (54.2)
Total	70 (100)	1927 (100)

with voiceless C at a much higher value than voiced C. Transitions from consonants to vowels were differentially affected by whether a voicing change was required or not.

8   Comparison of Japanese and English in Applied Domains

The main difference between Japanese and English is that whole-word repetitions are a less important symptom of stuttering in Japanese because there are few interstitial function words (functional properties are mainly signaled as particle endings on content words). The interstitial function words that are present tend to occupy positions that follow content words, which also gives function words a reduced likelihood of being repeated (Howell, 2010a). Also, as noted in section one, Nagafuchi (1985) advised against including whole-word repetitions as symptoms of stuttering in Japanese. This section examines what impact the low rates of whole-word repetitions and the advice to discard the few that are present on Japanese has on diagnosis and recovery rate of stuttering.

8.1   Diagnosis

If the advice to exclude whole-word repetitions is followed, then arguably diagnosis of stuttering will be improved. Whole-word repetitions occur frequently in the speech of typically developing children (Clark & Clark, 1977; Wingate, 2002). As such Wingate considers that they should not be used as a sign to diagnose stuttering. If whole-word repetitions are counted as stutterings, then stuttering will be diagnosed in cases where a child does not stutter. The Nagafuchi (1985) advice would preempt this problem. Even if the advice is not followed and whole-word repetitions are included, the risk of inappropriate diagnosis of stuttering would still be lower in Japanese compared to English because of their comparative rarity. Thus whether advice to exclude whole-word repetitions is followed or not, the likelihood of misdiagnosing stuttering in Japanese is lower than in English.

8.2   Recovery rates (and other epidemiological factors)

There are fewer statistics about prevalence and incidence of stuttering in Japan than in the US or UK. Therefore, nothing can be said about how these statistics compare with those from other countries where it is usually stated that prevalence is about 1% and incidence is about 5% (Guitar, 2006; Howell, 2010b). Symptoms always feature at some point in diagnoses subsequently intended to be used for estimating prevalence and incidence. Based on the argument in Section 8.1, it would be expected that misdiagnoses would be lower in Japanese than English and this would result in lower prevalence and incidence rates. This prediction ought to be examined in empirical research. Similarly, there is a lack of data on gender ratios in stuttering, but the better diagnosis of stuttering might be expected to reduce the changes in gender imbalance as age increases (Howell, 2010b). That is, gender ratio might be closer to even in Japan than in other countries. Again this is a prediction that could be tested empirically.

If stuttering is over-diagnosed in countries outside Japan relative to Japan because the former include whole-word repetitions, then recovery rate ought to appear lower in Japan (Wingate, 2002). Consistent with this, natural recovery rates in Japan have been reported to be 40–45% of stutterers (Tsuzuki, 2001). According to Ujihira (2006), the recovery rate is 66.7% in a small-sized sample. These rates are much lower than the rates reported in other countries where rates of 80% and above are commonly reported (Yairi & Ambrose, 2005).

9   Discussion: Drawing the Findings Together and Examining the Direction They Suggest for Theory

One important finding was the way that the main classes of disfluency (repetition, prolongation and block) appeared in complementary distribution (if a person repeated a sound, they did not prolong it etc.). An important question is whether this is linked to particular language structures (whole-word repetitions are linked to function words in English, but this cannot apply to Japanese for reasons discussed below in Section 9.3). One possibility is in the nature of the transitions that have to be made within words where analyses showed that speakers who stuttered had problems (high rates of repetition at the transition point) when the transitions were phonologically difficult.

Different elements are predominantly repeated in Japanese (CV) and English (C). CV repetition is one category of mora which massively dominates the pattern of repetition in Japanese (90%). It was also noted that there was a significant percentage of mora-based repetitions in English (43.1%). An explanation was offered of why Japanese shifts from

C to CV, namely Japanese has no consonant strings and fewer developmentally late-emerging consonants, both of which are structures that could potentially block the forward flow of speech. This idea is consistent with multiple interruption points such as in Kolk and Postma's (1997) work.

When stutterers and non-stutterers disfluency rates were compared, it was noted that there was a higher rate on C and a lower rate on CV in stutterers than non-stutterers. This could be explained on the basis that people who stutter were affected to some extent by consonant onsets and that this appeared to reduce the rate of repetition on CV for these individuals (although repetition rate on CV was at a high level).

Section 7 concerned language determinants and stuttering and looked in depth at which phonetic transition led to difficulty in people who stutter from different language groups and in comparison to non-stutterers. When CV repetitions were examined, for both languages vowel-plosive was difficult (for people who stutter only) and vowel-nasal were easy for the stutterers but led to disfleucny for the non-stutterers.

For C repetitions (only examined for English speakers), vowel-plosive and vowel-trill transitions were difficult for stutterers (approximant-vowel transitions were difficult for non-stutterers). Additional analyses, just on stutterers disfluencies, showed that they had trouble with articulation, whereas non-stutterers violated the Obligatory Contour Principle, OCP (Goldsmith, 1979). OCP is the principle governing phonological representations that prohibits or at least disfavors, the occurrence of identical feature specifications on adjacent autosegments. The adjacent segments that the non-stutterers have most disfluency have the same main features. So they would be disfavored by OCP.

Section 8 discussed data that showed recovery rate was lower for speakers who stuttered and spoke Japanese than for those who spoke English. This was attributed to potentially better diagnosis of stuttering for speakers of Japanese because whole-word repetitions necessarily feature less in diagnostic decisions and estimates of recovery rate. Further predictions were made, which can be tested empirically (e.g. that misdiagnoses may be lower in Japanese and the gender imbalance may differ from English).

9.1 Symptom distribution

An account that was offered for a general principle that led to stuttering and explained the different patterns in the different languages was that segmentally simpler material allowed forward movement of the position of disfluency. This would be compatible with models such as the covert repair hypothesis (Kolk & Postma 1997), which proposes that difficulty determines whether parts of language are stuttered or not and that examination of the ensuing symptoms allows the different points where disfluency arose to be located (in this theory, based on the amount of auditory feedback that was received before the forward flow of speech was interrupted). Another theory that proposes language difficulty leads to stuttering that would also allow speech segments to be interrupted at different points is Howell's (2004, 2010a) EXPLAN theory. This theory maintains that stuttering arises when a speaker starts an utterance based on an incomplete plan. It allows variable points of interruption as it proposes that part-planning of words will have proceeded to different points before they are required for output (Howell, 2010a). Although this finding can be accommodated by some existing theories, it is useful to have converging evidence about variable points of interruption (here from cross-linguistic data) to support these ideas.

9.2 Structural features of Japanese

An obvious alternative approach to accounting for the Japanese-English differences in terms of patterns of repetition is in terms of morae. Although these are not exclusive to Japanese, they are used much more widely in Japanese and would have a differential impact on the two languages. The main problems in using morae as a basis for cross-linguistic differences are: (1) that there is no agreed definition of mora; (2) judgment reliability may not be good. In addition, it would be difficult to introduce this perspective to researchers on English.

A point that has been made earlier is that the function-content word distinction which has been popular in work on English does not apply to Japanese. According to some viewpoints, function words are distinct from content words. Other research has emphasized the heuristic value of dividing words into these two distinct classes because they divide words along a number of dimensions, all of which relate to difficulty (see Howell & Rusbridge, this volume). Thus function words are short, rarely start with consonant strings, do not carry stress and occur frequently in speech, all of which make them easy to produce (and any of them may be a single or joint mediator of difficulty). Howell and Rusbridge also propose that lexical-free ways of defining difficulty could be developed. Such development for Japanese would need to incorporate simpler phonology (few consonant strings and absence of some developmentally difficult manners like /r-l/), mora principles and possibly higher level linguistic factors that might also impact on difficulty.

One possibility is that the particle endings that signal functional properties of words may be a source of difficulty for Japanese speakers. Table 6.8 shows data from 396 verbs which were selected from the

Table 6.8 Contingency table between type of conjugation (irregular, regular C-stem, V-stem) and stuttering and occurrence rates for Japanese speakers who stutter. The association between conjugation and stuttering/occurrence rates was not significant

Type of Conjugation	*Stuttering rate*	*Occurrence rate*
Irregular	57 (14.4%)	83 (18.7%)
Regular; C-stem	233 (58.8%)	278 (62.8%)
V-stem	106 (26.8%)	82 (18.5%)
Total	396 (100%)	443 (100%)

stuttering samples. Fifty-seven of the 396 verbs had irregular conjugations and 339 were regular. From the non-stutterers' samples 443 verbs were selected and 83 of the 443 had irregular conjugations and 360 were regular. As mentioned in Section 3.2, irregular verbs are the most complex conjugations, next are C-stem verbs that have endings of the inflections, and V-stem verbs are the simplest. Correlation of the complexity of conjugations with occurrence of stuttering is low. Details are provided in Table 6.8. For the irregular verbs, incidence rate in the stuttered materials was lower that in the fluent base rate material. The more complex particles did not produce higher rates of stuttering, against what was hypothesized above. Consequently, particle endings seem an unlikely factor that leads to difficulty that surfaces as stuttering.

Although the differences in stuttering between Japanese and English have been emphasized, there are some notable similarities. Thus, evidence was provided that speakers who stutter are affected by difficult articulation (making difficult phonetic transitions) and there was a small but significantly higher rate of disfluency on C-word repetitions for stutterers over non-stutterers in Japanese. Also many CV repetitions are seen in English disfluency as is true of Japanese.

9.3 Predictions from applied domains

The structural properties of Japanese that lead to fewer whole-word repetitions than in English allowed predictions about whether this symptom class should be considered a sign of stuttering, and whether these symptoms have a role in facilitating fluency to be tested. Specifically, if whole-word repetition is not a sign of stuttering, then there should be less chance of misdiagnosis in Japanese and recovery rate should appear lower. Available evidence was examined that seems to support these predictions. Other predictions were made where there is no available evidence. Further research is required to see whether or not these predictions about Japanese are confirmed.

10 Conclusions

The purpose of this chapter was to introduce non-Japanese researchers to some of the unusual features of that language and to pinpoint ways this challenges existing theories and suggest ways of reformulating and testing future theories. The diversity of the world's languages suggests that comparisons like that of Japanese-English are needed to inform future theories on stuttering.

References

Allen, W.S. (1973) *Accent and Rhythm*. Cambridge: Cambridge University Press.

Bernstein Ratner, N. and Sih, G.G. (1987) Effect of gradual increases in sentence length and complexity on children's dysfluency. *Journal of Speech and Hearing Disorders* 52, 278–287.

Bernstein Ratner, N. and Wijnen, F. (2007) The Vicious Cycle: Linguistic encoding, self-monitoring and stuttering. In J. Au-Yeung (ed.) *Proceedings of the Fifth World Congress on Fluency Disorders* (pp. 84–90). Dublin: International Fluency Association.

Bloodstein, O. (1995) *A Handbook on Stuttering*. San Diego: Singular Group.

Bloodstein, O. and Bernstein Ratner, N. (2007) *A Hand Book of Stuttering*. New York: Delmar Tompson Learning.

Brown, S.F. (1945) The loci of stutterings in the speech sequence. *Journal of Speech Disorders* 10, 181–192.

Clark, H.H. and Clark, E.V. (1977) *Psychology and Language: An Introduction to Psycholinguistics*. New York: Harcourt Brace Jovanovich.

Conture, E.G. (1990) *Stuttering*. Englewood Cliffs: Prentice-Hall.

Dejoy, D.A. and Gregory, H.H.(1985) The relationship between age and frequency of disfluency in preschool children. *Journal of Fluency Disorders* 10, 107–122.

Dworzynski, K. and Howell, P. (2004) Cross-linguistic factors in the prediction of stuttering across age groups: The case of German. In A. Meltzer, H.F.M. Peters (eds) *Theory, Research and Therapy in Fluency Disorders* (pp. 382–388). Nijmegen: Nijmegen University Press.

Fromkin, V. (1973) The non anomalous nature of anomalous utterances. In V. Fromkin (ed.) *Speech Errors as Linguistic Evidence* (pp. 215–242). The Hague: Mouton.

Gaines, N.D., Runyan, C.M. and Meyers, S.C. (1991) A comparison of young stutterers' fluent versus stuttered utterances of length and complexity. *Journal of Speech and Hearing Research* 34, 37–42.

Goldsmith, J. (1979) *Autosegmental Phonology*. New York: Garland.

Guitar, B. (2006) *Stuttering*. Tokyo:Gakuensha.

Hayes, B. (1989) Compensatory lengthening in moraic phonology. *Linguistic Inquiry* 13, 227–276.

Howell, P. (2004) Assessment of some contemporary theories of stuttering that apply to spontaneous speech. *Contemporary Issues in Communicative Sciences and Disorders* 31, 122–139.

Howell, P. (2007) Signs of developmental stuttering up to age eight and at 12 plus. *Clinical Psychology Review* 27, 287–301.

Howell, P. (2010a) Language processing in fluency disorders. In J. Guendouzi, F. Loncke and M. Williams (eds) *The Handbook on Psycholinguistics and Cognitive Processes, Perspectives on Communication Disorders* (pp 437–464). London: Taylor & Francis.

Howell, P. (2010b) Stuttering from the view of phonetics and support to schoolchildren who stutter. A handout for the lectures in Japan 2010.

Howell, P. and Au-Yeung, J. (2007) Phonetic complexity and stuttering in Spanish. *Clinical Linguistics and Phonetics* 21, 111–127.

Howell, P., Au-Yeung, J. and Sackin, S.(1999) Exchange of stuttering from function words to content words with age. *Journal of Speech, Language, and Hearing Research* 42, 345–354.

Howell, P., Bailey, E. and Kothari, N. (2010) Changes in the pattern of stuttering over development for children who recover or persist. *Clinical Linguistics & Phonetics* 24, 556–575.

Howell, P., Hamilton, A. and Kyriacopoulos, A. (1986) Automatic detection of repetitions and prolongations in stuttered speech. *Speech Input/Output: Techniques and Applications* (pp. 252–256). London: IEE Publications.

Howell, P., Au-Yeung, J., Yaruss, S.E. and Eldridge, K. (2006) Phonetic difficulty and stuttering in English. *Clinical Linguistics and Phonetics* 20, 703–716.

Howell, P., Au-Yeung, J., Charles, N., Davis, S., Thomas, C., Reed, P., Sackin, S. and Williams, R. (2001) Operant procedures that increase function word repetition used with children whose speech had not improved during previous treatment. In H-G. Bosshardt, J.S. Yaruss and H.F.M. Peters (eds) *Fluency Disorders: Theory, Research, Treatment and Self-Help. Proceedings of the Third World Congress of Fluency Disorders* (pp. 133–137). Nijmegen: Nijmegen University Press.

Hyman, L. (1984) *A Theory of Phonological Weight*. Dordrecht: Foris.

Iori, I. (2001) *The Guide to New Linguistics in Japanese Grammar*. Tokyo: Three A Net work.

Kindaichi, K. (1976) *Changes of Japanese Language*. Tokyo: Kodansya.

Kloth, S.A.M., Kraaimaat, F.W., Janssen, P. and Brutten, G.J. (1999) Persistence and remission of incipient stuttering among high-risk children. *Journal of Fluency Disorders* 24, 253–265.

Kolk, H. and Postoma, A. (1997) Stuttering as a covert repair phenomena. In R.F. Curlee and G.M. Siegal (eds) *Nature and Treatment of Stuttering* (pp. 182–203). Needham Height: Allyn & Bacon.

Kubozono, H. (1985) Speech errors and syllable structure. *Linguistics and Philology* 6, 220–243.

Kubozono, H. (1992) As to the independence of special morae in Japanese songs. *The Research Report 5; Japanese Speech Sound*, 63–66.

Kubozono, H. (1995) Perceptual evidence for the mora in Japanese. In B. Comri and A. Arvaniti (eds) *Phonology and Phonetic Evidence: Papers in Laboratory Phonology IV* (pp. 141–156). Cambridge: Cambridge University Press.

Kubozono, H. (1999a) Mora and syllable. In Natsuko Tsujimura (ed.) *The Handbook of Japanese Linguistics* (pp. 31–62). Malden: Blackwell Publishers Inc.

Kubozono, H. (1999b) *Japanese Phonetic Sound*. Tokyo: Iwanamisyoten.

Kubozono, H. and Honma, T. (2002) *Syllable and Mora*. Tokyo: Kenkyusha.

Martinet, A. (1960) *Elements of General Linguistics*. London: Faber & Faber.

Mikami, A. (1960) *Zoowa hanaga nagai*. Tokyo: Kurosiosyuppan.

Mihara, K. (1994) *Syntactic Structure in Japanese*. Tokyo: Shohakusya.

Moriyama, H., Ozawa, E. *et al.* (1981) The Test of Stutttering (Version I). *The Japan Journal of Logopedics and Phoniatrics* 22, 194–208.

Nagafuchi, M. (1985) *An Outline of Language Disorder*. Tokyo: Taisyukan.

Noda, H. (1989) Constituents of sentences. In Y. Miyaji, *et al.* (eds) *Japanese and Japanese Language Teaching* 1 (pp. 67–95). Tokyo: Meiji Syoten.

Prince, A. and Smolensky, P. (1993) *Optimality Theory: Constraint Interaction in Generative Grammar*, Technical Report2, Rutgers Center for Cognitive Science, Rutgers University. {To appear from MIT Press}

Reed, P., Howell, P., Davis, S. and Osborne, L. (2007) Development of an operant procedure for content word dysfluencies in persistent stuttering children: Initial experimental data. *Journal of Stuttering Therapy, Advocacy and Research* 2, 1–13.

Sander, E. (1972) Do we know when speech sounds are learned? *Journal of Speech & Hearing Disorders* 37, 55–63.

Selkirk, E.O. (1984) On the major class features and syllable theory. In M. Aronoff and R.T. Oehrle (eds) *Language Sound Structure* (pp. 107–136). Cambridge: MIT press.

Riley, G. (1994) *Stuttering Severity Instrument for Children and Adults*. Austin: Pro-Ed.

Suzuki, J. (1972) *Japanese Grammar • Morphology*. Tokyo: Mugi-syobo.

Suzuki, T. (1989) Constituent units of sentence and parts of speech. In Y. Miyaji, *et al.* (eds) *Japanese and Japanese Language Teaching* 4 (pp. 53–72). Tokyo: Meiji Syoten.

Takebayashi, S. (1996) *English Phonetics*. Tokyo: Kenkyusya.

Trask, R.L. (1996) *A Dictionary of Phonetics and Phonology*. NewYork: Routledge.

Tsuzuki, H. (2001) *Stuttering*. Tokyo: Kenpakusha.

Uchisugawa, H. (1990) *Language Disorder*. Tokyo: Hosodaigakukyoikushinkokai.

Ujihira, A. (1995) The analysis of stuttering as a phonetic transition deficit. *Proceeding of the National Convention of the Phonetic Society of Japan in 1995*, 92–97.

Ujihira, A. (1996a) Special morae in Japanese songs. *Phonological Studies-Theory and Practice*, Tokyo: Kaitakusya, 71–76.

Ujihira, A. (1996b) Songs and Special morae, the words to songs. *The Research of Japanese and Japanese Culture* 4, 14–25.

Ujihira, A. (1997) The trigger of stuttering in Japanese and in English. *Nihongakuho* 16, 49–67.

Ujihira, A. (1999) On Disfluencies of Stutterers and Nonstutterers in Japanese. *Journal of the Phonetic Society of Japan* 3, 65–75.

Ujihira, A. (2000) Linguistic and Phonetic Research on Disfluency. Unpublished thesis for a doctorate, Osaka University.

Ujihira, A. (2004) Phonetic and phonological analysis of disfluency in Japanese and English. *The Report of the Research on Prosodic Variations and Universalities* 2, 23–30.

Ujihira, A. (2006) Stutterer's voice and Natural Recovery of stuttering. *Larkhill* 28, 1–11.

Ujihira, A. (2008) From linguistic analysis to speech therapy for stuttering. *The Japanese Journal of Communication Disorders* 25, 129–136.

Ujihira, A. (2010) Disfluency and tone in Beijing dialect, A handout for The 5th Phonology Festa on Biwako sponsored by TCP and PAIK.

Ujihira, A. and Kubozono, H. (1994) A phonetic and phonological analysis of stuttering in Japanese. *Proceedings of ICSLP 94* 3, 1195–1198.

Van Riper, C. (1992) *The Nature of Stuttering*. Prospect Heights: Waveland Press Inc.

Wall, M.J., Starkweather, C.W. and Cairns, H.S. (1981) Syntactic influences on stuttering in young child stutterers. *Journal of Fluency Disorders* 6, 283–298.

Wingate, M.E. (1962) Evaluation and stuttering; part II: Environmental stress and critical appraisal of speech. *Journal of Speech and Hearing Disorders* 27, 244–257.

Wingate, M.E. (1964) A standard definition of stuttering. *Journal of Speech and Hearing Disorders* 29, 484–489.

Wingate, M.E. (1979) The loci of stuttering: Grammar or prosody? *Journal of Communication Disorders* 12, 283–290.

Wingate, M.E. (1988) *The Structure of Stuttering*. New York: Springer Verlag.

Wingate, M.E. (2002) *Foundations of Stuttering*. San Diego, CA: Academic Press.

Yairi, E. and Ambrose, N. (2005) *Early Childhood Stuttering*. Austin: Pro-Ed, Inc.

Zec, D. (1995) The role of moraic structure in distribution of segments within the syllable. In J. Durand and F. Katamba (eds) *Frontiers of Phonology* (pp. 149–179). New York: Longman.

Chapter 7

Disfluent Speech Characteristics of Monolingual Spanish-Speaking Children

JENNIFER B. WATSON, COURTNEY T. BYRD AND EDNA J. CARLO

Summary

The paucity of empirical study of stuttering in Spanish is alarming given the number of Spanish-speakers in the world, including in the United States. Spanish, which has been reported to be the second most frequently used language in the world (e.g. Lewis, 2009), was spoken at home by 23.4 million US residents in 2007, representing a 211% increase since 1980 (United States Bureau of the Census, 2010b). Despite these growing demographics, the number of reports describing stuttering in Spanish speakers is disproportionately low. In this discussion, reports of studies describing the disfluent speech and stuttering of young, monolingual Spanish-speaking children are reviewed. Specifically, the frequencies and types of disfluencies in the spontaneous speech of preschool, Spanish-speaking children who do and do not stutter are examined. Descriptions of the loci of stuttering in the speech sequence of young Spanish-speaking children along with the characteristics of stuttered word in Spanish are discussed. In addition, preliminary explorations examining the possible impact of syntactic complexity and length on stuttered speech in young Spanish speakers are presented. Reported outcomes, as might be expected, reveal both similarities and differences with reports of English-speaking children, including those who stutter. Suggestions for additional study of Spanish speakers are presented.

1 Introduction

Many investigators have noted the theoretical and clinical value of understanding communication disorders, including stuttering, in other languages (e.g. Anderson, 2007; Anderson & Centeno, 2007; Bernstein Ratner, 2004; Boey *et al.*, 2007; Carias & Ingram, 2006; Centeno *et al.*, 2007; Roberts & Shenker, 2007; Van Borsel *et al.*, 2001). Cross-linguistic comparisons of stuttering may be helpful in identifying common characteristics across languages and clarifying underlying attributes of stuttering. In addition, investigations of stuttering in languages other than English would allow us to assess the appropriateness of English-based models used to diagnose and treat stuttering in linguistically diverse populations. Although a number of studies have been completed examining disfluencies and stuttering in other languages, including German (e.g. Dworzynski & Howell, 2004; Dworzynski *et al.*, 2003, 2004; Natke *et al.*, 2006), Dutch (e.g. Boey *et al.*, 2007) and Mandarin (e.g. Lim *et al.*, 2008), reports describing stuttering in Spanish remain relatively few.

The paucity of empirical studies of stuttering in Spanish is particularly disconcerting given the number of Spanish-speakers in the world, including in the United States. Spanish has been reported to be the second most frequently used language in the world (Lewis, 2009). At estimates of 329 million, the number of Spanish speakers world-wide is considerably less than the 1213 million Chinese speakers, but exceeds the estimated 328 million English speakers. While other reports suggest that estimates of Spanish use actually may be higher than those just stated (e.g. Government of Spain, 2010), it is acknowledged that Spanish is the official language of 21 countries in North, Central and South America, the Caribbean and Europe (Lewis, 2009). In the United States, 20% of the residents in 2007 spoke a language other than English at home, with roughly 60% of these individuals speaking Spanish (United States Bureau of the Census, 2010a). The number of individuals 5 years and older in the United States who spoke Spanish at home rose to 23.4 million in 2007, a 211% increase since 1980 (United States Bureau of the Census, 2010b). This growth in numbers of Spanish speakers will undoubtedly continue in light of projections that in 2050 one in every three United States residents will be Hispanic (United States Bureau of the Census, 2008).

The prevalence of stuttering in Spanish speakers has been reported to be slightly above the 1% rate reported for English speakers, with similar reported sex ratios of male to female ranging from 2.9:1 to 5:1 (Almonte *et al.*, 1987; Ardila *et al.*, 1994; Bloodstein & Bernstein Ratner, 2008; Leavitt, 1974; Pelaz *et al.*, 1995; Pelaz *et al.*, 1997). However, the number of empirical studies of fluency and stuttering in Spanish is disproportionately low, particularly given the frequency of Spanish use. The following is a review of studies which have examined the disfluent speech, including stuttering, in monolingual Spanish-speaking children. While there are additional reports describing a variety of aspects of stuttering in monolingual Spanish-speaking adults (e.g. Carlo, 2006; Carlo & Watson, 2009; Garaigordobil & Ignacio Perez, 2007; Rodríguez & Silva, 1985), the focus of this discussion is young children, the age at which stuttering onset is most frequently observed (Yairi & Ambrose, 2005). Specifically, the frequencies and types of disfluencies in the spontaneous speech of preschool, Spanish-speaking children who do and do not stutter are reviewed. This discussion will be followed by a review of reports that describe the loci of stuttering in the speech sequence of young Spanish-speaking children. Characteristics of the stuttered word in Spanish and the possible impact of syntactic complexity and length on stuttered speech also will be explored.

It is important prior to this review to understand the context in which this information is presented and discussed. First, the outcomes of these studies of monolingual Spanish-speaking children cannot be generalized to bilingual, Spanish-English-speaking children. As noted by many, bilingualism is not simply the sum of two languages (e.g. Grosjean, 1989). Just as one must be cautious about applying guidelines developed through the study of monolingual English-speaking children to bilingual Spanish-English-speaking children, similar care must be exercised when considering monolingual Spanish-speaker reports. Young bilingual children learn multiple languages in a variety of ways, including through: (a) consistent dual-language (e.g. English and Spanish) exposure from birth, referred to as bilingualism as a first language (Centeno, 2007); and (b) exposure to a single language at home (e.g. Spanish) with the introduction of a second language (e.g. English) once preschool begins, referred to as preschool successive (Kayser, 2002) or early sequential bilinguals (Kohnert & Kan, 2007). It has been proposed that in this latter group, language development of the child's first language will be similar to that of typically developing monolingual children (Kohnert & Kan, 2007). This observation lends support for examining communication development, including fluency patterns of young monolingual Spanish-speaking children. However, when the second language is introduced to a child, language patterns are quite different from monolingual learners, simultaneous bilinguals and those who acquire a second language later in life (Kohnert & Kan, 2007). As a result, it is inappropriate to assume that the findings about monolingual children described below can be generalized to children who are bilingual. Study of both *monolingual* and *bilingual* Spanish-speaking children is needed to enhance speech and language clinicians' abilities to establish linguistically and culturally appropriate assessment and treatment strategies for these two unique populations (Anderson, 2007).

Also, it is important to remember that this review presents, at best, preliminary thoughts based on limited samples of children. Further, the children included in these investigations were from different regions and countries and spoke a variety of Spanish dialects (e.g. Caribbean, Mexican, Peninsular Spanish). In order to fully understand stuttering in monolingual Spanish-speaking children, additional investigations of greater depth and breadth are needed. Nevertheless, the following discussion provides an opportunity to raise issues for further consideration and should be regarded as an *exploration* rather than a *confirmation* of our understanding of the disfluent speech of Spanish-speaking children.

2   Frequencies and Types of Disfluencies in Spanish-Speaking Children

The type and frequency of speech disfluencies in monolingual Spanish-speaking children with normal communication skills have been examined in a series of studies (Carlo & Watson, 2003; Watson & Anderson, 2001; Watson & Carlo, 1998). In these investigations, the fluency of a total of 63 preschoolers (29 males and 34 females; 2;1 to 5;5) who were born and lived in Puerto Rico was examined. All participants, their family members and preschool teachers spoke only Spanish (Caribbean dialect) at home and at school. All children's speech and language skills were within normal limits based on speech and language screenings and parent and/or teacher report. Spontaneous speech samples were collected during play with a Puerto Rican adult examiner and were analyzed to determine the frequency of disfluent speech and presence of a variety of disfluency types. In addition, a similar, albeit much smaller, sample of monolingual Spanish-speaking children from Puerto Rico who stuttered (N = 8; 3;5 to 4;6) was examined (Watson & Byrd, 2005). These children had no communication difficulties with the exception of stuttering, which was identified by the parents and confirmed by a Puerto Rican examiner. Since no standardized Spanish severity scale is available, an adaptation of the *Stuttering Severity Instrument-3* (Riley, 1994) was completed by a bilingual (Spanish-English) speech-language pathologist to explore the speech variability across the youngsters. Picture description and conversational tasks were examined and scores included all behaviors considered to be stuttering behaviors as outlined in the instrument.[1] Severity ratings, based on the English-speaking norms and instrument modifications, ranged from very mild to moderate. The outcomes of these investigations are summarized in the following sections.

2.1   Frequency of disfluencies

The mean number of disfluent syllables per 100 syllables in the speech of all of the young Spanish-speaking children who did not stutter was 5.20 (*SD* = 3.1) (Watson & Carlo, 1998), with significantly more disfluencies observed in the 3-year-olds when compared with the 2-year-olds (Watson & Anderson, 2001) and no differences in disfluency rates between children aged 3;5 to 4;0 and 5;0 to 5;5 (Carlo & Watson, 2003) (see Table 7.1). Cross-linguistic comparisons of averages (accounting for

Table 7.1 Mean (SD) and ranges of frequencies of disfluent syllables in Spanish-speaking children who do not stutter

	2;1–2;11 *N = 18*	*3;0–4;0* *N = 28*	*5;0–5;5* *N = 17*	*All ages* *N = 63*
Watson and Anderson (2001)	3.59 (2.45) 0.70–11.04	5.52 (2.41) 1.43–10.18		
Carlo and Watson (2003)		5.36 (1.99) 1.60–8.93	6.65 (4.09) 2.98–18.89	
Watson and Carlo (1998)				5.20 (3.1) 0.70–18.89

different study metrics [i.e. syllable vs. word]) examining only studies with comparable participant inclusionary criteria (i.e. based on parent, educational, and/or examiner reports and perceptions and *not* based on specific disfluent speech criteria) suggest that the frequencies of disfluencies of Spanish-speaking children are similar to those reported for some English-speaking children (e.g. Haynes & Hood, 1977; Yairi & Lewis, 1984) and lower than averages reported for others (e.g. DeJoy & Gregory, 1985; Wexler, 1982; Wexler & Mysak, 1982). Further, the decrease in number of disfluencies reported for English speakers between 3 and 5 years (DeJoy & Gregory, 1985; Wexler, 1982; Wexler & Mysak, 1982; Yairi, 1997) was not observed in these Spanish speakers. However, similar to reports of English-speaking children (Ambrose & Yairi, 1999; Haynes & Hood, 1977; Kools & Berryman, 1971; Yairi & Lewis, 1984), no gender differences were found in the disfluency amounts for the Spanish speakers (Carlo & Watson, 2003). When examining the total disfluencies across children, marked variability was noted, with disfluencies ranging from 0.70 to 18.89 per 100 syllables.

Examination of the frequencies of disfluencies in the speech of the monolingual Spanish-speaking children who stuttered revealed similar means and variability ($M = 6.25$; $SD = 2.69$; range = 3.5 to 11.70) when compared with the children who did not stutter. It is interesting to note that total disfluency rates for many of the nonstuttering children exceeded those of the children who stuttered. This finding may reflect the mild severity of stuttering (and corresponding lower total disfluencies) in some of the children and/or the decreased role of disfluency frequency in the identification of stuttering in these children. That is, increased numbers of disfluencies alone may not be perceived as atypical (i.e. stuttering) by the community, including family members. Since the purpose of these studies was to examine the nature of the children's speech, no exclusionary speech criteria for fluency levels were used when selecting the children who do not stutter. These criteria are in contrast to those employed in studies of English-speaking children where nonstuttering children must exhibit less than three part-word repetitions, monosyllabic word repetitions and/or dysrhythmic phonations (i.e. prolongations and/or blocks) per 100 syllables (e.g. Yairi & Ambrose, 2005) or two or fewer within-word repetitions per 100 words (e.g. Zebrowski, 1991). Adoption of these English-speaking criteria would have resulted in excluding several of the Spanish-speaking children who were considered fluent (or typically disfluent) by their parents and other community members. It may be that the use of frequency of disfluencies as a diagnostic guideline for identifying stuttering in children who speak Spanish may lead to increased false positives and over-identification of stuttering in this population. Indeed, the presence of increased disfluencies in the speech of normally developing Spanish-speaking children has been reported by others. Bedore *et al.* (2006) found that 4- to 6-year-old monolingual Spanish-speaking children produced a significantly higher amount of mazes (i.e. grammatical revisions) than their monolingual English-speaking peers. They interpreted this finding as being a reflection of the complexity differences between the two languages, particularly in terms of the morphosyntactic structure. For example, Bedore and colleagues noted that in Spanish, when using an article, the speaker must choose the form with the appropriate level of definiteness, gender and number (e.g. *el, la, un, una, los, las, unos, unas*). By comparison, in English, the speaker only needs to be concerned about definiteness (e.g. *a* vs. *the*). It is possible that for monolingual speakers, aspects of the Spanish language may present more challenging linguistic contexts to maintain fluency.

2.2 Disfluency types

While frequency of all disfluency types may not differentiate Spanish-speaking children who do and do not stutter, the types and proportions of different disfluencies may prove to be more helpful. For both stuttering and nonstuttering Spanish-speaking children, a wide range of disfluency types were observed in their spontaneous speech (see Table 7.2). However, as might be expected, not all children produced all types. When looking at the children who do not stutter, monosyllabic word repetitions (e.g. *La – la niña* [The – the girl]) were the most frequently observed disfluency behavior, accounting for 21% of all disfluencies (see Table 7.2). Using a criterion of at least an average of 0.5 occurrences per 100 syllables, this repetitive behavior was the only disfluency type observed across all age levels of 2, 3 and 5 years (see Table 7.2). The mean frequencies of monosyllabic word repetitions (1.07 [*SD* = 0.72] for 3-year-olds and 1.50 [*SD* = 1.3] for 5-year-olds, Carlo & Watson, 2003; 0.86 [*SD* = 0.13] for 2-year-olds and 1.54 [*SD* = 1.22] for 3-year-olds, Watson & Anderson, 2001) were

Table 7.2 Mean (SD) and ranges of disfluency type/total disfluencies observed in Spanish-speaking children who do not stutter

	2;0–5;5[1]	2;0–2;11[2]	3;0–3;11[2,3]	5;0–5;5[3]
	N = 63	N = 18	N = 28	N = 17
Monosyllabic word repetitions	.21 (.12) .00–.45	+	+	+
Revisions	.14 (.08) .00–.37		+	+
Interjections	.12 (.09) .00–.34		+	+
Syllable repetitions	.09 (.07) .00–.27		+	
Phrase repetitions	.07 (.08) .00–.50		+	
Prolongations	.06 (.10) .00–.57			
Grammatical pauses	.06 (.04) .00–.25			+
Ungrammatical pauses	.06 (.05) .00–.21			+
Multisyllabic word repetitions	.05 (.05) .00–.19			
Incomplete phrases	.05 (.05) .00–.17			
Unfinished words	.04 (.05) .00–.22			
Sound repetitions	.03 (.04) .00–.13			
Broken words	.02 (.03) .00–.17			
Blocks	.01 (.02) .00–.09			

[1]From Watson and Carlo (1998).
[2]From Watson and Anderson (2001).
[3]From Carlo and Watson (2003).
+ Disfluency type in ≥ 0.50 syllables per 100 syllables.

greater than the means reported for some English-speaking children who are 3 years old (e.g. Yairi & Lewis, 1984) and 5 years old (e.g. DeJoy & Gregory, 1985). Cross-linguistic comparisons with studies that used the frequency of monosyllabic word repetitions as exclusionary criteria for study participation (e.g. Ambrose & Yairi, 1999; Yairi & Ambrose, 2005) were not completed. In addition to monosyllabic word repetitions, revisions (e.g. *La niña estaba – está comiendo* [The girl was – is eating]) (similar to the findings of Bedore *et al.* previously described) and interjections (e.g. *La niña (um) es bonita*. [The girl (um) is pretty]) were most frequent in the speech of 3- and 5-year-olds. Unique to the 3-year-olds was an increase in syllable repetitions (e.g. *La ni – niña* [The girl]; *La ti – tierra* [The ground]; *Ma – más* [More]) and phrase repetitions (e.g. *La niña – la niña es bonita* [The girl – the girl is pretty]), whereas the 5-year-olds exhibited more grammatical and ungrammatical pauses.

When examining the disfluencies observed in the speech of the Spanish-speaking children who do and do not stutter, the proportional relationships of the types were revealing. Specifically, the total number of sound, syllable and monosyllabic word repetitions, prolongations, blocks and broken words was divided by the total number of disfluencies. According to Yairi and Ambrose (2005), these specific types of disfluencies (i.e. stuttering-like disfluencies; SLD) are the most common behaviors noted in the speech of young English-speaking children who stutter and are the behaviors most apt to be perceived as stuttering. In their review of studies examining these relationships, Yairi and Ambrose conclude that these proportions are typically below 50% for children who do not stutter and above 65% for English-speaking children who do stutter. In the Spanish-speaking children examined in these studies, the proportions of these stuttering-like disfluencies were 42% in the children who do not stutter and nearly 70% in the children who stutter. It appears, then, that while behaviors that have been classified as stuttering-like in English-speaking children are present in both Spanish-speaking children who do and do not stutter, the proportional amount of these behaviors is much greater in the children who stutter. It should be noted, however, that unlike the reports of Ambrose and Yairi (1999), in these current studies, no exclusionary behavioral fluency criteria were used in the identification of children who do and do not stutter. Despite these differences in participant selection, the proportions were quite similar to those reported by Yairi and Ambrose.

The conceptualization of monosyllabic word repetitions as a 'stuttering-like' disfluency in English speakers has received considerable attention. Some investigators have suggested that these behaviors differ from the other SLDs and should not be included when defining stuttering (e.g. Anderson, 2007; Howell, 2007; Howell *et al.*, 2010). Others suggest that monosyllabic word repetitions are common events observed in the speech of children who stutter and are perceived as stuttering by listeners, meriting its classification as 'stuttering-like' (Yairi & Ambrose, 2005). When no exclusionary disfluency behaviors are used to identify those who do and do not stutter, monosyllabic word repetitions were a common disfluency observed in the speech of both stuttering and nonstuttering Spanish-speaking children. As is the case with English-speaking children, additional systematic study is needed as is the to examine the role of this disfluency type in predicting stuttering in Spanish-speaking children and its potential to facilitate differential diagnosis in the clinical process.

In addition to the disfluency types just described, multisyllabic word repetitions (e.g. *Pero – pero no queiro ir* [But – but I don't want to go]) were noted in the speech of a number of children who both did and did not stutter. Examination of this specific disfluency type, which has been categorized along with phrase repetitions in English (e.g. Yairi & Ambrose, 2005), may be prudent when assessing and describing the speech of Spanish-speaking children. For example, it was found that for some Spanish-speaking children who stuttered, severity levels increased when multisyllabic word repetitions were included in their weighted SLD severity measurement (a metric that considers frequency, type and extent of disfluencies; Yairi & Ambrose, 2005) (Watson & Byrd, 2007). The occurrence of multisyllabic word repetitions, which are rare in the speech of English-speaking children (Yairi & Ambrose, 2005), may be related to the increased frequency of multisyllabic words in Spanish. Spanish words often are longer than words in English, with two- and three-syllable words accounting for 90% of Spanish tokens (Vitevitch & Rodríguez, 2004) in contrast to one- and two-syllable words representing roughly 80% of English tokens (Zipf, 1935). In addition, increased stuttering has been observed on function words in both Spanish and English (to be discussed further later). Many of the single-syllable function words in English are multisyllabic in Spanish, including conjunctions (e.g. *pero* [but]; *sino* [but], *como* [as]), articles (e.g. *una* [a]; *unos* [some]), and prepositions (e.g. *para* [for]; *desde* [from]). To ensure that descriptions of stuttering are accurate and support the diagnosis and monitoring of stuttering in Spanish, inclusion of multisyllabic word repetitions in stuttering measurements may merit additional study.

2.3 Summary of Disfluency Frequencies and Types

These preliminary explorations of the disfluent behaviors of young Spanish-speaking children suggest that for the children included in these samples: (a) averages and variability of the total disfluency frequencies were similar in the children who do and do not stutter; (b) monosyllabic word repetitions is the most common disfluency type observed in nonstuttering children; and (c) proportions of disfluencies considered to be stuttering-like in English speakers (i.e. part-word repetitions, monosyllabic word repetitions and dysrhythmic phonations) were greater in the stuttering children than in the nonstuttering children. Additional study examining larger groups, including children who have a greater range of stuttering severity, is needed to clarify and/or confirm these observations. These studies should include the systematic examination of specific disfluency types, including monosyllabic and multisyllabic word repetitions, in predicting stuttering. Further, future investigations with young Hispanic children should consider using a variety of sampling techniques to obtain a full range of speech samples. For example, a recent study by Restrepo *et al.* (2005) (cited in Restrepo & Castilla, 2007) examining young Spanish-speaking Mexican-Americans revealed that utterances tended to be longer during picture descriptions tasks when compared with interview or adult-led conversations. Adult-led conversations, on other hand, yielded more utterances, while story-telling tasks resulted in samples with the most grammatical errors. These findings suggest that, in addition to being mindful of the cross-cultural appropriateness of the interaction, examiners need to recognize that different sampling techniques may alter utterance length and grammatical correctness, linguistic features related to increased disfluencies in the speech of young Spanish-speaking children who stutter.

3   Loci of Disfluencies and Stuttering in Spanish-speaking Children

The loci of stuttering has been explored extensively in monolingual English speakers with results lending support to the notion that the linguistic complexity of the language he/she is speaking contributes to the difficulty the person who stutters has in maintaining fluent speech production. Exploration of the loci of stuttering (i.e. function vs. content word, position of the stutter in the clause and word, the length of the disfluent word and the initial phoneme of the stuttered word) in monolingual Spanish-speaking children appears to lend additional support to the hypothesized link between stuttering and the grammatical structure of the language the person is speaking.

The phenomena that, early on, stuttering is more frequently observed on function words and, with development, shifts to a higher rate on content words has been documented with monolingual English-speaking children (e.g. Au-Yeung *et al.*, 1998; Bloodstein & Gantwerk, 1967; Bloodstein & Grossman, 1981; Howell *et al.*, 1999). This pattern also has been explored in the output of monolingual Spanish-speaking children. Au-Yeung *et al.* (2003) completed a cross-sectional analysis of the speech of 46 monolingual Spanish-speaking children in the following age groups: 3- to 5-years-old (N = 7); 6- to 9-years-old (N = 11); 10- to 11-years-old (N = 10); 12- to 16-years-old (N = 9); 20- to 68-years-old (N = 9). Results were similar to that of monolingual English children, with stuttering occurring more frequently on those function words that occurred prior to a content word as compared to the function words that occurred after a content word. Also similar to the English data, results revealed that children stuttered more frequently on function words when they occurred at the beginning of the sentence, but no utterance position effect was found for content words. Finally, there appeared to be the same trend with development that has been reported for monolingual English speakers with the rate of stuttering decreasing on function words and increasing on content words. Thus, these findings indicate that the 'exchange relation' between function and content words may be the same across these two languages.

However, Howell *et al.* (2004) further analyzed the conversational samples of the same participants examined in the Au-Yeung *et al.* study and found that, in contrast to monolingual English speakers, these monolingual Spanish-speaking children produced higher rates of stuttering on function words as compared to content words across all age groups, despite the trends of decreased stuttering on function words and increased stuttering on content words noted in the previous study. Closer study of the nature and linguistic complexity of function words in Spanish may provide insights about their role in fluency breakdown. It is possible that increased fluency breakdown on function words may be reflecting of the complexity of these structures rather than linguistic learning. Many function words are more complex in Spanish when compared with English. This complexity may be phonetically based (Howell & Au-Yeung, 2007) and/or the result of the unique linguistic features of Spanish. For example, articles (e.g. *el* [the], *una* [a]) and demonstratives (e.g. *ese* [that], *este* [this]) must agree with the noun in both gender and number. Clitics, or unstressed reflexive and nonreflexive pronouns that occur adjacent to verbs, may be free morphemes (e.g. <u>Me</u> peina el pelo [He/she brushes my hair]) or bound morphemes (e.g. *Peiname el pelo* [Brush my hair] (Villanueva Reyes, 2001). Placement of the clitic may alter the utterance meaning, as seen in the previous example, or not change the meaning (e.g. *Yo queiro tomar<u>lo</u>* or *Yo <u>lo</u> queiro tomar* [I want to take it]). The phonetic complexity of the function vs. the content words also may play a role in the speech of Spanish-speaking individuals but additional research is warranted. The linguistic complexity of these structures has been linked to increased disfluencies in the speech of normal developing Spanish-speaking children, with increased grammatical revisions occurring on both articles and clitics (Bedore *et al.*, 2006).

Watson (2002) analyzed the stuttering-like disfluencies of 11 monolingual Spanish-speaking children (2;11 to 6;1) who stutter to determine their position in the clause and word, the length of the disfluent word, the initial phoneme of the word, and whether it was a content or function word. Results revealed significantly greater proportions of stuttering on the following loci characteristics: (a) on or immediately prior to the initiation of a sentence or a clause; (b) on the initial phoneme of the word; (c) on one-syllable words; (d) on words beginning with consonants; and (e) on function words. These findings are similar to what has been reported for monolingual English-speaking children, with the exception of increased stuttering on one-syllable words. In addition, Watson also noted that there was a trend for an equal amount of stuttering to occur on vowel-initiated as compared to consonant-initiated words for almost half of the participants (5/11). This outcome may reflect differences in vowel inventories and is discussed further below.

Given that research examining monolingual, English speakers has shown that the loci of stuttering in some areas shifts with development, Watson *et al.* (2007) extended the Watson (2002) study to analyze the loci characteristics of the stuttering-like disfluencies produced in the spontaneous speech of younger (N = 9; mean age = 4;0) versus older monolingual Spanish-speaking children who stutter (N = 5; mean age = 7;4). Similar to Watson (2002), each instance of stuttering was analyzed in terms of its position in the clause and word, the length of the disfluent word, the initial phoneme of the word, and whether it was a content or function word. For the position in a clause, results revealed that both the younger and older children stuttered on words that occurred at both the onset and within a clause, with the older children stuttering more on words within a clause. These data conflict with what has been reported for monolingual English-speaking children, who tend to stutter more at the onset of a clause (e.g. Bernstein Ratner, 1981; Wall *et al.*, 1981.); a conflict that may reflect the differences between these two languages.

It is possible that the word-order flexibility observed in Spanish along with the pro-drop nature of the language may account for these disparate findings between English and Spanish speakers. First, in Spanish, the subject, object and verb constituents may occur in various locations within a sentence. Changes in the order of noun and verb phrases (e.g. *Mi abuelo me dio muchos dulces. Me dio muchos dulces mi abuelo. Me dio, me abuelo, muchos dulces.* [My grandpa gave me a lot of candy]), as well as alterations of the combinations of nouns and verbs with their modifiers (e.g. noun-adjective, *estrella brillante/brillante estrella* [bright star]; verb-adverb, *viene siempre/siempre viene* [s/he always comes]), are possible without changing the meaning of utterances (Anderson, 1995; Bedore, 2004). Also, Spanish is a pro-drop language where subject pronouns are frequently omitted since the sentential context and inflected verb form provide adequate information to identify the subject. Subject pronouns may be included, however, for emphasis (e.g. <u>Yo</u> *juego contigo* or *Juego contigo* [I played with you]; ¡*Qué mentiroso es él!* or ¡*Qué mentiro<u>so es</u>!* [He is such a liar!]) (Anderson, 1995; Anderson & Centeno, 2007). As a result, many utterances are verb initiated, in contrast to noun initiated as observed in English. It has been suggested that the pro-drop feature of Spanish led to increased verb-initiated utterances and more stuttering in the Spanish of a bilingual Spanish-English adult (Bernstein Ratner & Benitez, 1985). Both flexible word order and the inclusion/exclusion of a subject pronoun by the Spanish speaker may lead to initial word variability in an utterance, with these changes not altering the utterance meaning. Further, Spanish is a highly inflected language that has several inflectional affixes that designate a variety of syntactic and semantic functions in noun and verb phrases (Anderson & Centeno, 2007). This increased inflectional complexity is in marked contrast to the eight inflectional affixes found in English (e.g. plural, possessive, past) (Anderson & Centeno, 2007). It is possible that other linguistic features, such as the highly inflected verb forms common in Spanish, could 'trump' the effects of word position in an utterance and lead to increased stuttering. Additional research is needed to examine the potential role of each of these linguistic variables in fluency breakdown in Spanish. By studying the interactions of word order, noun and verb inflections, function vs. content and other linguistic variables, our understanding of stuttering in Spanish would be greatly enhanced.

Regarding the location of stuttering within the word itself, both younger and older groups stuttered the most on the initial sound of words, but the older children again displayed a slightly different pattern than the younger groups, producing more instances of stuttering in other positions within the word. The finding that stuttering occurred more frequently on the initial phoneme in words is similar to what has been reported for English-speaking children who stutter (e.g. Wingate, 1988). However, the increased occurrence of stuttering in other positions within the word has not been reported in English-speaking children. This onset versus within-word difference between monolingual English and monolingual Spanish speakers may be related to linguistic differences in word stress. For the majority of words in Spanish, stress occurs on the next to last syllable, that is, the penultimate (e.g. *necesita* [s/he needs]) (Goldstein, 2004). As a result, one- and two-syllable words would have initial syllable stress, with words of three more syllables having within word stress. Given the high number of multisyllabic words in Spanish (Vitevitch & Rodríguez, 2004), more syllables within the word are likely to be stressed. In contrast, the location of stress in English depends on factors such as the nature of the vowel (i.e. long or short) and the number of consonants that follow the vowel (Goldstein, 2004). The role of syllabic and lexical stress in stuttering has been examined in English, with findings suggesting that stuttering occurs more frequently around increased stress peaks (e.g. Wingate, 1984). If this pattern holds true for Spanish speakers, increased within-word stuttering, where the stressed syllable occurs, could be predicted. Once again, the inter-relationships among these variables (e.g. stressed syllables, linguistic function and structure of the word, word position) must be considered in future study of Spanish speakers.

Results from this study also revealed that both age groups stuttered more frequently on words of one syllable. This is not surprising given the morphosyntactic structure of the Spanish language. As Howell *et al.*

(2004) noted, in the Spanish language the mere production of function words appears to be much more frequent than in English and arguably the majority of function words are monosyllabic. Thus, it is possible that monolingual Spanish-speaking children would stutter more frequently on words comprised of one syllable as they may overlap with function words – a relationship requiring additional systematic study.

When examining the initial phoneme of the stuttered word, Watson *et al.* (2007) found no differences between the younger and older Spanish-speaking children who stuttered. Stuttering occurred to a similar degree on words that begin with both vowel and consonants. In contrast, monolingual English speakers tend to stutter more frequently on words that begin with consonants (e.g. Brown, 1938). There are large differences in the size of vowel inventories for Spanish and English with the Spanish inventory much smaller and consisting of five primary vowels (Anderson & Centeno, 2007; Bradlow, 1995). Spanish vowels are considered tense in contrast to the both tense and lax vowels in English. Whether or not specific features unique to Spanish vowels are contributing to the disruption of fluency or vowel-initiated words are associated with other disruptors (e.g. word position, highly inflected verbs) is yet to be determined.

Finally, relative to function versus content words, results revealed that for both older and younger Spanish-speaking children, stuttering occurred more frequently on function words. In contrast, the older children stuttered more frequently on content words than did the younger children. Thus, the observations of more frequent stuttering on function words in younger children are consistent with reported findings of English-speaking children who stutter (Bloodstein & Gantwerk, 1967; Bloodstein & Grossman, 1981; Howell *et al.*, 1999). These outcomes also are similar with the findings of the previously described research examining monolingual Spanish-speaking children (Au-Yeung *et al.*, 2003; Howell *et al.*, 2004). They are not, however, consistent with the later report of Howell *et al.* (2004) where a shift in stuttering from function to content words was not observed with increased age.

To date, loci research in monolingual English speakers has been limited to people who stutter perhaps with the assumption being that the locations in the utterance and words that contribute to speech breakdowns in persons who stutter are likely similar for persons who do not stutter. Preliminary research with monolingual Spanish-speaking children who do not stutter supports this assumption. Carlo *et al.* (2003) examined the within- and between-word disfluencies of 32 (ages 3;5 – 5;5) monolingual, Spanish-speaking, typically developing children who were born and raised in Puerto Rico. Disfluent words in spontaneous speech samples were described in terms of whether it was a content or function word, whether the disfluent word was initiated with a consonant or vowel, and the position of the stuttered word in the utterance (i.e.

initial, medial or final). Results were similar to what has been reported for monolingual English speakers (and for monolingual Spanish speakers as is discussed earlier in this section) in that the children produced a significantly higher number of within- and between-word disfluencies in or before function words than in content words. However, in contrast to English, but similar to the findings of Spanish-speaking children who stutter (Watson, 2002; Watson *et al.*, 2007), disfluencies occurred on words starting with both vowels and consonants, with no differences noted for either the within-word or the between-word disfluencies. In addition, both within- and between-word disfluencies occurred significantly more often on or before words within the utterance, finding consistent with the Spanish-speaking children who stutter (Watson *et al.*, 2007).

Taken together, these findings suggest that, similar to English-speaking persons who stutter, linguistic processing contributes to the difficulties monolingual Spanish-speaking persons who do and do not stutter have in maintaining fluent speech production. Further, results support the notion that these difficulties are closely tied to the structure of the language that the person is speaking. Additional study of the phonetic features, as well as lexical characteristics (e.g. word frequency, word familiarity, neighborhood density), of the stuttered Spanish word is needed.

4 Length and Complexity of Stuttered Utterances in Spanish-speaking Children

The relationship between disfluencies, utterance length and syntactic complexity has been examined extensively in English-speaking children who stutter. Outcomes of these studies are equivocal, with some studies suggesting that increased syntactic complexity, and in some cases utterance length, is related to increased fluency breakdown (e.g. Bauerly & Gottwald, 2009; Bernstein Ratner & Sih, 1987; Brundage & Bernstein Ratner, 1989; Gaines *et al.*, 1991; Kadi-Hanifi & Howell, 1992; Logan, 2003; Logan & Conture, 1995, 1997; Melnick & Conture, 2000; Sawyer *et al.*, 2008; Weiss & Zebrowski, 1992; Yaruss, 1999; Yaruss *et al.*, 1999). Further, it has been suggested that in English, syntactically more complex utterances relative to a child's overall syntactic proficiency may compromise fluency in children who both do and do not stutter (Bauerly & Gottwald, 2009; Zackheim & Conture, 2003). Whether or not the relationships among length, complexity and stuttering exist in Spanish has received limited systematic study.

Watson *et al.* (2010) examined the influence of utterance length, clause number and complexity, and grammatical correctness on the stuttering of 11 monolingual Spanish-speaking children from Puerto Rico, aged 35–70 months. Spontaneous speech samples were analyzed to identify stuttered and fluent utterances, number of syllables, clause number (including independent and subordinate clauses), clause complexity (no clause, simple clause or complex clause) and grammatical correctness (i.e. containing no syntactic or morphological errors). Results revealed that stuttered utterances in Spanish tended to be longer, more often grammatically incorrect, and contain more clauses, including more complex clauses, when compared with fluent utterances. When controlling for the inter-relatedness of syllable number and clause number, only utterance length and grammatical incorrectness were significant predictors of stuttering. In other words, the use of more complex clauses alone did not seem to lead to fluency breakdown in these Spanish-speaking children. However, grammatical incorrectness was associated with increased stuttering. The assessment of grammatical correctness is often used in the morphosyntactic analysis of Spanish-speaking children (Gutierrez-Clellen *et al.*, 2000; Restrepo, 1998) and may provide insights as to relative linguistic demands unique to each child. In this study, this metric suggested a link between these demands, which may have resulted in morphosyntactic errors, and disruption of the child's fluency. The importance of considering the relativity of syntactic measures when examining the relationship between stuttering and syntactic complexity has been raised in the study of English-speaking children (Bauerly & Gottwald, 2009; Zackheim & Conture, 2003).

Throughout the completion of this study, the importance of dialectal familiarity was evident. The diversity found across Spanish dialects (e.g. Caribbean, Andinan, Amazonic, Iberian) is extensive in comparison to English which is considered by some to be a more unified language (Butt & Benjamin, 2004). Both languages' lexicon may vary considerably from region to region. Dialectal variations in Spanish syntax and sound production, however, are pronounced. Hence, in contrast to the 'creeping homogenization' of American, British and other varieties of English (Butt & Benjamin, 2004), the dialectal differences of Spanish observed from country to country and from region to region must be considered in the completion of Spanish studies. In the Watson *et al.* (2010) study, the Caribbean dialect used by the young participants demonstrated how phonological differences may impact grammar (e.g. omission of postvocalic /s/, marking plurality only once in a noun phrase). These variations could have resulted, without examiner knowledge, in over-identification of grammatical errors.

In a follow-up to the Watson *et al.* (2010) study, the relationship between specific syntactic functions (e.g. declarative, interrogative) and forms (e.g. questions, simple, complex) and fluency while controlling for relative length was examined in the same children (Watson *et al.*, 2009). In order to address potential length effects when examining the syntactic functions and forms, the 50 percentile of syllable numbers was identified for each child and used to determine the relative utterance length for each participant. Utterances were then divided as shorter or longer and analyzed separately. The fluency of both the shorter and longer utterances containing the following grammatical functions that met inclusionary criteria was examined: declaratives, imperatives and interrogatives. In addition, the fluency of the shorter and longer utterances with the following syntactic forms was assessed: question forms (i.e. *qué, quién, dónde, cuál, cómo, cuándo, por qué, con qué, con quién, para qué, para quién, para dónde, cuánto*), utterance structure (i.e. elliptical, simple, complex); simple utterance forms (i.e. copula, intransitive, transitive), and complex coordinated utterance forms. Results revealed that shorter utterances tended to be fluent regardless of the function or form used. The longer utterances that contained declaratives, complex utterances, intransitives, transitives and coordination were stuttered as often as they were fluent – suggesting that these functions and forms may contribute to fluency breakdown. However, the shorter utterances that contained these same functions and forms were predominantly fluent. That is, for the functions and forms that appeared in both shorter and longer utterances, stuttering was present only when the utterances were longer. These preliminary findings suggest that length, rather than the syntactic functions and forms examined in the study, was the primary fluency disruptor for these Spanish-speaking children.

The results of these preliminary, exploratory studies suggest that, as observed in English, both syntactical complexity and length may play a role in disrupting fluency in young Spanish-speaking children who stutter. Further study is needed to both clarify and confirm these potential relationships. These investigations should include both descriptive and experimental paradigms and address a full array of linguistic features, including several of the variables previously mentioned.

5 Conclusion

As our efforts to better understand stuttering in Spanish speakers continue, several issues merit consideration and possible collaborations. Our ability to complete cross-linguistic comparisons of disfluent speech, and stuttering specifically, would be facilitated if we were able to find the appropriate balance between convergent and divergent study strategies. First, in order to enhance comparisons across languages it would be helpful to develop protocols that clarified sources of extraneous variance that *must* be controlled for, studied or otherwise addressed in order for us to conduct meaningful explorations of a variety of languages. Guidelines related to participants (e.g. age, time since onset, family history of stuttering, presence of additional communication disorders) and procedures (e.g. sample size, metrics employed) may improve our abilities to complete comparisons. That said, it is imperative to consider the cultural and linguistic features unique to each language, including Spanish, that may impact empirical procedures and, ultimately, investigative outcomes. Achieving this balance is challenging and requires purposeful and sustained efforts. The end result, however, should be an enriched understanding of stuttering across languages, including Spanish.

Note

1. Monosyllabic word repetitions were included in stuttering severity scores. See further discussion of the controversial nature of monosyllabic word repetitions as a stuttering behavior later in this chapter.

References

Almonte, C., Lecaros, S., Schwalm, E. and Salen, A. (1987) Aspectos clínicos y psicopatológicos de la tartamudez precoz patológica [Clinical and psychopathological aspects of early pathological stuttering]. *Revista Chilena de Pediatría* 58(6), 456–460.

Ambrose, N.G. and Yairi, E. (1999) Normative disfluency data for early childhood stuttering. *Journal of Speech, Language, and Hearing Research* 42(4), 895–909.

Anderson, R.T. (1995) Spanish morphological and syntactic development. In H. Kayser (ed.) *Bilingual Speech-language Pathology: An Hispanic Focus* (pp. 41–76). San Diego, CA: Singular.

Anderson, R.T. (2007) Cross-linguistic research: The convergence of monlingual and bilingual data. In J. G. Centeno, R.T. Anderson and L.K. Obler (eds) *Communication Disorders in Spanish Speakers: Theoretical, Research and Clinical Aspects* (pp. 82–90). Clevedon: Multilingual Matters.

Anderson, R.T. and Centeno, J.G. (2007) Contrastive analysis between Spanish and English. In J.G. Centeno, R.T. Anderson and L.K. Obler (eds) *Communication Disorders in Spanish Speakers: Theoretical, Research and Clinical Aspects* (pp. 11–33). Clevedon: Multilingual Matters.

Ardila, A., Bateman, J., Niño, C.R., Pulido, E., Rivera, D.B. and Vanegas, C.J. (1994) An epidemiologic study of stuttering. *Journal of Communication Disorders* 27(1), 37–48.

Au-Yeung, J., Gomez, I.V. and Howell, P. (2003) Exchange of disfluency with age from function words to content words in Spanish speakers who stutter. *Journal of Speech, Language, and Hearing Research* 46(3), 754–765.

Au-Yeung, J., Howell, P. and Pilgrim, L. (1998) Phonological words and stuttering on function words. *Journal of Speech, Language, and Hearing Research* 41(5), 1019–1030.

Bauerly, K.R. and Gottwald, S.R. (2009) The dynamic relationship of sentence complexity, childhood stuttering, and grammatical development. *Contemporary Issues in Communication Sciences and Disorders* 36, 14–25.

Bedore, L. (2004) Morphosyntactic development. In B. Goldstein (ed.) *Bilingual Language Development & Disorders in Spanish-English Speakers* (pp. 165–166). Baltimore, MD: Paul Brookes.

Bedore, L., Fiestas, C., Peña, E. and Nagy, V. (2006) Cross-language comparisons of maze use in Spanish and English in functionally monolingual and bilingual children. *Bilingualism, Language and Cognition* 9(3), 233–247.

Bernstein Ratner, N. (1981) Are there constraints on childhood disfluency? *Journal of Fluency Disorders* 6, 345–350.

Bernstein Ratner, N. (2004) Fluency and stuttering in bilingual children. In B.A. Goldstein (ed.) *Bilingual Language Development & Disorders in Spanish-English Speakers* (pp. 287–308). Baltimore, MD: Paul H. Brookes.

Bernstein Ratner, N. and Benitez, M. (1985) Linguistic analysis of a bilingual stutterer. *Journal of Fluency Disorders* 10, 211–219.

Bernstein Ratner, N. and Sih, C.C. (1987) Effects of gradual increases in sentence length and complexity on children's dysfluency. *Journal of Speech and Hearing Disorders* 52(3), 278–287.

Bloodstein, O. and Bernstein Ratner, N. (2008) *A Handbook on Stuttering* (6th edn). Clifton Park, NY: Delmar.

Bloodstein, O. and Gantwerk, B.F. (1967) Grammatical function in relation to stuttering in young children. *Journal of Speech and Hearing Research* 10(4), 786–789.

Bloodstein, O. and Grossman, M. (1981) Early stutterings: Some aspects of their form and distribution. *Journal of Speech and Hearing Research* 24(2), 298–302.

Boey, R.A., Wuyts, F.L., Van de Heyning, P.H., De Bodt, M.S. and Heylen, L. (2007) Characteristics of stuttering-like disfluencies in Dutch-speaking children. *Journal of Fluency Disorders* 32(4), 310–329.

Bradlow, A. (1995) A comparative acoustic study of English and Spanish vowels. *Journal of the Acoustical Society of America* 97(3), 1918–1924.

Brown, S.F. (1938) A further study of stuttering in relation to various speech sounds. *Quarterly Journal of Speech* 24, 390–397.

Brundage, S.B. and Bernstein Ratner, N. (1989) Measurement of stuttering frequency in children's speech. *Journal of Fluency Disorders* 14(5), 351–358.

Butt, J. and Benjamin, C. (2004) *A New Reference Grammar of Modern Spanish* (4th edn). New York: McGraw-Hill.

Carias, S. and Ingram, D. (2006) Language and disfluency: Four case studies on Spanish-English bilingual children. *Journal of Multilingual Communication Disorders* 4(2), 149–157.

Carlo, E.J. (2006) *Speech Rate of Non-stuttering Spanish-speaking Adults.* Paper presented at the Fifth World Congress on Fluency Disorders Dublin, Ireland.

Carlo, E.J. and Watson, J.B. (2003) Disfluencies of 3- and 5-year old Spanish-speaking children. *Journal of Fluency Disorders* 28(1), 37–53.

Carlo, E.J. and Watson, J.B. (2009) *Disfluency Behaviors of Non-stuttering Spanish-speaking Adults.* Paper presented at the American Speech-Language-Hearing Association, New Orleans, LA.

Carlo, E.J., Irene, R. and Villanueva Reyes, A. (2003) *Linguistic Characteristics of Normal Disfluencies of Puerto Rican Spanish-speaking Preschoolers.* Paper presented at the Fourth World Congress on Fluency Disorders, Montreal, Canada.

Centeno, J.G. (2007) Bilingual development and communication: Implications for clinical language studies. In J.G. Centeno, R.T. Anderson and L.K. Obler (eds) *Communication Disorders in Spanish Speakers: Theoretical, Research and Clinical Aspects* (pp. 46–56). Clevedon: Multilingual Matters.

Centeno, J.G., Anderson, R.T. and Obler, L.K. (eds) (2007) *Communication Disorders in Spanish Speakers: Theoretical, Research and clinical Aspects.* Clevedon: Multilingual Matters.

DeJoy, D.A. and Gregory, H.H. (1985) The relationship between age and frequency of disfluency in preschool children. *Journal of Fluency Disorders* 10, 107–122.

Dworzynski, K. and Howell, P. (2004) Predicting stuttering from phonetic complexity in German. *Journal of Fluency Disorders* 29(2), 149–173.

Dworzynski, K., Howell, P. and Natke, U. (2003) Predicting stuttering from linguistic factors for German speakers in two age groups. *Journal of Fluency Disorders* 28(2), 95–113.

Dworzynski, K., Howell, P., Au-Yeung, J. and Rommel, D. (2004) Stuttering on function and content words across age groups of German speakers who stutter. *Journal of Multilingual Communication Disorders* 2(2), 81–101.

Gaines, N.D., Runyan, C.M. and Meyers, S.C. (1991) A comparison of young stutterers' fluent versus stuttered utterances on measures of length and complexity. *Journal of Speech and Hearing Research* 34(1), 37–42.

Garaigordobil, M. and Ignacio Perez, J. (2007) Autoconcepto, autoestima y sintomas sicopatologicos en personas con y sin disfemia: Un analisis descriptivo y comparativo. *International Journal of Psychology and Psychological Therapy* 7(2), 285–298.

Goldstein, B. (2004) Phonological development and disorders. In B. Goldstein (ed.) *Bilingual Language Development and Disorders in Spanish-English Speakers* (pp. 259–285). Baltimore: Paul H. Brookes.

Government of Spain. (2010).*The President Claimed that the Spanish Language is 'a source of wealth and development'* Retrieved 28 April 2010. from http://www.lamoncloa.es/IDIOMAS/9/ActualidadHome/29012009_CongresoLengua.htm.

Grosjean, F. (1989) Neurolinguists, beware! The bilingual is not two monolinguals in one person. *Brain and Language* 36(1), 3–15.

Gutierrez-Clellen, V.F., Restrepo, M.A., Bedore, L., Peña, E. and Anderson, R.T. (2000) Language sample analysis in Spanish-speaking children: Methodological considerations. *Language, Speech, and Hearing Services in the Schools* 31(1), 88–98.

Haynes, W.O. and Hood, S.B. (1977) Language and disfluency variables in normal speaking children from discrete chronological age groups. *Journal of Fluency Disorders* 2, 57–74.

Howell, P. (2007) Signs of developmental stuttering up to age eight and 12 plus. *Clinical Psychology Review* 27, 287–306.

Howell, P. and Au-Yeung, J. (2007) Phonetic complexity and stuttering in Spanish. *Clinical Linguistics and Phonetics* 21(2), 111–127.

Howell, P., Au-Yeung, J. and Sackin, S. (1999) Exchange of stuttering from function words to content words with age. *Journal of Speech, Language, and Hearing Research* 42(2), 345–354.

Howell, P., Bailey, E. and Kothari, N. (2010) Changes in the pattern of stuttering over development for children who recover or persist. *Clinical Linguistics and Phonetics* 24(7), 556–575.

Howell, P., Ruffle, L., Fernández-Zuniga, A., Gutiérrez, R., Fernandez, A., O'Brien, M., *et al.* (2004) Comparison of exchange patterns of stuttering in Spanish and English monolingual speakers and a bilingual Spanish-English speaker. In A. Packman, A. Meltzer and H.F. Peters (eds) *Theory, Research and Therapy in Fluency Disorders* (pp. 415–422). Nijmegen, The Netherlands: Nijmegen University Press.

Kadi-Hanifi, K. and Howell, P. (1992) Syntactic analysis of the spontaneous speech of normally fluent and stuttering children. *Journal of Fluency Disorders* 17(3), 151–170.

Kayser, H.R. (2002) Bilingual language development and language disorders. In D.E. Battle (ed.) *Communication Disorders in Multicultural Populations* (pp. 205–232). Boston, MA: Butterworth-Heinemann.

Kohnert, K. and Kan, P.F. (2007) Lexical skills in young children learning a second language: Methods, results, and clinical applications. In J.G. Centeno, R.T. Anderson and L.K. Obler (eds.) *Communication Disorders in Spanish Speakers: Theoretical, Research and Clinical Aspects* (pp. 156–168). Clevedon: Multilingual Matters.

Kools, J.A. and Berryman, J.D. (1971) Differences in disfluecny behavior between male and female nonstuttering children. *Journal of Speech and Hearing Research* 14, 125–130.

Leavitt, R.R. (1974) *The Puerto Ricans: Cultural Change and Language Deviance.* Tucson, AZ: University of Arizona.

Lewis, M.P. (ed.) (2009) *Ethnologue: Languages of The World* (16th edn). Dallas, TX: SIL International, Online version: http://www.ethnologue.com/.

Lim, V.P.C., Lincoln, M., Chan, Y.H. and Onslow, M. (2008) Stuttering in English-Mandarin bilingual Speakers: The influence of language dominance on stuttering severity. *Journal of Speech, Language, and Hearing Research* 51(6), 1522–1537.

Logan, K.J. (2003) Language and fluency characteristics of preschoolers' mutliple-utterance conversational turn. *Journal of Speech, Language, and Hearing Research* 46(1), 178–188.

Logan, K.J. and Conture, E.G. (1995) Length, grammatical complexity, and rate differences in stuttered and fluent conversational utterances of children who stutter. *Journal of Fluency Disorders* 20(1), 35–61.

Logan, K.J. and Conture, E.G. (1997) Selected temporal, grammatical, and phonological characteristics of conversational utterances produced by children who stutter. *Journal of Speech, Language, and Hearing Research* 40(1), 107–120.

Melnick, K.S. and Conture, E.G. (2000) Relationship of length and grammatical complexity to the systematic and nonsystematic speech errors and stuttering of children who stutter. *Journal of Fluency Disorders* 25(1), 21–45.

Natke, U., Sandrieser, P., Pietrowsky, R. and Kalveram, K.T. (2006) Disfluency data of German preschool children who stutter and comparison children. *Journal of Fluency Disorders* 31(3), 165–176.

Pelaz, M., Gil Verona, J.A., Pastor, J.F., Bodega, B., and Aguilar, S. (1997) Alteraciones del lenguaje en una muestra de pacientes en edad infantil (<6 años) [Language alterations in a sample of young children (<6 years)]. *Boletín de Pediatría,* 37, 226–229.

Pelaz, M., Gil Verona, J.A., Pastor, J.F., and Coca, J.M. (1995) Tartamudez en la infancia: Estudio de 30 niños [Stammering in childhood: Study of 30 children]. *Boletín de Pediatría,* 36, 307–312.

Restrepo, M.A. (1998) Identifiers of predominantly Spanish-speaking children with language impairment. *Journal of Speech, Language, and Hearing Research* 41(6), 1398–1411.

Restrepo, M.A. and Castilla, A.P. (2007) Language elicitation and analysis as a research and clinical tool for Latino children. In J.G. Centeno, R.T. Anderson and L.K. Obler (eds) *Communication Disorders in Spanish Speakers: Theoretical, Research and Clinical Aspects* (pp. 127–141). Clevedon: Multilingual Matters.

Restrepo, M.A., Youngs, C. and Castilla, A.P. (2005) Evaluation of three language elicitation techniques with Spanish-speaking children. Manuscript in preparation.

Riley, G.D. (1994) *Stuttering Severity Instrument for Children and Adults* (3rd edn). Austin, TX: Pro-Ed.

Roberts, P. and Shenker, R. (2007) Assessment and treatment of stuttering in bilingual speakers. In E.C.R. Curlee (ed.) *Stuttering and Related Disorders of Fluency* (3rd edn) (pp. 183–210). New York: Thieme.

Rodríguez, P.R. and Silva, C. (1985) Perfil de la tartamudez y del tartamudo [Stuttering and stutterer's profile]. *Revista Latinoamericana de Psicología* 17(1), 87–112.

Sawyer, J., Chon, H. and Ambrose, N.G. (2008) Influences of rate, length, and complexity on speech disfluency in a single-speech sample in preschool children who stutter. *Journal of Fluency Disorders* 33(3), 220–240.

United States Bureau of the Census (2008) *An Older and More Diverse Nation by Midcentury.* http://www.census.gov/Press-Release/www/releases/archives/population/012496.html. Retrieved 18 May 2009.

United States Bureau of the Census (2010a) *Language use in the United States: 2007.* http://www.census.gov/prod/2010pubs/acs-12.pdf. Retrieved 29 April 2010.

United States Bureau of the Census (2010b) *New Census Bureau Report Analyzes Nation's Linguistic Diversity.* http://www.census.gov/Press-Release/www/releases/archives/american_community_survey_acs/014737.html. Retrieved April 28, 2010.

Van Borsel, J., Maes, E. and Foulon, S. (2001) Stuttering and bilingualism: A review. *Journal of Fluency Disorders* 26, 179–205.

Villanueva Reyes, A. (2001)*Categorías Semántico-Sintácticas de los Verbos Utilizados por Niños Puertorriqueños de Tres a Cinco Años de Edad del Area Metropolitana de San Juan de Puerto Rico: Aplicaciones Educativas [Semantic-syntactic categories of verbs used by three and five year-old Puerto Rican children from the San Juan, Puerto Rico Metropolitan Area: Educational applications.].* Unpublished doctoral dissertation, University of Puerto Rico.

Vitevitch, M.S. and Rodríguez, E. (2004) Neighborhood density effects in spoken word recognition in Spanish. *Journal of Multilingual Communication Disorders* 3(1), 64–73.

Wall, M.J., Starkweather, C.W. and Cairns, H.S. (1981) Syntactic influences on stuttering in young child stutterers. *Journal of Fluency Disorders* 6, 283–298.

Watson, J.B. (2002) *Loci of Disfluencies in Spanish-speaking Children Who Stutter.* Paper presented at the American Speech-Language-Hearing Association, Atlanta, GA.

Watson, J.B. and Anderson, R. (2001) Disfluencies of 2- and 3-year-old Spanish-speaking children from Puerto Rico. *Contemporary Issues in Communication Sciences and Disorders* 28, 140–150.

Watson, J.B. and Byrd, C.T. (2005) *Disfluencies of Monolingual Spanish-speaking Children Who Stutter.* Paper presented at the American Speech-Language-Hearing Association, San Diego, CA.

Watson, J.B. and Byrd, C. (2007) Influence of multisyllabic word repetitions on severity measures of monolingual Spanish-speaking children who stutter. In J. Au-Yeung and M. M. Leahy (eds) *Research, Treatment, and Self-Help in Fluency Disorders* (pp. 68–75). New Horizons: International Fluency Association.

Watson, J.B. and Carlo, E.J. (1998) *Disfluent Behaviors of Spanish-speaking Children Aged Two through Five Years.* Paper presented at the American Speech-Language-Hearing Association, San Antonio, TX.

Watson, J.B., Byrd, C. and Carlo, E.J. (2007) *Characteristics of Stuttered Words in Older and Younger Spanish-speaking Children.* Paper presented at the American Speech-Language-Hearing Association, Boston, MA.

Watson, J.B., Byrd, C.T. and Carlo, E.J. (2010) Effects of length, complexity, and grammatical correctness on stuttering in Spanish-speaking preschool children. Unpublished manuscript under review.

Watson, J.B., Carlo, E.J., Villanueva-Reyes, A. and Byrd, C. (2009) *Influence of Syntactic Complexity on the Stuttering of Spanish-speaking Children.* Paper presented at the IFA 2009 World Congress, Rio de Janeiro, Brazil.

Weiss, A.L. and Zebrowski, P.M. (1992) Disfluencies in the conversations of young children who stutter: Some answers about questions. *Journal of Speech and Hearing Research* 35(6), 1230–1238.

Wexler, K.B. (1982) Developmental disfluency behavior in 2-, 4-, 6-year old boys in neutral and stress situations. *Journal of Speech and Hearing Research* 25, 229–234.

Wexler, K.B. and Mysak, E.D. (1982) Disfluency characteristics of 2-, 4-, and 6-year old males. *Journal of Fluency Disorders* 7, 37–46.

Wingate, M.E. (1984) Stutter events and linguistic stress. *Journal of Fluency Disorders* 9, 295–300.

Wingate, M.E. (1988) *The structure of stuttering.* New York: Springer-Verlag.

Yairi, E. (1997) Disfluency characteristics of childhood stuttering. In R. Curlee and G. Siegel (eds) *Nature and Treatment of Stuttering: New Directions* (2nd edn) (pp. 181–188). Boston, MA: Allyn & Bacon.

Yairi, E. and Ambrose, N.G. (2005) *Early Childhood Stuttering: For Clinicians, by Clinicians.* Austin, TX: Pro-Ed.

Yairi, E. and Lewis, B. (1984) Disfluencies in the onset of stuttering. *Journal of Speech and Hearing Research* 27, 154–159.

Yaruss, J.S. (1999) Utterance length, syntactic complexity, and childhood stuttering. *Journal of Speech, Language, and Hearing Research* 42(2), 329–344.

Yaruss, J.S., Newman, R.M. and Flora, T. (1999) Language and disfluency in non-stuttering children's conversational speech. *Journal of Fluency Disorders* 24(3), 185–207.

Zackheim, C.T. and Conture, E.G. (2003) Childhood stuttering and speech disfluencies in relation to children's mean length of utterance: A preliminary study. *Journal of Fluency Disorders* 28(2), 115–142.

Zebrowski, P. (1991) Duration of the speech disfluencies of beginning stutterers. *Journal of Speech and Hearing Research* 34, 483–491.

Zipf, G.K. (1935) *The Psycho-biology of Language: An Introduction to Dynamic Philology.* New York: Houghton.

Chapter 8

Characteristics of Developmental Stuttering in Iran

HAMID KARIMI AND REZA NILIPOUR

Summary

In this chapter, some aspects of developmental stuttering among monolingual and bilingual Persian-speaking populations living in Iran are reviewed. Prevalence, whether stuttering is associated with linguistic factors, and its symptoms in Persian language are discussed. Bilingualism prevails in some regions of Iran. Thus, data from both monolingual and bilingual populations with Persian as the national language are considered.

1 Introduction

1.1 Languages spoken in Iran

The population of Iran is around 70 million. It is a polyglot country. The official and educational language of the country is Persian, which is a member of the Indo-European group of languages. In addition to Persian, several other languages are spoken within the borders of Iran. Azari, as a member of the agglutinated family of languages in which affixes are added to the base of a word, is the second most frequently spoken language with roughly 10 million speakers. Kurdish, Arabic, Turkeman, Baluchi, Armenian and Asurian are other local languages spoken by ethnic groups from different parts of Iran. There are also two main dialects of Persian (Gilaki & Mazandarni) spoken by people who live along the Caspian coast (Katzner, 2002). A short description of major characteristics of Persian is given in order to permit cross-linguistic comparison and to identify relevant language-specific factors that affect stuttering.

1.2 Persian typology and major characteristics

Persian belongs to the Iranian branch of the Indo-European group of languages. Typologically, it is a Subject-Object-Verb (SOV) language and it has a rich morphology. It is an analytic SOV language, and most affixes are prepositional except for verb endings. The only postposition in Persian is the direct object marker /ra/. The word order is rather loose and all major constituents of the sentence (S, O and V) may be reshuffled for pragmatic purposes. The initial subject may be optionally omitted since the verb is inflected for person, number and tense. Direct object and indirect object are marked with post-posed /*ra*/ and preposed /*be*/ markers respectively. Adjectives follow the head noun and auxiliaries follow the main verb, but modals precede the main verb. Arabic, a Semitic and typologically unrelated language, is the source of many loan words and the alphabet. Arabic nouns typically retain their Arabic plural forms, which makes them irregular plural forms in Persian (Nilipour, 2000; Nilipour & Raghibdoust, 2001).

There is no gender and case in Persian, and hence no gender and case agreements. There is no number agreement for adjectives in prototypical noun phrase constructions (N+ADJ), although there is subject agreement with respect to person and number.

1.3 Syntax

The syntax of Persian is characterized by certain grammatical free morphemes, notably /*râ*/ as postposed direct (Example 2), and /*be*/ as preposed indirect object markers (Example 1). The postposition /*râ*/ is used primarily as the direct object marker (OBJ), as well as marking the specificity of the object (Example 3).

1-/*pul be man be-deh*/
money to me IMP*-give-you
'Give me some money'.
*imperative morpheme

2-/*pul râ be man be-deh*/
money OBJ to me IMP-give-you
'Give me the money'.

3- /reza ketab-ra be - ali dad/
Reza book-OBJ to-Ali gave
'Reza gave the book to Ali'

1.4 Word formation

1.4.1 Nouns

Persian has two major types of word forms: compounding and derivation. In compounding, two or more stems are joined to make a single lexical item (Examples 4 and 5). In derivation, a new lexical item is made using a stem plus bound derivational elements such as suffixes and prefixes (Example 6). A combination of the two forms is also possible, that is, compounding of stems plus a derivational suffix or prefix (Example 7). These patterns of word formation are applicable to all major lexical categories.

4- /âb mive/
water fruit
'fruit juice'

5- /ruz name/
day letter
'newspaper'

6- /xaste-gi/
tired-ness
'tiredness'

7. /dandân pezeški/
tooth physician-*i*
'dentistry'

Derivational morphemes are a widespread source of new lexical items formed by attachment of a morpheme to the present (Examples 8 and 9) and past stems (Example 10) of verbs:

8- /xor-âk/ = present stem + /-âk/   'food'
9- / xor-eš/ = present stem + /-eš/   'dish'
10- / xord-an-i/ = past stem + Infin marker + /-i/   'eatable'

Definite nouns are generally unmarked in Persian, while indefinite nouns are marked with the suffix /-i/ (Examples 11, 12 and 13).

Nouns are pluralized by adding the plural morpheme (/-hâ/ as unmarked morpheme for all nouns, /-ân/ as marked morpheme for some animate nouns) to the singular base form (Examples 11, 12 and 13):

11- / zan-i/   /zan-hâ/   /zan-ân/
a woman   the women   the women

12- / medâd-i/   /medâd-ha/
a pencil   the pencils

13 -/deraxt/   /deraxt-hâ/   /deraxt-ân/
tree   trees   trees

A noun denoting a specific direct object may also be followed by the specific direct object marker /râ/ (Example 14).

14- /deraxt-hâ râ bor-id-and/
tree-s 'the' cut-ed-they
'They cut the trees'.

1.4.2 Verbs

Persian verbs are either simple or compound. The verbal element is derived from a base form called the infinitive, consisting of the past stem plus an infinitive suffix marker. Each verb has a present stem and a past stem. The present stem of regular verbs is derived from the past stem by deleting the past marker /-an/ (Example 15):

Infinitive	PRESENT STEM	PAST STEM
Regular Verb		
15-/xor-d-an/	/xor/	/xor-d/
eat-PAST- Infin marker		ate
'to eat'		
Irregular Verb		
16- /âmad-an/	/â/	/âmad/
came-Infin marker		came
17- /did-an/	/bin/	/did/
saw-Infin marker		saw

1.4.2.1   Compound verb

A compound verb consists of a noun or adjective followed by a light verb (Examples 18 and 19). Compound verb construction is very widespread and frequent in Persian and may be a target for stuttering.

18- /zamin xordan/
ground to beat
'to fall down'

19-/bime kardan/
insurance to do
'to insure'

A conjugated verb is morphologically as well as semantically a complex lexical unit and a possible candidate for stuttering. The past stem yields the forms of the past tense (both simple and progressive) and the present stem yields the present, future and imperative. Every conjugated verb carries person and number by adding the personal endings to the present or past stem.

20- **Present**		**Past**	
/ mi-xân-am/	I am reading	/xând-am/	I read
PROG-read-I	I read		read-PAST-I
/ mi-xân-i/	you are reading	/xând-i/	you read
/ mi-xân-ad/	he/she/it reads	/xând-0/	he/she/it read
/mi-xân-im/	we read	/xând-im/	we read
/mi-xân-id/	you read	/xând-id/	you read
/mi-xân-and/	they read	/xând-and/	they read

Verb construction is made more complex by adding two major verb prefixes to the base form of the verb to mark aspect: Prefix /mi /indicates the duration and progression of the action (Examples 20 and 21), and /be-/ is affixed to the verb in subjunctive and imperative forms (Example 22).

21- /*sib mi-xor-i*/
apple PROG-eat-you
'Are you eating the apple? / Do you eat the apple?'

22- /*sib râ be-xor*/
apple-the IMP-eat
'Eat the apple.'

1.4.3 Pronouns

The personal pronouns have six independent forms for first-, second- and third-person singular and plural, without any sex distinction. Aside from the independent personal pronouns, there are personal inflectional endings attached to the verb that denote the person and number of the subject. Pronominal enclitics (-*m*, -*t*, -*š*, -*mân*, -*tân*, -*šân*) are attached to the preceding word, functioning as attributes (Examples 23 and 24).

23- /*man sib-aš râ xord-am*/
I apple-his OBJ ate-I
'I ate his apple.'

24- /*u sib-am râ xord*/
he apple-my OBJ ate
'He ate my apple.'

There are also demonstrative pronouns (/*in*/ 'this' and /*ân*/ 'that') as well as reflexive pronouns functioning as independent attributes (Examples 25 and 26):

25- /*in ketâb râ be-xân*/
this book-the read
'Read this book.'

26-/*ketâb-e xod-am râ be u dâd-am*/
book-of myself OBJ to he gave-I
I gave him my own book.

1.4.4 Prepositions

Persian has eight basic prepositions. They can be divided into two categories according to meaning: (1) those used to express spatial relationships (Example 27), and (2) those used to express other syntactic relationships (Example 28):

27- /*az*/ 'from', /*be*/ 'to', /*dar*/ 'in', /*bâ*/ 'with', /*tâ*/ 'as far as' or 'until'

28- /*bâ*/ 'with', /*barâye*/ 'for', /*joz*/ 'except', /*bi*/ 'without'

The *ezafe* morpheme /-*e*/ as syntactic marker is used to link a head noun to its complements or modifiers; it can often be translated as 'of', e.g. /*eyd-e now ruz*/ 'holiday of new day' (New Year's Day). The *ezafe* construction is the universal type of attributive construction in Persian; i.e. it allows various lexical items to be combined as noun attributes, such as nouns, adjectives, pronouns (personal, reflexive, interrogative and demonstrative) and ordinal numbers. If a lexical item has several modifiers, they are placed one after another following the modified word, each pair connected with an *ezafe* marker /*-e*/ (Example 29).

29- /*kif-e siyâh-e bozorg-e pedar-e pir-e to*/
bag-of black-of big-of father-of old-of you
'Your old father's large black bag.'

Word order in an *ezafe*(/-e/) construction chain is semantically highly significant, but does not have a grapheme representation in writing and has to be deciphered by the reader in context. The modified item is always directly followed by the qualitative modifier, then by the modifier of possession linked by ezafe /-e/ morpheme (Example 30):

30- /*divâr-e siyâh-e otâq*/
wall-of black-of room
'The black wall of the room.'

Since there is no grapheme representation for Ezafe construction it may be considered as a language-specific candidate for stuttering when used in written tasks (Examples 29 and 30).

In the next sections, we will review documented studies on prevalence and linguistic factors affecting stuttering.

2   Prevalence of Stuttering

In general, research concerning the prevalence, onset and natural history of stuttering is limited and difficult to interpret (Packman & Onslow, 1998). One reason is that the data regarding the prevalence of stuttering are derived from a limited number of studies. The overall prevalence of stuttering is usually estimated at slightly under 1% in the United States and somewhat above 1% in European populations (Craig *et al.*, 2002). Higher prevalence rates were reported for younger children and lower prevalence rates were claimed for adolescents and adults. It is also generally accepted that stuttering prevalence is higher in males than females with a ratio of about 3 to 1.

Although there is general consensus on prevalence of about 1% in different US and European studies, its prevalence in other countries and cultures are not well documented, especially in countries which have markedly different forms of language to English and where there are multilingual populations and various ethnic groups who speak different pairs of languages.

Iran is an example of a multilingual country. Although there are several studies on prevalence on large groups of monolingual and bilingual stuttering population in Iran, some of the documented studies are limited in scope and methodology. Zeynali (2001) studied the prevalence of stuttering among 6262 monolingual school–age boys in the province of Qom in Iran. Zeynali's initial data were derived from a questionnaire sent to all school teachers who were asked to identify those children who stuttered. Then a speech and language pathologist (SLP) was assigned to test these children. A 100-word passage was read by each child and was recorded and transcribed to check the number of disfluency events and to confirm the teacher's initial diagnosis and avoid any possible misinterpretation of stuttering with other forms of disfluency. Based on his report the highest prevalence rate was for second graders around the age of 8 (1.3%) and the lowest rate was among fourth graders, around the age of 10 (0.68%). This study on the prevalence of stuttering was based on monolingual elementary school boys in Qom and did not include girls. Another shortcoming was that there was no way of checking whether school teachers had missed any children who stuttered.

A recent prevalence study on 11,425 bilingual Kurdish–Persian students living in the city of Javanroud in the west of Iran was conducted by Mohammadi *et al.* (2008b). This study covered all students in elementary, guidance and high schools in Javanrood. The students were initially identified by their teachers as children who stutter. The teachers were first informed about different types of speech disorders to minimize any misinterpretation of stuttering. Subsequent to teacher identification, an SLP screened the candidate children based on stuttering measures indicated in DSM-IV. The highest rate (2.06%) was found among the primary school students while the prevalence rates of stuttering among guidance school and high school students were lower and estimated at 0.87% and 0.5%, respectively. With respect to gender, more males were reported to stutter (1.35%) than females (0.88%). The male to female ratio was reported as 1.3:1 among the primary school students, 3.25:1 in guidance school and 1.76:1 among high school students. The primary school starts at age 6, the guidance school starts at age 12 and the high school education starts at age 15 and continues for 4 years.

Based on this study the prevalence of stuttering among Kurdish-Persian children was higher than that reported for monolinguals (1%), but it is still lower than reported in some studies on bilingual populations (Van Borsel *et al.*, 2001). In Mohammadi *et al*'s. report the discrepancy was attributed to Persian and Kurdish linguistic and cultural differences leading to higher rates compared to monolinguals (Mohammadi *et al.*, 2008a). To explain the lower rate in these bilinguals relative to other bilingual studies, the authors argued that stuttering prevalence among the bilingual population with two similar languages could have decreased the chance of stuttering as compared to populations who spoke two structurally distant languages. This conclusion is in agreement with Van Borsel *et al.* (2001), who assumed that the prevalence of stuttering among bilinguals may be influenced by the degree of similarity between the languages involved.

Molahosseini (2000) also studied the prevalence of stuttering among 6000 Kurdish-Persian bilingual students and reported an overall rate of 1.48% among school-aged children. In his study 2.16% of boys stuttered as compared to 0.8% of girls giving a gender ratio of about 2.7 to 1. The problem with this study is that the diagnosis was based on untrained teachers' and/or family reports and there was no SLP confirmation on the initial diagnosis. Einarsdottir and Ingham (2008) have indicated that preschool teachers displayed, on average, above 80% accuracy in identifying stuttering events, even prior to training. However, the term 'stuttering' is sometimes used by non-specialists for various types of speech and language disorders in Iran. Consequently Einarsdottir and Ingham (2008) observations may not apply in this country.

A more methodologically sound study was conducted by Karimi (2006). He investigated the prevalence of stuttering among monolingual and bilingual Arab-Persian-speaking school-aged children living in Ahwaz in the south of Iran. Reading and spontaneous speech tasks were used to assess their stuttering. Initially, trained SLP students went to different schools and recorded speech samples of children who were suspected to stutter. Subsequently each child's stuttering was checked by a speech-language pathologist based on his/her recorded speech sample. A child was confirmed as a stutterer if s/he exhibited three or more within-word incidences of disfluency (i.e., sound prolongations, sound/syllable repetitions, monosyllabic whole-word repetitions or broken words) per 100 words in either his/her spontaneous speech or in the reading task. Karimi reported an overall prevalence of 1.02%. In his study 55% of 7700 children were monolingual and the rest were bilingual. The bilingual children were identified as those who were born in Arab families and spoke mostly Arabic at home but received formal education in Persian at school. The results indicated that 1.08% of monolingual and 1.15% of bilingual students were stutterers. The difference was not statistically significant. Also, the ratio of boys who stuttered as compared to girls was about 3 to 1 (1.32% boys stuttered versus 0.47% girls). The highest prevalence rate was for the first-grade students at about 1.57% (the rates for the second-, third-, fourth- and fifth-graders were 1.07%, 1.02%, 0.66% and 0.88% respectively). These findings are in general agreement with Zeynali who reported the highest stuttering rate among the second graders and the lowest among the fourth graders (It is worth mentioning that Zeynali's participants were boys).

The limitation of Karimi's study was that all of the trained SLP students who participated in this research except one were monolingual Persian speakers. This shortcoming made it difficult for them to assess stuttering in both languages of the bilingual students. According to Van Borsel *et al.*'s (2001) review on bilingualism and stuttering, bilinguals usually stutter in both languages and bilinguals who stutter in only one language are rare. Cases where bilingual children stuttered in the language other than Persian would be missed (though the impact of this would be minor if Van Borsel *et al.* are right that stuttering usually affects both languages).

The general conclusion drawn from the present studies on the prevalence of stuttering in Iran is that the rate is around the same value as reported in other countries. Similarly, the rate of stuttering among male and female children and amongst young children and older children and adults were within the same range as in other reports. Furthermore, in Karimi's study the difference in prevalence of stuttering between monolinguals and bilingual Persian-Arab speaking children was not significant. However, differences have been reported when Persian is paired with other languages in bilinguals. For example, Mohammadi's study revealed that stuttering is more prevalent among Kurdish-Persian bilingual primary school children. Zeynali reported a prevalence of less than 1.3% in monolingual primary school boys whereas Molahosseini and Mohammadi reported 2.16% and 2.06% for Kurdish-Persian bilingual stuttering children, respectively. Consequently, based on these reports Kurdish-Persian bilingual children stuttered more than monolinguals. More clinical data are needed to support the results of prevalence with other bilingual groups such as Azari, Turkemans, Baluchi, Armenian and Asurians living in Iran. Also, if the reports are confirmed, specific ways in which the languages differ which may impact on stuttering (e.g. differences in syntax and phonology) need to be examined which may pinpoint specific aspects of language structure that trigger stuttering.

The difference in prevalence rates between monolinguals and bilinguals and between the bilinguals in Iran and other countries is marginal at best. This is somewhat surprising from the point of view that language factors lead to stuttering, given that Persian is very different to languages like English that have been more extensively studied. Many of the initial identification of cases of stuttering and assessment of bilinguals were based on non-expert-report and there were other procedural differences between all these studies. The cautious conclusion is that there is little unequivocal evidence for higher incidence and prevalence of stuttering in bilinguals than monolinguals in the Iranian work. Again this would seem to suggest that language factors may have little impact on stuttering.

3 Linguistic Factors that Affect Stuttering

Although the summary of the previous section suggested that the impact of language factors on stuttering may not be dramatic, some researchers working on English have reported that linguistic factors can lead to stuttering and to variations in severity (Bernstein Ratner, 1997; Seery *et al.*, 2007). In this section, the studies that document whether such effects of linguistic factors occur in Persian-speaking children who stutter are reviewed.

3.1 Syntactic factors

Some studies have reported a higher incidence of stuttering on longer than shorter utterances (e.g. Logan & Conture, 1995; Yaruss, 1999) and on complex than simple utterances (e. g. Logan & LaSalle, 1999). Other studies have found that both longer and more complex utterances play a comparable role to shorter and simpler utterances with respect to the rate of stuttering (Gaines *et al.*, 1991; Zackheim & Conture, 2003). These reports are exclusively on English. As seen earlier in this chapter, heavy reliance on morphology, complexity of verb morphology, verb compounding, and *ezafe* marker and loose syntax as a result of postpositional marker /*ra*/ in Persian give it a very different syntax to English. Thus, the rest of this section is a short review of the documented reports on the effects of some aspects of Persian syntax on stuttering.

Haresabadi *et al.* (2010) investigated the effect of length of utterance on disfluency in 4–6-year-old stuttering and non-stuttering Persian-speaking children. The subjects were asked to repeat 10 sets of simple and complex sentences. Morphemes were added one by one to sentences in each set in order to assess the impact of utterance length on disfluency. SSI-3 was used as a measure to diagnose stuttering children. They reported that speech disfluency increased with utterance length in both stuttering and non-stuttering children ($p = 0.001$). Increasing the length of utterance of both simple and complex sentences resulted in more stuttering. However, a limitation is that the researchers did not specify what events were considered to be stutters.

Kalashi (2003) also studied the effects of length of utterance as well as syntactic complexity in 6–12-year-old children who do and do not stutter. In her study repetition of sound, part or whole-word pause, prolongation and blocks were specified as stuttering events. All children were required to repeat 40 sentences with eight levels of syntactic complexity. The complexity of the sentence was based on the length and complexity of the major components as well as the embedded clauses in each sentence. The results of her study revealed that the increase in length of utterance led to more disfluency for both groups of speakers. Similarly, syntactic complexity was reported to result in more disfluency in this age group. Thus, the results were almost the same as those of Haresabadi *et al.* (2010) who worked with the younger, 4- to 6-year-old, children.

Vahab (2004) studied the impact of syntactic complexity in 18 stuttering and 38 non-stuttering adults aged 20–25. She used two different tasks.

One task included 30 sentences, with three levels of syntactic complexity based on 10 basic sentences. The number of syllables was kept the same in each sentence to eliminate any length effect. Syntactic complexity was defined as the number of nodes involved according to the generative grammar method of sentence analysis (Chomsky, 1965). The second task included 75 sentences based on five basic sentences of different lengths and 15 levels of syntactic complexity. In this task, syntactic complexity was fixed but the number of syllables varied. Vahab reported no effect of syntactic complexity in speakers who stutter or controls, but did find an effect of utterance length on disfluency for both groups of speakers albeit to a lesser degree in the control group. In her study, results were given as percentage of syllables stuttered, but the events included were not specified. The results were different from what Haresabadi *et al.* (2010) and Kalashi (2003) reported for younger age groups. All these reports concluded that there was an effect of utterance length at different rates for speakers who stutter and controls. Thus, the impact of utterance length on stuttering does not change with age in Persian although the effect of syntax on stuttering may do.

None of the above except for Kalashi (2003) indicated what events were counted as stuttering, which makes it difficult to compare their results. If it is assumed that similar events were counted, the Persian studies referred to indicate syntactic complexity and length of utterance affect young speakers who stuttered and speakers who did not stutter. From the Vahab (2004) study, it appears that there is more effect of utterance length for speakers who stutter as they get older (but no differential effect of syntactic complexity in these speakers).

Other studies have focused on particular syntactic constructions. For example, Shafiei (1998) studied subject agreement in 4- to 5-year-old stuttering and non-stuttering children. He wanted to establish whether there was any delay in syntactic development of young children who stutter. The results indicated that there were no differences between stuttering and non-stuttering children in subject-noun-verb, subject-pronoun-verb and subject-crossed-verb agreement sentence structures. The only significant difference was on the imperative reflexive pronoun-verb agreement in which stuttering children performed significantly poorer than controls. An example is given below of reflexive pronoun-verb agreement in Persian:

31- /xodat sib ra bardashti/
Yourself apple OBJ picked up
'You yourself picked up the apple'

It is not clear what was counted as stuttering incidence in their report which may have affected the results. Shafiei suggested that more research on the effect of syntactic factors in younger developing children who stutter is needed.

3.2 Lexical factors

The two major lexical classes are content and function words (Brown & Fraser, 1963). These have different organizational roles in the syntactic structure of the language and carry different types of information (Kucera & Francis, 1967; Landau & Jackendoff, 1993). Some researchers have reported higher incidence of stuttering frequency on content words rather than function words in English-speaking adults (Au-Yeung *et al.*, 1998), whereas others report no differences (Griggs & Still, 1979; Koopmans *et al.*, 1991). There seems to be a developmental pattern in grammatical class and stuttering. With increasing age, there is an increase in content-word stuttering and a decrease in function-word stuttering (Au-Yeung *et al.*, 1998; Bloodstein & Gantwerk, 1967; Bloodstein & Grossman, 1981; Dworzynski *et al.*, 2003; Howell *et al.*, 1999; Rommel, 2001).

There are a few reports on the effect of different word classes in Persian-speaking stutterers. Samadi (2000) studied the behavior of 6–10-year-old children who stutter when using function and content words in descriptive speech, and he reported that stuttering occurred more often on content words rather than function words. In his study part-/whole-word repetition, pause, prolongation and blocks were assumed as stuttering events.

Bakhtiar *et al.* (2009) studied lexical characteristics of stuttered words among 46–70-month-old Persian-speaking children. Sound prolongations, sound/syllable repetitions, monosyllabic whole-word repetitions and broken words were assumed as stuttering events in this study. In contrast with Samadi´s results, they did not find any differences in the behavior of the children when using function and content words. The difference in the results of two reports may be due to their methodological procedures. Samadi's results were based on counting the number of stuttered function and content words, whereas Bakhtiar *et al.* reported on the results of stuttered content/function words out of all content/function words produced. Since content and function words are not used equally in the same corpus, simply counting the number of stuttered function or content words without taking the total number of uttered words in each category into consideration might be misleading. On the other hand, it might be argued that a stuttering incidence on a function or a content word reflects a single locus of difficulty and not the relative rate of occurrence of each type.

Mokhlesin (2006) studied the incidence of disfluency on function and content words in the spontaneous speech of children and adults.

Her results indicated that Persian-speaking stutterers of different ages exhibited different patterns of disfluency. The pattern of disfluency changed from predominantly function to content words as age increased. The dominant symptoms were reported as silent prolongation, interjection and revision patterns in the older population. The pattern of stuttering on function words and content words in children and adults who stuttered was function word plus content word (FC) and function word plus function word plus content word contexts (FFC). They rarely stuttered on both content and function words in either FC or FFC, suggesting a reciprocal relationship between stuttering on function and content words.

The results for Persian-speaking populations are similar to what has been already reported in English and German (Dworzynski *et al.*, 2003; Howell *et al.*, 1999). Howell and Au-Yeung (2002) proposed an account of the etiology of stuttering events based on these findings, which may also be applicable to Persian based on Mokhlesin's findings.

More research on Persian is needed on the role of different lexical categories (function/content words) to see how it affects stuttering on different parts of speech given that these categories do not coincide with those in English and that function word position varies from those occupied in English. Also, factors that are confounded with content and function words need examining. For example, word frequency is confounded with word type (content words are statistically less likely to be high frequency than are function words). Studying each lexical category (e.g. content words: verbs, nouns, adjectives, adverbs) and even different lexical items (e.g. nouns: derivation, compounding) would be interesting to examine.

Since stuttering usually occurs on the first words of the sentence, and given that Persian is an SOV language, nouns might be more susceptible to stuttering. On the other hand, verbs convey an important aspect of the meaning of the sentence and they occupy terminal positions in sentences for Persian. However, as we mentioned before, word order is rather loose in Persian and all major constituents of the sentence (S, O and V) may be reshuffled for pragmatic purposes. In reading tasks, the SOV order is dominant, but not necessarily in the spoken mode. Therefore, more research is needed in languages with different syntactic patterns such as Persian, Arabic, Turkish and Hindi to compare the effect of different types of content words in different positions, especially for languages where the verb can occupy different positions. Persian places verbs at the end of sentences which might reduce their chance of being stuttered, but the verb forms are more complex that should make them more likely to be stuttered. Cross-linguistic word might help deconfound these influences. Also worthy of study is what effect moving a verb around in a sentence for pragmatic purposes (which is allowed in Persian) has on stuttering rate.

3.3 Phonological factors

Howell and Rusbridge's chapter summarizes the prevalence of phonological disorders among children not identified as having a stuttering problem, as ranging between 2% and 13%. In contrast, it is commonly reported that 30–40% of children who stutter have a co-occurring phonological disorder (Conture, 2001; Melnick & Conture, 2000; Wolk *et al.*, 2000). The relationship between phonological disorders and stuttering calls for attention. However, the evidence for such factors affecting stuttering in English is weak (Howell & Rusbridge, this volume; Nippold, 2002). There are a few recent clinical reports on this topic in Persian. Bakhtiar *et al.* (2007) examined phonological encoding in 5–8-year-old children who stutter (CWS) during a non-word repetition task to test the covert repair hypothesis (CRH) and phonological skills of Persian-speaking children. They compared 12 CWS with 12 non-stuttering children (CWNS). A list of 40 bisyllabic and trisyllabic non-words was used in a repetition task to collect information about (a) reaction times (RTs) and (b) the number of phonological errors (PEs). The stimulus presentation and data recording were operated using DMDX software (DMASTR Web site: http://www.u.arizona.edu/~kforster/dmastr/dmastr.htm.) on a laptop with millisecond accuracy. The Persian version of the Test of Language Development-I: 3 (TOLD) (Newcomer & Hammill, 1997) was used to exclude children with developmental language disorders. The results indicated that CWS had a slightly poorer performance than CWNS but there was no significant weakness in their phonological skills. In addition, TOLD results on phonological analysis also did not confirm the existence of a significant difference in phonological ability between CWS and CWNS groups.

Initial consonant clusters are absent from Persian. The permitted syllable patterns are as follows: CV, CVC and CVCC, and there are no V-onsets. Consequently, there is no way to compare words with initial vowels and consonants. Interestingly, it has been reported that words with the initial glottal stop consonant /?/, that is considered by some phoneticians to have vowel-like properties, are more susceptible to be stuttered (Karimi Javan, 2003).

3.4 Acoustic factors

High-precision temporal coordination of oral and laryngeal movements is considered critical for the fluent and accurate production of connected speech, and several authors have proposed discoordination of these actions as a specific version of the general hypothesis that stuttering is a disorder of timing (Adams, 1999; Boutsen, 1995; Conture *et al.*, 1985;

Perkins *et al.*, 1976; St. Louis, 1979, Van Riper, 1982 as cited in Max & Gracco, 2005).

To produce voicing contrasts, speakers need to be able to coordinate their speech production systems (respiration, phonation and articulation). Such speech-motor activities that require coordination may be poor in people who stutter. One aspect that has been examined is Voice Onset Time (VOT) of voiceless consonants which distinguishes minimal contrasts like /b/ (short VOT) and /p/ (longer VOT). In the majority of VOT studies, significant differences between stutterers and non-stutterer's VOT have been found in selected conditions (De Nil & Brutten, 1991).

A small number of reports on acoustic features are available for Persian-speaking stutterers. Forutan (2000) studied VOT in 11-year-olds and older stutterers and compared the results with a matched non-stuttering group. The participants were 30 males and 4 females in each group. The subjects were asked to read 18 four-syllable words each of which began with one of the voiceless plosive consonants (/p, t, k/) or a voiced plosive consonants (/b, d, g/) and the data were analyzed by spectrogram. The first and third syllables were the same in every word in the task. The results indicated that the mean VOTs of the first and third syllables in subjects who stuttered were significantly longer than in non-stuttering subjects ($p < 0.05$). Also, the mean VOTs of the first syllables were longer than those of the third syllables in both stuttering and non-stuttering subjects ($p < 0.05$). Forutan did not report any significant difference between males and females within each group. He argued that longer VOT in the first syllables was due to discoordination between speech subsystems (respiration, phonation and articulation) and caused most of the stutterers' longer VOT on the first syllable. In a replication, Yadegari and Salehi (2000) conducted a similar study in children under 5 years of age and reported similar results. The VOTs of stuttering children were significantly longer than that of the non-stuttering children.

Shaker Ardekani (2006) examined fundamental frequency, jitter (variation in frequency between successive vibratory cycles) and shimmer (variation in amplitude between successive vibratory cycles) among Persian adults who do and do not stutter using Dr. Speech software (Tiger Electronics, Neu-Anspach, Germany). Stromsta (1986) believed that if the magnitude of vocal perturbation, as indicated by either jitter or shimmer, in the fluent phonatory behaviors of stutterers was shown to be significantly greater than that of non-stutterers, this would provide additional support to the hypothesis that stutterers demonstrate generally less-competent neurophysiologic regulatory control over their peripheral mechanisms of phonation and respiration. The tasks in the Shaker Ardekani (2006) study consisted of sustained phonation of vowels /a/ and /i/, reading 20 sentences, and rhythmic counting (counting digits 1 to 20). There were no significant differences between the two groups in F0 and standard deviation of F0 in performing the three speech tasks. No differences were reported in jitter and shimmer between the two groups either.

Rezaie-Aghbash *et al.* (1999) compared the VOTs of five Persian and five English speakers whose stuttering was mild to severe. The VOT measurements were obtained from both stuttered and fluent productions of speech for voiceless plosives /p, t, k/ and voiced plosives /b, d, g/. In contrast to the English group the VOT patterns for the Persian group were consistent with Viswanath and Joullian's (1994) research. Viswanath and Joullian reported that mean VOT values in stuttered speech increase from bilabial to alveolar to velar. In Rezaie-Aghbash's results for the Persian group, both voiced and voiceless plosives showed an increase from bilabial to alveolar to velar for both the stuttered and fluent voiceless plosives. Inter-language-group comparisons of both the stuttered and fluent VOT data indicated that the Persian group had longer VOT values for the voiceless plosives /p, k/ compared to the English group. Conversely, the voiced plosives for the English group were more aspirated and had longer VOT values compared to those for the Persian group. The researchers stated that differences may be due to the heterogeneity of the Persian speakers who like the English speaker group, included mild to sever stutterers. A larger scale study that looks more systematically at whether severity affects VOT production would be merited.

In conclusion, coordination problems in people who stutter (reflected in VOT measures) were observed in two studies on Persian. Measures of F0 or measures based on F0 failed to reveal differences between adults who stutter and controls in Persian.

4 Psycholinguistic Factors

Differences in semantic processing have also been investigated in people who stutter in Persian. Karimi Javan (2003) used Osgood's semantic differential technique. 'This technique was designed to measure the connotative meaning of different concepts (Osgood *et al.*, 1957) and requires participants to rate each words as "adequate-inadequate", "good-evil" or "valuable-worthless" on a seven point scale to measure the subjects' attitudes on different concepts'.

In Karimi Javan's study, 20 people who stuttered (PWS) aged between 17 and 25 years participated and their performances were compared with those of 20 controls subjects (PWNS). They were matched for age, sex and education. The participants were asked to read a 200-word passage designed for the study that included all Persian phonemes and had words from different concepts and categories. Disfluently uttered words were identified by an experienced SLP. Two fluent and disfluent words were selected at random from the passage (for example, if a participant stuttered on 20 words, the tenth and eleventh disfluent words were selected). Then PWS subjects were asked to complete Osgood's semantic differential test for the two disfluent and fluent uttered words. PWNS also completed the same task using the same words as stuttering adults. The results revealed that there was no difference between PWS and PWNS in semantic processing. Indeed, both groups rated the meaning of these words the same. Therefore, based on the results it seems that the emotional aspects of meaning of the words do not interfere with the performance of PWS.

Instead, the important issue for participants was the phonological features of the selected words, specially the initial consonant in each word. Most participants stuttered on words with initial glottal stop (/?/). As was mentioned before, all Persian words start with an initial consonant and there are no initial consonant clusters. Interestingly, words initiated with the consonant /?/ as a glottal stop had the highest incidence of stuttered words (speaking with an open glottis is sometimes used as a way of inducing fluency).

In a further study, Karimi *et al.* (2007) investigated implicit and explicit memory in adults who stutter using cued recall and word-stem completion tasks. Cued recall is a task designed to measure explicit memory and refers to the process in which a person is given a list of items to remember and then is asked to recall the cued words. Cues act as a facilitator for the person to recall the word. In contrast to free recall, the person is prompted to remember certain items on the list or remember the list in a certain order (Bower & Gordon, 2000). The word stem completion task (WSC) is a verbal test of perceptual implicit memory. In this task the participant is presented with the first few letters of a word and asked to complete the word stem with the first word he/she can recall (Graf *et al.*, 1982). The participants are usually unaware that they have to complete these tasks using words they have been previously exposed to. This task calls on implicit memory because at the time of word presentation participants have merely been exposed to the items and have not been asked to consciously memorize them.

Their task used 30 words from three different categories. There were 10 positive, 10 negative and 10 emotionally neutral words in the task, based on Denny and Hunt's (1992) study. The inter-group analysis results revealed that adults who stutter remembered fewer emotionally positive words compared to non-stuttering control subjects while performing the explicit memory task. Also, in implicit and explicit tasks, stutterers (intra group analysis) remembered more words with negative emotional meaning (p < 0.05) than words with positive meaning.

5 Conclusions

The general conclusion we can draw from the present documented reports on the prevalence of stuttering is that rates among Persian speakers in Iran is similar to that found elsewhere where other languages are used. Although some new reports have indicated differences in prevalence between monolingual and bilingual Persian-speaking populations (Mohammadi *et al.*, 2008b; Molahosseini, 2000), the present data are not yet comprehensive and more research is needed to confirm the results. With respect to symptoms of stuttering among Persian-speaking children and language-specific confounding factors on stuttering, more solid data are needed to make a conclusive judgment on language-specific factors related to stuttering in Persian-speaking population. The present results indicate that both syntactic complexity and length of utterance have effects on rate of stuttering. Some studies have also been reported on the role of function and content words. Mokhlesin's data (2006) presented the developmental evidence in Persian. While children stuttered more on function words, adults tended to stutter on content words. This observation is in agreement with reports in English, Spanish and German and is in line with EXPLAN theory (Howell, 2004).

From a phonological point of view, it seems that more research must be done on both phonological development of Persian children who stutter and the prevalence of concomitant articulation disorders in PWS. Although some Iranian clinicians have reported that some of their stuttering clients suffer from other concurrent speech and language disorders, there are no systematic studies to support this claim. Stuttering is more probable in the first two words of utterances and on words starting with glottal stop consonants in Persian. With respect to acoustic features, stutterers are not different from other people in features such as F0, standard deviation of F0, jitter or shimmer. The only reported difference was longer VOTs in Persian speakers who stutter as compared to non-stuttering speakers. Further solid clinical data with more extended scope and larger samples as well as systematic pairing of languages (Persian with Arabic and so on) are needed to confirm the present results and to look at other possible language-specific confounding factors for cross-linguistic purposes.

Acknowledgments

We are very grateful to Professor Peter Howell who read the previous drafts of this chapter and gave valuable and constructive comments. Any errors and misinterpretations are those of the authors.

References

Au-Yeung, J., Howell, P and Pilgrim, L. (1998) Phonological words and stuttering on function words. *Journal of Speech, Language, and Hearing Research* 41, 1019–1030.

Bakhtiar, M., Dehghan Ahmad Abadi, A. and Seif Panahi, M.S. (2007) Nonword repetition ability of children who do and do not stutter and covert repair hypothesis. *Indian Journal of Medical Sciences* 61, 462–470. Retrieved from http://www.indianjmedsci.org/text.asp?2007/61/8/462/33711

Bakhtiar, M., Salmalian, T., Ghandzade, M. and Nilipour, R. (2009, August) *Lexical Characteristics Effect of Stuttered Words in Persian-speaking Children*. Paper presented at the 6th World Congress on Fluency Disorders. Rio de Janeiro, Brazil.

Bernstein Ratner, N. (1997) Stuttering: A psycholinguistic perspective. In R.F. Curlee and G.M. Siegel (eds)*Nature and Treatment of Stuttering: New Directions* (2nd edn) (pp. 99–127). Boston, MA: Allyn & Bacon.

Bloodstein, O. and Gantwerk, B.F. (1967) Grammatical function in relation to stuttering in young children. *Journal of Speech and Hearing Research* 10, 786–789.

Bloodstein, O. and Grossman, M. (1981) Early stuttering: Some aspects of their form and distribution. *Journal of Speech and Hearing Research* 24, 298–302.

Bower, G.H. and Gordon, H. (2000) A brief history of memory research. In E. Talving and F.I.M. Craik (eds) *The Oxford Handbook of Memory*. Oxford: Oxford University Press.

Brown, R. and Fraser, C. (1963) The acquisition of syntax. In N.C. Cofer and B. Musgrave(eds) *Verbal Behavior and Learning: Problems and Processes* (pp. 158–201). New York: McGraw-Hill.

Chomsky, N. (1965) *Aspects of the Theory of Syntax*. Cambridge, MA: MIT Press.

Conture, E.G. (2001) *Stuttering: Its Nature, Diagnosis, and Treatment*. Needham Heights, MA: Allyn & Bacon.

Craig, A., Hancock, K., Tran, Y., Craig, M. and Peters, K. (2002) Epidemiology of stuttering in the communication across the entire life span. *Journal of Speech and Hearing Research* 45, 1097–1105.

De Nil, L.F. and Brutten, G.J. (1991) Voice onset time of stuttering and nonstuttering children: The influence of externally and linguistically imposed time pressure. *Journal of Fluency Disorders* 16, 143–158.

Denny, E.B. and Hunt, R. (1992) Affective valenca and memory in depression. *Journal of Abnormal Psychology* 10(1), 575–580.

Dworzynski, K., Howell, P. and Natke, U. (2003) Predicting stuttering from linguistic factors or German speakers in two age groups. *Journal of Fluency Disorders* 28(2), 95–113.

Einarsdottir, J. and Ingham, R.J. (2008) The effect of stuttering measurement training on judging stuttering occurrence in preschool children who stutter. *Journal of Fluency Disorders* 33, 167–179.

Forutan, E. (2000). *The Comparison of Voice Onset Time Between Stuttering and Non Stuttering People*. (Unpublished Master's thesis). Iran University of Medical Sciences, Iran.

Gaines, N.D., Runyan, C.M. and Meyers, S.G. (1991) A comparison of young stutterers' fluent versus stuttered utterances on measures of length and complexity. *Journal of Speech and Hearing Research* 34, 37–42.

Graf, P., Mandler, G. and Haden, P. (1982) Simulating amnesic symptoms in normal subjects.*Science* 218, 1243–1244.

Griggs, S. and Still, A.W. (1979) An analysis of individual differences in words stuttered. *Journal of Speech and Hearing Research* 22, 572–580.

Haresabadi, F., Puladi, Sh., Mahmoudi Bakhtiari, B. and Kamali, M. (2010) Baresi asare tule gofte bar mizane naravanie goftare kudakane loknati va gheyre loknati farsi zaban [Effect evaluation of utterance length on speech dysfluency in stuttering and nonstuttering Persian-speaker children]. *Journal of Audiology* 19(1), 86–93.

Howell, P. (2004) Assessment of some contemporary theories of stuttering that apply to spontaneous speech. *Contemporary Issues in Communicative Sciences and Disorders* 31, 122–139.

Howell, P., Au-Yeung, J. and Sackin, S. (1999) Exchange of stuttering from function words to content words with age. *Journal of Speech Language Hearing Research* 42(2), 345–354.

Howell, P. and Au-Yeung, J. (2002) The EXPLAN theory of fluency control and diagnosis of stuttering. In E. Fava (ed.) *Current Issue in Linguistic Theory Series: Pathology and Therapy of Speech Disorders* (pp. 75–94). Amsterdam: John Benjamins.

Kalashi, M. (2003)*The Effects of Length of Utterance and Syntactic Complexity on Dysfluency of 6 to 12 Year Old Stuttering and Non Stuttering Persian Speaking Children.* (Unpublished Master's thesis). University of Social Welfare and Rehabilitation Sciences, Tehran, Iran.

Karimi, H. (2006) *The Prevalence of Stuttering among Monolingual and Bilingual Primary School Age Children in Ahwaz.* (Unpublished manuscript), Department of Speech & Language Therapy, Isfahan University of Medical Sciences, Iran.

Karimi Javan, G. (2003) *Semantic Processing of Fluent and Non Fluent Uttered Words in Stuttering and Non Stuttering Adults.* (Unpublished Master's thesis). Tehran University of Medical Sciences, Iran.

Karimi Javan, G., Nilipour, R., Ashayeri, H., Yadegari, F. and Karimlu, M. (2007) Naghshe hafeza ashkar va hafeze zemni dar afrade mobtala be loknat [The role of explicit and implicit memory in stutterers]. *Journal of Rehabilitation* 1(30), 69–72. Retrieved from http://www.jrehabilitation.com/browse.php?a_code= A-10-1-163&slc_lang=fa&sid=1&sw=%D9%84%D9%83%D9%86%D8%AA.

Katzner, K. (2002) *The Languages of the World*. New York: Routledge.

Koopmans, M., Slis, I. and Rietveld, T. (1991) The influence of word position and word type on the incidence of stuttering. In H.F.M. Peters, W. Hulstijn and C.W. Starkweather (eds) *Speech Motor Control and Stuttering* (pp. 333–340). Amsterdam: Elsevier.

Kucera, H. and Francis, W.N. (1967) *Computational Analysis of Present–day American English*. Providence, RI: Brown University Press.

Landau, B. and Jackendoff, R. (1993) 'What' and 'where' in spatial language and spatial cognition. *Brain and Behavioral Sciences* 16, 217–265.

Logan, K.J. and Conture, E. (1995) Length, grammatical complexity, and rate differences in stuttered and fluent conversational utterances of children who stutter. *Journal of Fluency Disorders* 20, 35–61.

Logan, K.J. and LaSalle, L.R. (1999) Grammatical characteristics of children's conversational utterances that contain disfluency clusters. *Journal of Speech, Language & Hearing Research* 42, 80–91.

Max, L. and Gracco, V.L. (2005) Coordination of oral and laryngeal movements in the perceptually fluent speech of adults who stutter. *Journal of Speech, Language, and Hearing Research* 48, 524–542.

Melnick, K. and Conture, E. (2000) Relationship of length and grammatical complexity to the systematic and nonsystematic speech error and stuttering of children who stutter. *Journal of Fluency Disorders* 25(1), 21–45.Doi: 10.1016/S0094-730X(99)00028-5.

Mohammadi, H., Nilipour, R. and Yadegari, F. (2008a) Stuttering prevalence among kurdish-Farsi students: Effects of the two language similarities. *Iranian Rehabilitation Journal* 6(7), 83–88. Retrieved from http://www.rehabj.ir/article- A-10-9-1-1-en.html.

Mohammadi, H., Yadegari, F., Nilipour, R. and Rahgozar, M. (2008b) Shoyue loknat dar daneshamuzane dozabane maghte mokhte tahsilie shahre Javanrood [Prevalence of stuttering in javanroud's bilingual students]. *Journal of Rehabilitation* 9(1), 43–48. Retrieved from http://www. jrehabilitation.com/browse.php?a_code=A-10-1-204&slc_lang=fa&sid=1& sw=%D9%84%D9%83%D9%83%D9%86%D8%AA.

Mokhlesin, M. (2006) *The Comparison of Dysflueny Patterns in Persian Speaking Children and Adults who Stutter* (Unpublished Master's thesis). Tehran University of Medical Sciences, Iran.

Molahosseini, M. (2000) *The Prevalence of Stuttering among Primary School Students in Kermanshah.* (M.D thesis), Kermanshah University of Medical Sciences, Iran.

Newcomer, P.L. and Hammill, D.D. (1997) *The Test of Language Development-I:3 (TOLD).* Austin, TX: Empiric Press.

Nilipour, R. (2000) Agrammatic language: Two cases from Persian.*Journal of Aphasiology* 14(12), 1205–1242.

Nilipour, R. and Raghibdoust, Sh. (2001) Manifestations of aphasia in Persian. *Journal of Neurolinguistics* 14(2), 209–230.

Nippold, M.A. (2002) Stuttering and phonology: Is there an interaction? *American Journal of Speech-Language Pathology* 11(2), 99–110.

Osgood, C.E., Suci, G.J. and Tannenbaum, P.H. (1957) *Measurement of Meaning.* Urbana: University of Illinois Press.

Packman, A. and Onslow, M. (1998) What is the take-home message from Curlee and Yairi? *American Journal of Speech-Language Pathology* 7, 5–6.

Rezaie-Aghbash, N., Whitesid, S.P. and Cudd, P.A. (1999, September) *Cross-language Analysis of Voice Onset Time in Stuttered Speech.* Paper presented at the Sixth European Conference on Speech Communication and technology (pp. 1079–1082), Budapest. Full paper retrieved from http://www.isca-speech. org/archive/eurospeech_1999/e99_1079.html.

Rommel, D. (2001) The influence of psycholinguistic variables on stuttering in childhood. In H.G. Bosshardt, J.S. Yaruss and H.F.M. Peters (eds) *Fluency Disorders: Theory, Research, Treatment and Self- help* (pp. 195–202). Proceedings of the Third World Congress of Fluency Disorders in Nyborg, Denmark. Nijmegen: Nijmegen University Press.

Samadi, M.J. (2000) *The Effects of Word Types and Position of Words in the Sentence on Dysfluency of 6 to 10 Year Old Stuttering and Non Stuttering Persian Speaking Children in Hamedan* (Master's thesis), Iran University of Medical Sciences, Iran.

Seery, C.H., Watkins, R.V., Mangelsdorf, S.C. and Shigeto, A. (2007) Subtyping stuttering II: Contributions from language and temperament. *Journal of Fluency Disorders* 32, 197–217.

Shafiei, R. (1998) *Subject-verb Agreement in the Speech of 4 to 6 Year Old Stuttering and Non Stuttering Persian Speaking Children* (Unpublished Master's thesis). University of Social Welfare and Rehabilitation Sciences, Iran.

Shaker Ardekani, M. (2006) *Some Acoustic Features of Stuttering and Non Stuttering People* (Unpublished Master's thesis). Tehran University of Medical Sciences, Iran.

Stromsta, C. (1986) *Elements of Stuttering.* Oshtemo, MI: Atsmorts publishing.

Vahab, M. (2004) *The Effects of Length of Utterance and Syntactic Complexity on Dysfluency of 20 to 25 Year Old Stuttering and Non Stuttering Persian Speaking Adults* (Unpublished Master's thesis), University of Social Welfare and Rehabilitation Sciences, Iran.

Van Borsel, J., Maes, E. and Foulon, S. (2001) Stuttering and bilingualism: A review. *Journal of Fluency Disorders* 26, 179–205.

Viswanath, N. and Joullian, A. (1994) Consequences of the relation between VOT and types of fragments in part-word repetition. *Proceedings of the 1st World Congress on Fluency Disorders*, Vol. 1 (pp. 60–63), 8–12 August 1994, Munich, Germany.

Wolk, L., Blomgren, M. and Smith, A. (2000) The frequency of simultaneous disfluency and phonological errors in children: A preliminary investigation. *Journal of Fluency Disorders* 25(4), 269–281. Doi: 10.1016/S0094-730X (00)00076-0.

Yadegari, F. and Salehi, A. (2000) Tashkhise efteraghie loknate avaliye va naravanie tabiei dar kudakan [Deferential diagnosis of primary stuttering and normal nonfluency in children referring to Saba clinic]. *Journal of Rehabilitation* 4(3), 57–63. Retrieved from http://www.jrehabilitation.com/browse.php?a_code= A-10-1-178&slc_lang=fa&sid=1&sw=%D9%84%D9%83%D9%86%D8%AA.

Yaruss, J.S. (1999) Utterance length, syntactic complexity, and childhood stuttering. *Journal of Speech, Language, & Hearing Research* 42, 329–344.

Zackheim, C. and Conture, E. (2003) Childhood stuttering and speech disfluencies in relation to children's mean length of utterance: A preliminary study. *Journal of Fluency Disorders* 28, 115–142. Doi:10.1016/S0094-730X(03)00007-X.

Zeynali, A. (2001) *The Prevalence of Stuttering among Primary School Age Boys in Qom* (Unpublished Master's thesis). Tehran University of Medical Sciences, Iran.

Chapter 9

Stuttering Research in Brazil: An Overview

MÔNICA DE BRITTO PEREIRA

Summary

The objective of this chapter is to offer an overview on stuttering research conducted in Brazil during the last 15 years. The chapter is divided into five sections: the first one describes studies about the knowledge of certain social groups about the disorder, the second is about studies on the prevalence of stuttering and the third and fourth on studies about linguistic, auditory and behavioral aspects of stuttering and the fifth on studies about assessment and treatment of stuttering, respectively. The chapter shows that there is a lack of research on intervention and on the development of therapy methods appropriate for the Brazilian population. The fact that the studies are mainly published in Brazilian journals hampers dissemination of research findings to international audiences.

1 Introduction

This chapter gives an overview of studies on stuttering in Brazil conducted in the last 15 years. Some general information about speech language pathology and audiology in the country are presented first.

Speech language pathology and audiology started in Brazil in the 1930s and their focus was the correction of speech and reading problems in school-aged children. The first two teaching programs in speech language pathology and audiology started in 1961, one at the Universidade de São Paulo which was conducted to the Otolaryngology Clinic of the Hospital of the Faculty of Medicine, and the other at the Catholic University of São Paulo which was delivered by the Psychology Institute. In 1972 the latter also started the first master's program in Brazil. In December 1981 law number 6965 was issued that regulated the profession and determined which competences were required by a practicing speech language pathologist/audiologist. Based on this law, a federal and regional council of professionals was founded to monitor the professional practice. The federal council also granted (and still grants) the title of 'specialist' in the area. The recognized areas of specialization in Brazil are audiology, language disorder, oromyofunctional disorders, voice and public health. The number of speech language pathologists/audiologists in the country is

214

34,468, and the greatest concentration is in São Paulo (10,795), followed by Rio de Janeiro (5466). Today there are 94 graduate programs in speech language pathology and audiology, eight master programs and four doctoral programs.

Scientific aspects of the profession are taken care of by the Sociedade Brasileira de Fonoaudiologia (SBFa) that was created in 1988 with the aim of stimulating research. The SBFa has a general directory, and departments that correspond to the areas of specialization recognized by the federal council. The SBFa also has committees that assess education and merit, and financial and administrative councils. In addition, the society publishes a quarterly journal (Revista da Sociedade Brasileira de Fonoaudiologia) and organizes a yearly congress. The area of fluency disorders comes under the specialization of language.

The country has two associations devoted to providing information and delivering services to persons who stutter. The first one established was Abra Gageira, a non-governmental non-profit organization of people who stutter, that promotes actions to improve the quality of life of people who stutter. It does this, not only by organizing support groups in the various states of the country, but also by organizing a yearly meeting and offering diverse types of information that may be relevant for people who stutter. The other association is the Instituto Brasileiro de Fluência – IBF, which has as its goal dissemination of knowledge about speech and its disorders for the benefit of persons with fluency disorders, their relatives and professionals who work in the area.

Although there is a large number of speech language pathologists/audiologists, there are few professionals who specialize in the study and treatment of stuttering. Specialist clinics are rare and are mainly found at universities, where research in the area is conducted. I present next an overview of research on fluency disorders and stuttering. The studies are organized in four categories. These are studies on: (1) knowledge of different social groups about the disorder; (2) prevalence of stuttering; (3) linguistic, auditory and behavioral aspects of stuttering; and (4) clinical aspects including assessment and treatment.

2 Studies on the Knowledge of Certain Social Groups about Stuttering

One of the first studies conducted on this issue was by Chiquetto (1996) who investigated the beliefs, ideas and knowledge of school teachers about stuttering and its causes. Participants were 28 teachers of first-year, elementary school classes. The schools were both public and private, in Florianopolis. A questionnaire was specifically designed for the study and this was filled out by the teachers. Results showed that teachers had difficulty distinguishing stuttering from other speech language disorders and that their attitude, although well intentioned, was not always adequate for the children's fluency requirements. For instance, they reported that they asked children to be calm, to speak slowly, and that they completed the utterances for the children.

Cibotto and Schiefer (2001), in a questionnaire study conducted in São Paulo, investigated level of knowledge about stuttering among 15 relatives of children who stuttered. The participants reported that stuttering is a behavior that was learned through imitation. They also thought that nervousness was not the cause of stuttering but could aggravate it, and confirmed that they considered that stuttering is not a disease and can be cured. They considered that stuttering is not hereditary, that it did not affect the intelligence of their children and that the parents were not guilty for the speech problem. They also expressed the opinion that in some cases stuttering could be triggered by environmental, physical or psychological factors and that their children suffered in their daily life from prejudices about stuttering. It was also observed that participants adhered to popular knowledge and stereotypes about stuttering (e.g. that children who stutter do so because they are anxious and nervous), which can influence in a negative way the person who stutters in all aspects of life. As such the study further reflects the importance of the speech language pathologist for disseminating accurate scientific knowledge about stuttering.

Calais *et al.* (2002) interviewed 43 teachers from four public schools in Bauru in São Paulo about stuttering and the way they dealt with it when they encountered cases. They concluded that although the teachers correctly defined stuttering as a speech disorder, they believed that emotional issues were most important and also that stuttering can be cured. According to the authors, analysis of the results indicated that teachers do not have sufficient information to be able to deal adequately with pupils who present with stuttering.

In a questionnaire study conducted in private schools in the city of Recife, Silveira *et al.* (2002) studied knowledge about childhood disfluency among the parents and teachers of children in the early stages of language acquisition. The study also investigated whether it was necessary to make clear the role of the speech language pathologist in the school. The participants consisted of 40 parents and 40 teachers of children aged 2–5 years; half of them were from schools that had a speech language pathologist in the team (the other half did not have one). Results showed that both the parents and teachers did not know about normal disfluencies and for the majority of them the task of the speech language pathologist in the school was not clear. Importantly, this was true of schools with and without a speech language pathologist. It should be noted that the study was conducted in private schools and as such it is unknown whether these findings would apply to public schools as well.

Ferriolli *et al.* (2005) investigated knowledge and attitudes about stuttering in teachers of public and private elementary schools in the city of São Paulo. They collected 55 questionnaires. Among the teachers who responded, 72.7% indicated that they had lay-knowledge about stuttering and that this led to uncertainty when they had to deal with a pupil who stuttered. The authors concluded that teachers must be better informed in order to acquire better skills in a class that has pupils who stutter. Based on the information obtained from the questionnaire the authors also concluded that the development of a preventive program in schools is necessary.

Oliveira *et al.* (2007) distributed questionnaires to 57 professionals and 50 speech language pathology students. They investigated comprehension by working professionals and third- and fourth-year students in speech language pathology about aspects of fluency and disfluency, what factors the respondents thought affected fluency and the types of disfluencies observed, using both open and closed questions. On the question 'What are the components of fluent speech for you?' speech rate was mentioned most often. Psychological factors such as anxiety and introversion-extraversion were among the most-cited factors that were considered to influence the degree of fluency. The types of disfluencies identified most often were blocks, initial prolongations and associated behaviors. There were no statistically significant difference in the response patterns of students versus professionals, but the number of years of professional practice influenced certain answers. For instance, the respondents who had more years of experience used terms like 'speech without prolongations', 'speech without pause', 'efficient speech' more often as characteristics to describe fluency. On the other hand, the more-experienced participants used terms like 'speech without breaks', 'speech without blocks' less often than less-experienced colleagues. The participants, irrespective of experience, tended to believe that being fluent meant having 'speech without disruption' and considered disfluency as an abnormal speech phenomenon. They were also of the opinion that speech rate and not the disfluencies themselves were the component that most affected the degree of fluency. They considered that affective factors, primarily anxiety, most influenced the degree of fluency (the net effect of this is to attribute a secondary role to linguistic, cognitive and genetic factors as influences on stuttering). The classification of types of disfluencies into normal and stuttered disfluencies by the participants was in line with the literature.

St Louis *et al.* (2005) ran a pilot study in Brazil using POSHA (Public Opinion Survey of Human Attributes). This involved 50 graduate students in speech language pathology in the cities of São Paulo and Alfenas, in the state of Minas Gerais. The main findings were that stuttering was considered a serious disorder in Brazil but that Brazilians were not well-informed about the disorder.

Britto Pereira *et al.* (2008) investigated the knowledge of the lay person about stuttering in the city of Rio de Janeiro. The instrument used was a questionnaire that had been developed and used in previous studies in Belgium and China, with questions about prevalence, onset, gender distribution, occurrence in different cultures, cause, treatment, intelligence and hereditability (Van Borsel *et al.*, 1999). Data that were collected on 606 participants showed that although stuttering is a disorder that was known about by the majority of the participants, knowledge was limited for certain aspects (including prevalence, age of onset, gender distribution and the cause of stuttering). Knowledge also differed according to gender, age and educational level. Comparison of the results with the studies conducted in Belgium and in Shanghai, China showed several similarities but also some differences. For example, Brazilian lay-participants, like those in Belgium and Shanghai, generally estimated the prevalence of stuttering at too high a rate, they were unrealistically optimistic about the possibilities of treatment, and were not sufficiently aware of the hereditary and neurogenic basis of stuttering. Results in Rio de Janeiro were clearly different: For example, over 20.8% of the respondents in Brazil situated the onset of stuttering before age 2 (compared to 9.8% and 5.7% in the Belgian and Chinese studies, respectively), where over 22.8% thought that stuttering does not occur in all races (compared to 8% and 2% in the Belgian and Chinese study respectively). Also, whereas over 23.8% of the Brazilian participants thought that intelligence was higher in people who stutter than in people who did not stutter, only 4.8% of the Belgian and 8.42% of the Chinese participants expressed this opinion.

Although results from questionnaire studies should be treated with caution, the studies described in this section suggest that knowledge about stuttering is limited not only among teachers and the general population, but also among speech and language pathologists and students.

3 Studies on the Prevalence of Stuttering

One of the few studies on the prevalence of stuttering in Brazil is that of Andrade (1997). She examined a group of 2980 children aged between 1.0 to 11.11 years enrolled in a health center in a neighborhood of São Paulo. Among these, 4.19% presented with a communication disorder and 2.9% presented specifically with stuttering.

Graça (2001), in a study in the neighborhood Mangueira in Rio de Janeiro, found an overall stuttering prevalence of 5.1% in 196 children aged 4–11 years. Prevalence in boys and girls was comparable (5.7% and 5.3% respectively) which is unlike what is seen in most studies in the international literature. The reasons for this intriguing finding are not clear.

Britto Pereira *et al.* (2007) assessed 203 children in a public school in the neighborhood of Tijuca in Rio de Janeiro. Six of the children (i.e. 2.9%) presented with a fluency disorder. Of these six children, three showed stuttering only when reading, one child presented with a disfluency that was reminiscent of cluttering (the child only showed normal disfluencies, had a high speaking rate and showed evidence of disordered articulation), another child was classified with normal childhood disfluency, and the last one showed stutter-like disfluencies (i.e. blocks, prolongations, syllable and sound repetitions). Five of the six children were male (which is consistent with the gender imbalance usually reported).

Except for the equal gender ratio reported in one study (Graça, 2001), the prevalence data found in the above studies are in agreement with the literature for other languages (Bloodstein & Ratner, 2008). To the best of our knowledge, there are no studies on the prevalence of stuttering in adults in Brazil.

4 Studies about Linguistic, Auditory and Behavioral Aspects of Stuttering

4.1 Linguistic aspects

Andrade reported three qualitative studies on the natural history of stuttering in childhood about: (1) fluency patterns; (2) the oromyofunctional system and its functions; (3) vocabulary, phonology and pragmatics. The purpose was to compare children with and without a family history of stuttering on all these aspects. Participants in the first study (Andrade, 2002a) were five children, two with and three without ancestors who stuttered. Dividing the small samples that were started with in this way would reduce power further. Age ranged between 24 and 60 months of age. Two hypotheses were formulated: (1) that children of the group with a family history of stuttering would present with a greater impairment of fluency than those without a family history; (2) that the degree of genetic relatedness of relatives who stuttered would be related to the degree of impairment in fluency. The study partially confirmed the first hypothesis: the children with family members who stuttered showed a greater number of stuttered and non-stuttered disfluencies but they did not differ from those without family members who stuttered with respect to speech rate. The second hypothesis was not confirmed. A limitation of this study was the small sample size.

The second study (Andrade, 2002b) used a similar small sample in which ages ranged between 30 and 60 months. The goal was to investigate whether children with and without genetic antecedents differed in the acquisition and development of aspects of the oromyofunctional system (sucking, swallowing, chewing and feeding). No differences were observed between the two groups but again it should be noted that the sample size was low.

In the third study (Andrade, 2002c), performed on the same participants as in study two, the purpose was to compare the two groups for lexical, phonologic and pragmatic aspects. Again no differences were found.

Degiovani *et al.* (1999) analyzed the types and frequency of disfluencies (see below) in the speech of 49 children according to age and gender. Participants were 23 boys and 26 girls aged between 3 and 5.11 years. The most frequently observed disfluencies were filled pauses, word and phrase repetitions. Least frequent were blocks, broken words, prolongations and part-word repetitions. No age differences were observed. The boys presented with more disfluencies than the girls but the difference was small (21.17% versus 19.58%), and was probably not statistically significant (no further information was provided).

Andrade *et al.* (2003) evaluated 70 individuals who had been diagnosed as stutterers at the University of São Paulo with the aim of investigating the relationship between stuttering severity and speech rate. All participants were above the age of 18 years and there were 51 males and 19 females. Fluency (stuttering severity) was determined using a translation of the SSI-3 (Stuttering Severity Instrument, Riley, 1994). Speech rate was measured in terms of both the number of words per minute (as an index of 'information production') and the number of syllables per minute (as an index of 'articulation transition ability'). There was a significant positive correlation between stuttering severity and speech rate, both in terms of words per minute and in terms of syllables per minute. The more severe the stuttering was, the fewer the number words produced per minute and the lower was the person's articulation ability.

Souza and Andrade (2004) investigated speech fluency and language of children who were born preterm. Fourteen neurologically normal children between 2 and 3 years of age who had a birth weight below 2500 g were examined. They analyzed type of disfluencies, speech rate and frequency of disfluencies. Results on subgroups of the sample (divided by gestational age and birth weight) were compared and results were also compared with reference norms for Brazilian children. Statistically significant differences on frequency of disfluencies were found according to gestational age and birth weight. The rate of disfluencies was significantly higher in the group with a gestational age between 32 and 33 weeks than in the group with a gestational age between 34 and 36 weeks and was also higher in the group with 'extreme' or 'very low' birth weight when compared to the group with 'low' birth weight. The overall sample in this study had means that were significantly low according to Brazilian norms for both normal and stuttered disfluencies and for speech rate. The authors concluded that preterm children showed an unbalanced fluency pattern in comparison with full-term children, and considered that this would have implications on discourse abilities and articulatory aspects of speech control.

Juste and Andrade (2006) studied the influence of type of disfluency and grammatical class on the occurrence of disfluencies in stuttering and fluent children. There were 80 children, 40 in each group. Both the stuttering and the fluent group consisted of 29 boys and 11 girls, aged between 4 and 11.11 years. There was no difference between the two groups for normal disfluencies (hesitations, interjections, revisions, unfinished words, word and phrase repetitions) but stuttered disfluencies (sound and syllable repetitions, prolongations, blocks, tense pauses, sound intrusions) occurred significantly more often in the stuttering children. Both groups had more disfluencies on function words. It was also observed that normal disfluencies occurred mainly on function words whereas stuttered disfluencies occurred equally often on lexical words as function words. This led to the conclusion that normal disfluencies seem to be influenced by grammatical class whereas stuttered disfluencies are not since they occurred in both word classes.

Martins and Andrade (2008) studied the fluency pattern of 392 fluent speakers of both genders (100 preschoolers and school children each, 130 adolescents, four groups of adults between 18 and 60 each with 34 participants, and four groups from 60 till 99 years with 36, 48, 31 and 13 participants respectively). The age range was an impressive 2–99 years (the intention was to study variation of fluency across the lifespan). Spontaneous speech samples were collected and analyzed following the procedure of Andrade (2004), looking at type and frequency of disfluencies and speech rate (syllables and words per minute). The study concluded that the pattern of disfluencies did not show much variation across this age span, whereas speaking rate appeared to be lower in childhood (<12.0 years), increased in adolescence (12.0 to 17.11 years) and adulthood (18.0 to 59.11) and decreased again at old age (>80 years). In 2010 the same authors investigated the variation of fluency in 128 elderly above the age of 60 and observed an increase in speech disruptions and confirmed a decrease in speaking rate above the age of 80 (Andrade & Martins, 2010).

As this section shows, studies on stuttering characteristics in speakers of Brazilian Portuguese have looked at a variety of aspects. These include type and frequency of disfluencies, speech rate, variation according to age, gender, genetic factors and medical status (gestational age, birth weight). The relationship between stuttering severity and speech rate and the distribution of disfluencies among grammatical classes have also been studied. Most studies so far have examined children. There are no studies that directly compared disfluency characteristics in speakers of Brazilian Portuguese with those seen in speakers of English. From the studies discussed above it would seem that patterns in Brazilian Portuguese do not differ substantially from what has been found for English but, of course, this needs confirmation.

4.2 Auditory aspects

Studies that investigated the auditory performance of people who stutter were initiated in Brazil by Andrade and Schochat (1999). They compared data from a fluency analysis (Campbell & Hill, 1994) and an analysis of auditory processing (dichotic digits and non-verbal test, frequency and duration pattern sequences test) in 10 adults (aged between 20 and 40 years) with developmental stuttering who had no concomitant disorders (no auditory, cognitive or neurological disorders). They reported that the impairment of fluency was accompanied by alterations in auditory processing. Participants that presented problems in the duration pattern sequences test showed high rates of pauses and prolongations. Participants that presented problems in the frequency pattern sequences test presented not only high rates on pause and prolongations, but also on repetitions. The two participants with the most severe stuttering were the only ones that had problems on the three auditory processing tests. The degree of alteration was also linked to the degree of stuttering. For instance, the more severe the stuttering the more difficulty they exhibited in the frequency patterns sequence test.

Schiefer *et al.* (1999) also conducted a study on the relationship between stuttering and central auditory disorders. In their 120 participants they too found a correlation between stuttering and a functional alteration of hearing (as demonstrated in a series of tests of central auditory processing developed at the Speech and Language Pathology and Audiology Department of the Federal University of São Paulo). However, they did not find that the degree of alteration in auditory processing deficit was linked to the degree of stuttering. Some years later another study, this time by Andrade *et al.* (2008d), investigated performance of the right and left ear separately. They used an extensive battery of tests of auditory processing developed by Pereira and Schochat (1997), in 56 individuals aged 4–34 years with different severity of stuttering (as assessed by the translated SSI-3). It was observed that in tests with verbal material overall, the performance of the right ear was better, but that stuttering severity had no influence.

Angrisani *et al.* (2009) sought possible correlations between auditory aspects and fluency. The study employed auditory evoked potentials (short and middle latency response and P300) in people who stutter and a documented history of the speech therapy the participants had received was available. Sixteen individuals aged between 18 and 30 years, eight of whom presented with developmental stuttering, participated in the study. The study showed a non-significant tendency towards altered evoked responses (shorter latency times) in the stuttering group at the end of the treatment which was interpreted by the authors as a sign of improvement or neural plasticity.

The studies presented in this section showed changes in auditory processing in people who stutter and apparently there is some relation between types of auditory processing difficulty and types of disfluencies. Thus far, these findings did not result in proposals for therapeutic approaches.

4.3 Behavioral aspects

In the following section we describe some studies that shed light on behavioral aspects of stuttering. The term 'behavioral' is used here in a broad sense to include a large variety of aspects not considered to now in this review.

There are a number of studies that used acoustic analysis for studying stuttering behavior. One was by Britto Pereira (2001) who performed an acoustic analysis of the disfluencies in the speech of 21 adults with developmental stuttering. The findings showed that persons who stutter do not produce 'repetitions' of sounds, syllables, words and phrases since from the phonetic point of view the repeated productions were different from the final word. This suggests that the repetitions in reality are attempts to produce a different word. These findings are contrary to those reported by Howell and Vause's (1986) study which was replicated by Viswanath and Neel (1995). Another interesting aspect that this study showed regards blocks and prolongations of plosives. In this sound class what is called a block is in reality a prolongation of the closed phase of the sound, as evidenced by an analysis of VOT.

Britto Pereira *et al.* (2003) analyzed the duration of consonants in samples of spontaneous speech in 20 adults and adolescents with developmental stuttering. For this analysis only perceptibly fluent words were selected for examination and the duration of the consonants in syllable-initial position was measured using the program WinPitch. The data were compared with reference values for normal consonant duration (Reis, 1995). It was reported that consonant duration in fluent words was less in people who stutter than in fluent speakers. One interpretation of these findings is that people who stutter increased speaking rate at fluent moments in order to compensate for non-fluent moments, maintaining in this way the balance of the prosodic structure of their utterances that some authors refer to as a local rate change (Howell & Sackin, 2000; Howell *et al.*, 1999; Viswanath, 1989).

To further examine phonetic properties of utterances, Arcuri *et al.* (2009) compared the speech rate in a sentence-repetition task in persons with different degrees of developmental stuttering. Three males and three females with a mean age of 26.2 years participated in the study. The participants with mild and moderate stuttering demonstrated similar and greater speech rates values than the group with severe stuttering, indicating that the more severe the stuttering is, the smaller the speech rate. In another study (Arcuri *et al.*, 2010), the same authors compared the duration of words in six adults with different degrees of developmental stuttering, also in a sentence-repetition task. The study showed that segment duration differed between stuttering and non-stuttering participants and also that the more severe the stuttering was, the longer the duration.

Oliveira *et al.* (2009) analyzed vocal characteristics in stuttering adults. There were 15 participants aged between 21 and 41 years. Acoustic parameters analyzed were quality and type of voice, vocal tension, resonance, speaking rate, vocal-respiratory coordination, vocal attack and pitch range. Variability of fundamental frequency was also measured. It was found that the most frequent parameters that changed during stutters were vocal tension, pitch range and vocal-respiratory coordination.

Brabo and Schiefer (2009) investigated verbal and non-verbal performance in individuals who stutter in order to determine whether early onset stuttering compromises non-verbal praxis. They assessed 40 adults, 20 who had no communication problems and 20 who stuttered. They found with respect to verbal praxis that the stuttering group, as expected, exhibited a greater number of stuttered and non-stuttered disfluencies than the control group. As far as non-verbal praxis was concerned, there was no difference between the stuttering and the non-stuttering participants, and as such the hypothesis that early onset stuttering may compromise non-verbal praxis was not confirmed.

Studies using external electromyography during speech tasks and non-speech tasks were conducted by Andrade *et al.* (2008a) so that muscle activity in fluent and stuttering individuals could be compared. The results showed that there was no difference at rest in electromyographic activity between the two groups. People who stuttered had longer reaction times than fluent speakers. Another finding was that laryngeal muscular activity during speech was not different in the two groups with the exception of the suprahyoid muscle which showed lower muscular activity during the reaction time in people who stutter. Muscular activity during non-verbal tasks at rest was similar to what was seen for all muscles at rest which was not the case with the fluent speakers. The latter group showed greater activity in the musculus orbicularis inferior (a lip muscle) in non-verbal tasks than at rest, suggesting a readiness of the motor system for this activity. The lack of such a readiness in stuttering individuals could be due to deficient timing between planning and motor processes in speech, reflecting an increased latency to start verbal activities, which in turn led to speech disruptions.

The temperament of children who stutter was investigated by Andrade *et al.* (2004). They compared the perception of temperament of the parents of stuttering and non-stuttering children. Participants were 40 fathers and/or mothers, 20 of stuttering children and 20 of non-stuttering children. Data were collected using a multiple-choice scale for temperament characteristics, composed of seven questions related to the family perception about the behavior of the children in relation to unknown objects and people, the distance of the parents, time needed to interact with strangers, behavior in group situations and fears in environmental changes. Results did not indicate differences between stuttering and fluently speaking children. The authors suggested that stuttering children and their parents suffer stereotypes held by the public in general and by professionals who are not up to date with current knowledge.

In order to investigate the influence of speaking ability on the life quality of fluently speaking individuals and people who stutter, Andrade *et al.* (2008b) studied 40 adults, divided into two groups matched for gender and age: a group of fluent speakers and a group of persons with developmental stuttering. All participants filled out the adult version of the Protocolo de Auto-Avaliação (Self Assessment Protocol, Campanatti & Andrade, 2000), that is composed of three thematic sections: one relating to affective aspects, one on behavioral aspects and one on cognitive aspects. In addition stuttering severity was assessed in the non-fluent group using the SSI-3. Results indicated differences between the two groups as to perception of speech and fluency and its functioning generating a negative impact on the life quality of people who stutter. Severity of the fluency disorder, however, did not influence the results.

5 Studies on the Assessment and Treatment of Stuttering

5.1 Assessment

A study by Van Borsel and Britto Pereira (2005) investigated whether persons who are knowledgeable about stuttering were able to judge disfluency in languages other than their own. The study was conducted in Belgium and Brazil. Twenty-eight final-year students in speech language pathology, 14 from a university in Rio de Janeiro who spoke Brazilian Portuguese, and 14 from a University in Gent who spoke Dutch were asked to identify and judge stuttering in individuals speaking Portuguese and Dutch. They had to watch two films, one of speakers of Dutch and one of speakers of Portuguese, which showed, at random, people who stuttered and people who do not stutter. The study showed that judges can make a similar judgment in a native and a foreign language, although both groups of judges were of the opinion that assessment in a foreign language was more difficult.

Van Borsel *et al.* (2008) investigated further the influence of the closeness to the listener's native language when identifying stuttering in an unfamiliar language. To that end the film showing speakers of Dutch was presented to a group of speakers of English and the results of that group were compared with those of the Dutch and Portuguese judges.

It was found that speakers of Dutch and English (both West Germanic Languages) performed better in identifying Dutch people who stutter and people who did not stutter than did the panel speaking Brazilian Portuguese (a Romance language). This suggests that closeness of the language does play a role in judging stuttering in a foreign language.

Studies on the assessment of behavior and attitude of people who stutter in speech situations are being developed in Rio de Janeiro, based on the *Behavior Assessment Battery* of Brutten and Vanryckeghem (2003, 2007). The test batteries for adults and children have been translated and adapted for Brazilian Portuguese and studies with stuttering and fluent children are running. As far as stuttering children are concerned, no correlation is seen between stuttering severity and the scores on the test battery, contrary to what was observed in studies in Belgium and the United States. There is, however, a correlation between attitude and emotions in communication situations indicating that the negative emotions experienced by stuttering children in speech situations can lead to a negative attitude towards communication (Moraes, 2010). The results with regard to fluent children indicate an increasingly worsening attitude with age but no gender differences (Britto Pereira *et al.*, 2009).

5.2 Treatment

In relation to childhood stuttering, Oliveira *et al.* (2010) investigated the possible contribution that advice to the family about speech fluency makes to children who stutter. Twenty children and their parents participated in the study. An initial assessment of the type and frequency of disfluencies was performed before giving advice. The advice was aimed at promoting fluency and included suggestions about how to interact with the child, how to model speech and how to react to the stuttering. The advice to the family was given in up to two sessions and a summary of the suggestions was provided on a flyer. After 30 days the children were re-evaluated using the same procedures as at the initial assessment. With respect to the type of disfluencies which were examined separately, comparison of the two evaluations showed that occurrence rate of four of six normal disfluencies and five of six stuttered disfluencies decreased. Seventy percent of the children demonstrated a significant reduction of the percentage of the disfluencies overall (normal and stuttered) and 80% showed a significant reduction in rate of stuttered disfluencies.

Andrade *et al.* (2008c) conducted a study to investigate the use of electromyography in the treatment of stuttering. The study involved four adults with developmental stuttering without co-morbid disorders. The treatment incorporated fluency-enhancing techniques such as negative practice, the use of smooth movements, timing control and flexibility of the parameters of speech, from the Programa Fonoaudiológico de

Promoção de Fluência (Andrade, 2003). The treatment consisted of 12 weekly sessions of 20 minutes during each of which fluency-enhancing techniques were used, and performance was monitored electromyographically. The results showed a significant reduction of both stuttered and normal disfluencies but no increase in speech rate. It was concluded that surface EMG provides a sensitive measure to assess the effects of treatment.

Van Borsel *et al.* (2010) investigated the use of delayed auditory feedback in a case of neurogenic stuttering in a 49-year-old Brazilian man who started to stutter after traumatic brain injury. Delayed auditory feedback did not have an unequivocal positive effect on speech fluency. The results suggested that delayed auditory feedback may have a different effect in individuals with neurogenic stuttering than in individuals with developmental stuttering. The study also concluded that further investigation of the effects of DAF in cases of neurogenic stuttering as compared to developmental stuttering is necessary.

6 Conclusion

The studies reported not only show the evolution of the research on stuttering conducted in Brazil, but also give rise to some reflections. Although the various studies investigating knowledge about stuttering in certain social groups show that knowledge is limited, there are no programs to instruct the Brazilian population to improve that knowledge. Considering that Brazil has 200 million inhabitants and that the estimated prevalence of stuttering is 1%, it is clear that there is a large number of people in the country who need advice and treatment. Unfortunately there are few centers specialized in the treatment of stuttering in the country and for the greater part they are to be found in the South East, in the state of São Paulo.

There is also a need for studies on the effectiveness of different therapy approaches in Brazil. There is only one study reporting the successful use of surface electromyography in treatment. However, due to the cost of the equipment and the special knowledge required, this approach is but seldom used. The treatment approaches for stuttering that are currently available were almost always developed in the United States and Europe and often are not compatible with the more casual lifestyle in Brazil. It is for instance not easy to motivate people who stutter to change their speech pattern and to use the techniques learned in therapy in everyday life, or to motivate parents to attend therapy with assiduity. This may be even more the case in more remote areas that have less access to health care facilities, to libraries or internet, and where illiteracy rate is still high.

We can also conclude from this overview that the vast majority of studies is published in national journals, which hampers dissemination of research findings internationally. A significant step forward was made, however, with the organization of the 6th World Congress of Fluency Disorders in 2009 at the Veiga de Almeida University in Rio de Janeiro. This event brought together 130 participants from 27 different countries.

References

Andrade, C.R.F. (1997) Prevalência das desordens idiopáticas da fala e da linguagem em crianças de um a onze anos de idade. *Revista Saúde Pública* 31(5), 495–501.

Andrade, C.R.F. (2002a) História natural da gagueira – estudo I: Perfil da fluência. *Pró-Fono Revista de Atualização Científica* 14(3), 351–360.

Andrade, C.R.F. (2002b) História natural da gagueira – estudo II: Sistema Miofuncional oral e funções. *Pró-Fono Revista de Atualização Científica* 14(3), 361–370.

Andrade, C.R.F. (2002c) História natural da gagueira – estudo III: Vocabulário, fonologia e pragmática. *Pró-Fono Revista de Atualização Científica* 14(3), 371–382.

Andrade, C.R.F. (2003) Programa Fonoaudiológico de promoção da fluência em adultosgagos: Tratamento e manutenção. In S.C.O. Limongi (organizador) *Fonoaudiologia informação para formação – procedimentos terapêuticos em linguagem.* Rio de Janeiro: Guanabara-Koogan.

Andrade, C.R.F. (2004) Fluencia. In C.R.F. Andrade, D.M. Befi-Lopes, F.D.M. Fernandes and H.F. Wertzner. *Teste de Linguagem infantile nas areas de fonologia, vocabulario, fluencia e pragmatic.* 2a ed (pp. 51–82). Barueri: Pro Fono.

Andrade, C.R.F. and Martins, V.O. (2010) Variação da fluência da fala em idosos. *Pró-Fono Revista de Atualização Científica* 22(1), 13–18.

Andrade, C.R.F. and Schochat, E. (1999) Comparação entre os achados neurolinguísticos e neuroaudiológicos nas gagueiras. *Pró-Fono Revista de Atualização Científica* 11(2), 27–30.

Andrade, C.R.F., Cervone, L.M. and Sassi, F.C. (2003) Relationship between the stuttering severity index and speech rate. *São Paulo Medical Journal* 121(2), 81–84.

Andrade, C.R.F., Sassi, F.C. and Meira, M.I.M. (2008a) Atividades de fala e não fala em gagueira: Estudo preliminar. *Pró-Fono Revista de Atualização Científica* 20, 67–70.

Andrade, C.R.F., Sassi, F.Q., Juste, F.S. and Ercolin, B. (2008b) Modelamento da fluência com o uso da eletromiografia de superfície: Estudo piloto. *Pró-Fono Revista de Atualização Científica* 20(2), 129–132.

Andrade, C.R.F., Sassi, F.Q., Juste, F.S. and Ercolin, B. (2008c) Qualidade de vida em indivíduos com gagueira desenvolvimental persistente. *Pró-Fono Revista de Atualização Científica* 20(4), 219–224.

Andrade, C.R.F., Sepulcre, A.S., Romano, M.V.R., Juste, F. and Sassi, F.C. (2004) Percepção de pais de crianças gagas e fluentes sobre as características de temperamento de seus filhos. *Revista da Sociedade Brasileira de Fonoaudiologia* 9(4), 205–210.

Andrade, N.A., Gil, D., Schiefer, A.M. and Pereira, L.D. (2008d) Processamento auditivo em gagos: Análise do desempenho das orelhas direita e esquerda. *Revista da Sociedade Brasileira de Fonoaudiologia* 13(1), 20–29.

Angrisani, R.M.G., Matas, C.G., Neves, I.F., Sassi, F.C. and Andrade, C.R.F. (2009) Avaliação eletrofisiológica da audição em gagos, pré e pós terapia fonoaudiológica. *Pró-Fono Revista de Atualização Científica* 21(2), 95–100.

Arcuri, C.F., Osborn, E., Schiefer, A.M. and Chiari, B.M. (2009) Taxa de elocução de fala segundo a gravidade da gagueira. *Pró-Fono Revista de Atualização Científica* 21(1), 45–50.

Arcuri, C.F., Osborn, E., Schiefer, A.M. and Chiari, B.M. (2010) Duração do *onset* vocálico da fala fluente de gagos. *Revista de Sociedade Brasileira de Fonoaudiologia* 15(1), 108–114.

Bloodstein, O. and Bernstein Ratner, N.B. (2008) *A Handbook on Stuttering* (6th edn). Clifton Park, NY: Thomson-Delmar.

Brabo, N.C. and Schiefer, A.M. (2009) Habilidades de praxia verbal e não-verbal em indivíduos gagos. *Revista CEFAC* 11(4), 554–560.

Britto Pereira, M.M. (2001) *Análise linguística da gagueira*. Tese de Doutorado. Programa de Pós Graduação em Estudos Linguísticos. Belo Horizonte: Universidade Federal de Minas Gerais.

Britto Pereira, M.M., Costa, C.A.S and Onofre, A.C. (2007) Prevalencia de alterações da fluencia em uma instituição publica. In 15 Congresso Brasileiro de Fonoaudiologia – 7 Congresso Internacional de Fonoaudiologia, Gramado. *Revista da Sociedade Brasileira de Fonoaudiologia – Suplemento Especial.*

Britto Pereira, M.M., Perni Rossi, J. and Van Borsel, J. (2008) Public awareness and knowledge of stuttering in Rio de Janeiro. *Journal of Fluency Disorders* 33, 24–31.

Britto Pereira, M.M., Ferrante, C., Cohen, C. and Carvalho, G.G.T. (2003) Análise da duração de consoantes na fala fluente de gagos. *Revista da Sociedade Brasileira de Fonoaudiologia* 2, 14–18.

Britto Pereira, M.M., Silva, F.H., Moraes, C.S., Esteves, T., Brutten G.J. and Vanryckeghem, M. (2009) Behavior assessment battery – normative data for Brazilian fluent children. New Orleans, ASHA Convention, November 2009.

Brutten, G. and Vanryckeghem, M. (2003) *Behavior Assessment Battery: A multidimensional and Evidence-Based Approach to Diagnostic and Therapeutic Decision Making for Adults Who Stutter.* Organization for the Integration of Handicapped People, Belgium & Acco Publishers, Netherlands.

Brutten, G. and Vanryckeghem, M. (2007) *Behavior Assessment Battery for School Age Children who Stutter.* San Diego: Plural Publishing.

Calais L.L., Jorge, T.M. and Pinheiro-Crenite, P.A. (2002) Conhecimento dos professores do ensino fundamental sobre a gagueira. *Pró-Fono Revista de Atualização Científica* 14(1), 23–30.

Campanatti-Ostiz, H. and Andrade, C.R.F. (2000) Gagueira: Manutenção, generalização e transferência. *Pró-Fono Revista de Atualização Científica* 12(2), 121–130.

Campbell, J.G. and Hill, D.G. (1994) *Systematic Dysfluency Analysis*. Evanston: Northwestern University.

Chiquetto, M.M. (1996) Reflexões sobre a gagueira: Concepções e atitudes dos professores. *Pró-Fono Revista de Atualização Científica* 8(1), 13–18.

Cibotto,T.E. and Schiefer, A.M. (2001) O conhecimento sobre a gagueira apresentado pelos pais de crianças gagas: Senso comum. São Paulo, *Fono Atual* 4, 16, 31–38.

Degiovani, V.M., Chiari, B.M. and Schiefer, A.M. (1999) Disfluencia: Caracterização dos tipos e frequência de ocorrência em um grupo de escolares. *Pró-Fono Revista de Atualização Científica* 11(1), 32–37.

Ferriolli, B.H.V.M., Leitão, P.M. and Pereira, E.L.F. (2005) O conhecimento e as atitudes dos professores frente à gagueira. JBF. *Jornal Brasileiro de Fonoaudiologia* 5(22), 321–330.

Graça, C.M.L. (2001) *Perfil epidemiológico dos usuários do projeto olímpico do programa social do grêmio recreativo escola de samba estação primeira de mangueira.* Dissertação de Mestrado. Rio de Janeiro: Mestrado Profissional em Fonoaudiologia, Universidade Veiga de Almeida.

Howell, P. and Sackin, S. (2000) Speech rate modification and its effects on fluency reversal in fluent speakers and people who stutter. *Journal of Developmental and Physical Disabilities* 12, 291–315.

Howell, P. and Vause, L. (1986) Acoustic analysis and perception of vowels in stuttered speech. *Journal of the Acoustical Society of America* 79, 1571–1579.

Howell, P., Au-Yeung, J. and Pilgrim, L. (1999) Utterance rate and linguistic properties as determinants of speech dysfluency in children who stutter. *Journal of the Acoustical Society of America* 105, 481–490.

Juste, F. and Andrade, C.R.F. (2006) Tipologia das rupturas de fala e classes gramaticais em crianças gagas e fluentes. *Pró-Fono Revista de Atualização Científica* 18(2), 129–140.

Martins, V.O. and Andrade, C.R.F. (2008) Perfil evolutivo da fluência da fala de falantes do Português Brasileiro. *Pró-Fono Revista de Atualização Científica* 20(1), 7–12.

Moraes, C.S. (2010) *Tradução, adaptação e padronização de instrumento de avaliação do comportamento e da atitude na comunicação em crianças que gaguejam.* Dissertação de Mestrado. Rio de Janeiro: Mestrado Profissional em Fonoaudiologia, Universidade Veiga de Almeida.

Oliveira, A.M.C.C., Ribeiro, I.M., Merlo, S. and Chiappetta, A.L.M.L. (2007) O que fonoaudiólogos e estudantes de fonoaudiologia entendem por fluência e disfluência. *Revista CEFAC* 9(1), 40–46.

Oliveira, B.F.V., Soares, E.Q.W., Azevedo, L.L. and Britto, D.B.O. (2009) Análise de parâmetros perceptivo-auditivos e acústicos em indivíduos gagos. *Revista da Sociedade Brasileira de Fonoaudiologia* 14(3), 323–331.

Oliveira, C.M.C., Yasunaga, C.N., Sebastião, L.T. and Nascimento, E.N. (2010) Orientação familiar e seus efeitos na gagueira infantil. *Revista da Sociedade Brasileira de Fonoaudiologia* 15(1), 115–124.

Pereira, L.D. and Schochat, E. (1997) *Processamento auditivo central: Manual de avaliação.* 1ª ed. São Paulo: Lovise.

Reis, C. (1995) *L'Interaction entre l'accent, l'intonation et le rythme en portugais brésilien.* These de Doctorat. Aix en Provence: Université de Provence.

Sassi, F.C. and Andrade, C.R.F. (2004) Eletromiografia de superfície e o tratamento da gagueira: Uma perspectiva neuromotora. *Revista da Sociedade Brasileira de Fonoaudiologia* 9(1), 55–60.

Schiefer, A.M., Barbosa, L.M.G. and Pereira, L.D. (1999) Considerações preliminares entre uma possível correlação entre gagueira e os aspectos lingüísticos e auditivos. *Pró-Fono Revista de Atualização Científica* 11(1), 27–31.

Silveira, P.C.M., Cunha, D.A., Fontes, M.L., Lima, E.A., Farias, P.S. and Lucena, J.A. (2002) A importância da prevenção à gagueira nas escolas. *Revista Fono atual* 5(22), 12–27.

Souza, R. and Andrade, C.R.F. (2004) O perfil da fluência de fala e linguagem de crianças nascidas pré-termo, *Pediatria* 26(2), 90–96.

St Louis, K.O., Andrade, C.R.F., Georgieva, D. and Troudt, O.F. (2005) Experiênciae relato pessoal sobre pesquisa de cooperação internacional – Brasil, Bulgária e Turquia – que avalia as atitudes em relação à gagueira. *Pró-Fono Revista de Atualização Científica* 17(3), 413–416.

Van Borsel, J. and Britto Pereira, M.M. (2005) Assessment of stuttering in a familiar versus unfamiliar language. *Journal of Fluency Diso*rders 30, 109–124.

Van Borsel, J., Drummond, D. and Britto Pereira, M.M. (2010) Delayed auditory feedback and acquired neurogenic stuttering. *Journal of Neurolinguistics* 23, 479–487.

Van Borsel, J., Leahy, M.M. and Britto Pereira, M.M. (2008) Judging stuttering in an unfamiliar language: The importance of closeness to the native language. *Clinical Linguistics and Phonetics* 22(1), 59–67.

Van Borsel, J., Verniers, I. and Bouvry, S. (1999) Public awareness of stuttering. *Folia Phoniatrica et Logopaedica* 51, 124–132.

Viswanath, N.S. (1989) Global-temporal and local-temporal effects of a stutteringevent in the context of a clausal utterance. *Journal of Fluency Disorders* 14, 245–269.

Viswanath, N.S. and Neel, A.T. (1995) Part-word repetitions by persons who stutter: Fragment types and their articulatory processes. *Journal of Speech and Hearing Research* 38, 740–750.

Chapter 10

A Survey on Traditional Treatment Practices for Stuttering in Sub-Saharan Africa

ANNE-MARIE SIMON

Summary

Animism is the idea that souls or spirits exist not only in humans and animals, but also in natural phenomena, like rocks and geographic features, as well as other entities in the natural environment. Humans are assumed to have souls that exist apart from their bodies before and after death. There is a triangular relationships between humans, animals and the saintly. Because of the widespread belief in animism, people who stutter in Africa may be considered to be damned, bring bad luck to the community, and to be possessed by evil spirits. These people are often excluded from their community. Stuttering is regarded in a different way, compared to the Western world. Treatments are preceded by rituals, magic spells and formulae that have been passed down from father to son. There are many different treatment approaches to stuttering in this area. Perhaps the most striking such treatments involve cruel and unusual practices, such as starvation, strangulation, cutting and burning.

1 Introduction

This chapter reports the results of a survey that was conducted in 2005. It is not concerned with language but cultural influences that may affect approaches to stuttering. The survey concerned traditional practices for the treatment of stuttering in sub-Saharan Africa. It is necessary to describe animism which is the framework within which the traditional practices occur before the results of the survey are reported, It is important to realize that I am not an ethnologist or a sociologist, but a qualified speech pathologist observing and reporting on these practices. With the risk of disappointing you, I will not offer an interpretation of the behaviors and the rites/rituals or practices that were reported. The intention is to describe the practices without value judgment where possible. No comparison or judgment is made about the practices with those usually practiced in the West. When this is done by other writers, it is often with a feeling of superiority with respect to the black world.

2 Animism

Animism is the philosophical, religious or spiritual idea that souls or spirits exist not only in humans but also in other animals, plants, rocks, natural phenomena such as thunder, geographic features like mountains or rivers, and other entities in the natural environment. The concept that humans possess souls and that souls have a life apart from human bodies before and after death are central to animism. Another tenet of animism is the ideas that animals, plants and celestial bodies have spirits. We will find this belief within the various treatments for stuttering. The practices that result use tools and plants, and assume that the plants have a spirit that is able to intervene in the disorder of stuttering.

It is estimated that about 40% of the world's population has perspectives that finds their origin in animism. Animism as a treatment for disease in general is widely practiced in many countries and is present, to some degree, in all cultures. Africa is the continent where animism is practiced most often (by 72 million people) followed by Asia (58 million) and South America (12.7 million).

In the animist universe, and thus in the black African universe, everything that is alive, even the simplest appearance or the slightest sign that one can feel, has a specific power. Every single being irrespective of age and status has a soul that gives it power (anima is the Latin word for soul). A widespread belief is that animists in Africa have a pre-logical mentality and their life is ruled by superstition, irrational beliefs, barbarian practices and meaningless rituals.

My first contact with animism was in Dogon country in Mali where I was very impressed by cosmogony. Cosmogony is the process in animism by which sacred places and concepts come into existence (e.g. the origin of the universe).This was described clearly by Marcel Griaule (Griaule, 1935a, 1935b, 1938a, 1938b; Griaule & Dieterlen, 1950). Reading this work changed my condescending perception towards African concepts and I became interested in the people of Africa, animist treatments of stuttering and so on, in their own right. This was a difficult transition for someone brought up in a Western culture to make. I tried to find out about traditional practice in the animist approach beginning with observations made in Douala. The first observation made in Douala was that the suffering caused by the disorder is as great in African, as it is in Western, countries.

Like other religions, traditional African religion explains the mysteries of life and death. Animism proposes that the soul exists independent of the physical body in order to explain the difference between a living thing and the same thing when it is dead.

The creator, or 'Great Spirit', as it is called in Benin, gives part of his own vital power that circulates in the universe to animals and objects. Life in the world is nothing but an exchange of powers. The creator does not intervene, and remains inaccessible and has no visible form. There are intermediate gods (both good and evil) who are divine beings, spirits or genies that inhabit the elements (the wilderness, the waters, the river, the earth, etc.). These gods are stronger than man and have specific functions that relate to their element. Animists feel related to the creatures of the world. All the objects, plants and animals are partners of man. *Hence one can consider animism as a triangular relationship between nature, human beings and the saintly.*

Knowledge about the saintly individuals is only accessible to certain persons who have been initiated. The Africans attribute this state to several types of person, for example, fortune-tellers, medicine men, healers and shamans. These persons can contact the gods and put in a good word for you with the Great Spirit. The word of the shamans etc. has weight and gives them powers over illness, the elements of nature and human beings and, because of the range of their abilities, they are consulted in many circumstances. They interpret the messages and present gifts to the gods for anyone who consults them. The spirits can be pleased by offerings, by practicing rituals or observing taboos. The initiated are consulted about the origin of the evil that affects a person or a village.

Thus, animism extends across living things, dead beings, genies and spirits. It has a strong social dimension insofar as the perspective influences the offspring, the village and even the community. It is an inherent part of the daily life of individuals and the communities in which they live. Numerous rites mark out the most important stages of life (birth, puberty, burial) with which the gods are associated. Every family has its own techniques to enter into contact with the deceased. Music, masks and costumes (worn by initiated dancers) facilitate the entrances of worshippers in the holy ceremonies, especially those involving initiation rights.

The secret forces are called on through contracts and agreements based on magic (white and black magic). One cannot, therefore, talk about animism without talking about magic. For instance, when an object has become a fetish, incarnated by a spirit that gives it its power, this power comes from magic substances which it contains (supernatural magic power which can be good or evil).

Sorcery, the intervention of evil magic and demons, is common in black Africa. A great many techniques of sorcery exist including casting spells, exorcism, hypnosis, magic fits and insertion of objects into the body. It will be seen that some of these magic practices are behind animist treatments for stuttering although it is not always possible to trace why they are considered effective.

3 The Survey

Two hundred people who stutter from all over black Africa contacted the author after three Radio France Internationale broadcasts (RFI). A questionnaire was designed to solicit information from them. Fifty of the 200 people who had contacted me returned the questionnaire. Additional questionnaires were obtained: (1) at the international conference of the International Stuttering Association (ISA) in Douala (2005); (2) at the school for speech therapy of Lomé (Togo) where students filled out the questionnaire; (3) from two speech therapists, one in Yaoundé (Claire Nkoué) and the other in Cotonou (Edith Ochoumaré. A copy of the questionnaire is included as Appendix A.

There were 69 questionnaires in total. Questionnaires from three children between 12 and 14 years of age were eliminated, one mother, one therapist and one incomplete questionnaire were also excluded. This left a total of 63 usable questionnaires.

There was a gender bias with 87.3% questionnaires from males (55 males, 4 females). All participants lived either in an urban area or close to such an area. The majority of the respondents sent the questionnaire by email (Internet access is not widespread in Africa and this suggests that the sample was biased to higher socio-economic groups). It is stressed that the samples are from particular populations and may not be generalizable to other groups (e.g. other socio-economic groups, to illiterate persons or to rural dwellers).

The participants were asked to specify their country, age, and whether they had other family members who stutter. All respondents lived in French-speaking African countries (Bénin, Burkina Fasso, Burundi, Cameroun, Congo Brazza, Côte d'Ivoire, Mali, Niger, RDC, Sénégal). The mean age of the respondents was 27 years. This ranged from 16 to 51 years with 84% (N = 54) between 18 and 38 years.

There was some reluctance to talk about treatments because they thought their forms were considered backward by Western people. Even the students from Togo experienced difficulty in giving responses on the subject of stuttering. This shows that stuttering is even more a taboo than it is in the West. It was emphasized on the questionnaire that respondents should not feel ashamed, that there were no taboos and answers were treated confidentially.

3.1 Traditional practices

Resulting from sorcery and being the object of superstition, stuttering brings about for those that undergo it mockery, disdain, injury and malediction because of not having made the sacrifices to the ancestors or the rites they deserve. Considered as damned, bringing bad luck for the community, people who stutter are sometimes excluded since they are considered as being possessed by an evil spirit. Stuttering is the work of sorcery, the result of an infringement or the wrath of an offended god.

3.2 Taxonomy of treatments

The responses about treatments were classified into the following categories: (1) Cruel practices; (2) Associated with fluids; (3) Associated with coverings; (4) Temporal factors (hour of the day, rhythm); (5) Involving plants and potions; (6) Rites or magic acts. These are discussed in the following sections.

3.2.1 Cruel practices

Uganda is an English-speaking country and, as such, it was excluded from the survey. However, one particularly horrific response to the occurrence of stuttering in that country needs to be reported. Based on testimony that I received, it appears that children are killed ritually if they have not stopped stuttering by the age of 7. Either they are strangled, suffocated or their parents let them die from hunger. The stuttering is seen as a spell put on the family and killing the child is considered to calm down the gods.

There are other forms of cruelty practiced in French-speaking African countries that can also lead to fatalities: One form is where children are not given food until they speak well and withdrawal of food has led to them dying from hunger. Another supposed cure involves burning the tongue with a hot knife. Children may be hit about the ears whilst they are sleeping. This has to be done in a way such that the children do not recognize who hit them; otherwise the person giving the beating will die within the year. Children were also reported to have to eat the droppings of an owl.

Some treatments force the child to speak in different ways. Children may be obliged to run 1 km every morning: The idea here is to make this unpleasant for the child so that he or she cries out and begs the parents to stop. Children's eyes have been covered with a bandage and they are then forced to call their friends so that they do not fall. Children have also been commanded to talk under the threat that, otherwise, they will be eaten by a lion or another wild animal (similar threats are made about wolves in French culture to get a child to do things that they do not wish to).

Children who stutter are grouped with the disabled such as those with amputated limbs, who are crippled or who are blind. These marginal groups are marginalized, ill-treated, beaten and even killed. They are isolated from their family and school environment and are kept apart from other children on the grounds that the others would imitate them. It was also reported that children who stutter are deprived from every contact with the outside world when the moon is full because of fear that their stuttering would increase and this is especially the case when the disorder has accompanying bodily movements.

The practice was also noted of violently throwing a wet cloth into the face of the one who stutters. The idea behind this is to pierce the person's skin. The guilt of having mocked other children who stutter appeared three times in the survey. Their own stuttering is then seen as a punishment. This punishment can be taken away by one of these abuses or by forces.

The frenulum is the flap of skin that lies on the midline under the tongue body. When children reach the age of 6 and are about to go to school, healers cut the frenulum if the child is still stuttering. This method was always reported to end in death due to hemorrhaging or blood-poisoning caused by traditional knifes.

3.2.2 Treatments associated with fluids

The association with running water is that fluent speech is seen to run as the water runs whereas stuttering does not. Several examples of this class were reported. One was to make the person suck stones drawn from a riverbed. A healer reported that he used seaplants and had stutterers drink seawater to cure their problem. Drinking water after rain showers where the water was collected in the cavity of a tree, or from a bend in the river where animal spirits are supposed to be strong, was also reported. It was also required that speakers should drink water that a rooster left after it had drunk (this involves an association between water and song), or to drink the rest of the dishwater in the kitchen. Other cures were to drink water that was put in the pot to facilitate cleaning after cooking a porridge of cereals the day after and similarly for water put in a tam-tam (a percussion instrument similar to a gong). The water was left in the open air and had to be drunk the next day.

A more complicated form involved the person bathing in a mixture of ashes and cooked guava leaves. They then have to drink part of it, and to throw the rest in the river so that it takes the curse with it. In this way, the forgiveness of the spirits is obtained. In order that fluency and water can be brought closer together, one of the healers told us to forbid sticky and gluey things to the patient during treatment.

Interestingly, for different reasons from the West, the idea of speaking whilst standing next to a waterfall is also advocated. The speaker shouts and by shouting the speaker drinks in certain words loudly to beg the god of the word that he comes and gives him back his lost words. In the West, the effects of speaking by a water fall are often attributed to masking of the person's voice.

3.2.3 Treatments associated with coverings

The tam-tam, pots, gourds, mortars, the shells of snails or turtles are all structures that are related to the notion of resonance and song. Resonance features more directly in treatments for stuttering as when stutterers have to speak in a loud voice into a mortar at moonlight, or to drink from a gourd following a certain rhythm dictated by the healers.

3.2.4   Hour, time, rhythm

In the preceding section involving water, it was often required that this must have stagnated, have rested for several days or at least overnight. All these had to be drunk at a later date, and, in that sense, involve time. The dregs of palm wine must have stayed a week in the vineyard before it is drunk. The idea that liquids must be dirty or foul is often repeated (water changes quickly because of the heat or has to be taken from dish-water or used for cleaning grains at the market that is then collected and consumed).

The drinks often have to be sipped in rhythm with musical instruments. The tam-tam was reported to be widely used and the healer specified the number of beats required between sips (typically every seventh or eighth beat). The rites often had to be performed at moonlight. Alternatively, the cure had to be taken according to a fixed schedule (several times a day). Again these cures have some similarities with techniques that involve speech rate control used in the West. Other forms of treatment that would achieve rate control involve the ubiquitous talking with pebbles in the mouth, and in a specifically African variant, speaking with pearls under the tongue.

Irregular breast-feeding (a form of biological rhythm) was considered to be the origin of one child's stuttering (the mother was a student that led to irregular timekeeping).

3.2.5   Treatments involving plants and potions

Some examples of potions used are a sauce made from ox-tongue, preparations based on medicinal herbs, salted papaya juice. Milk extracted from a boiled manioc tuber had to be drunk in small doses. A yellow flower that gives the imbiber the desire to drink it all the time (probably the Datura, a pendulous flower) was considered a way of getting the tongue into movement. Insects were commonly involved in potions too. For instance, grasshoppers were pressed and the juice that came out of them had to be drunk and grilled crickets had to be eaten.

One mother received ginger powder from a storyteller. The child was given one spoon to swallow each night just before going to sleep. Another spoonful of the ginger powder had to be taken the next morning before the child spoke to anyone or had anything put in their mouth.

One child had to search the forest with the father. A stem of a liana had to be found, cut and the bitter juice drunk. A child aged 12 had diffi-culty controlling his emotions. Every morning and evening he had to eat peanuts left by a parrot and had to repeat without thinking and without understanding the words that he found difficult.

During pregnancy to prevent having a child who stutters, the mother must search the market in the evening for grains of maize, broomcorn and peanuts. A potion is prepared from them that has to be taken every morning and evening until she gives birth. This treatment, like several others, involves several of the forms of classification (here time as well as a potion).

3.2.6   Treatments involving rites or magic

Traditional rites often involve chasing the evil spirits of stuttering from the person. Some of the rites reported were to have the person who stutters taste the food first each time a meal was prepared, to buckle up the storyteller's belt or extraction of a mystic thread from the person by the sorcerer.

One example of a rite that was reported was related to a dispute that occurred in the family's village at the time the mother was pregnant. When the child was 5 years old, he started to stutter and this was attributed to the past conflict. The witch doctor considered that the stuttered words were associated with a tree. He danced around the indicated tree and threw money into the river.

In another case, a father-in law and his son-in-law hated each other even though they did not know each other. No dowry was given, and this violated the rules of the people. This explained why the child stuttered when he reached 7 years of age.

Recall that a child is born with the spiritual principles of his ancestors, genies or other spirits. Consequently, if he is born with a malformation, or is different because he stutters, this may reflect a reincarnation of evil spirits, and this is a danger for the family. This should help the reader appreciate the difficulties that have to be overcome in many African families where a child with a disorder or a handicap is regarded as an insurmountable extra burden.

3.3   Answers to the other questions of the survey

Nine out of 60 persons who responded to the family history question indicated that there was no other person in the family that stutters. All the others pointed to a possible hereditary factor behind their stuttering. Number of affected relatives was reported to be between one and six and the affected relatives were predominantly male. It should be noted that the question did not delve deeply into the family history of the disorder.

Other indicators where more than one respondent reported features associated with stuttering were as follows (number out of the 63 respondents who indicated these associations is in brackets): Fear, tension, emotion, mockery (6); Imitation (15); A language or communication disorder (3); A psychological cause (2); Illness (2); Bilingualism (2); Having mocked others (2); Timidity (2).

It is surprising that persons who stutter seek traditional remedies when their personal responses indicate that they consider that they do not work, in the main. This is possible because as society develops, they have experience of practices that they perhaps had to undergo but in which they no longer believe.

Further from this, all the practices described had little effect on stuttering as indicated next: To the question 'How much credence do you give to these practices', out of 36 responses, 19 said no credence at all, 8 said total credence and 7 spoke of moderate credence. In the last case, there seemed to be a synthesis between animism and Christianity or Islam. To give one example, a person who stuttered reported that the second time he went to see a magician, he was given a medication that had to be mixed with tea and drunk over nine successive days. The treatment worked for 2 weeks and then his stuttering started again.

In addition to the traditional practices 19 responses mentioned Western practices: Relaxation and breathing control techniques were mentioned most often (Mac Guire), as well as self-assurance training and so on. This may reflect the fact that the respondents were from urban populations and were well informed thanks to the internet.

The mother was mentioned most often as the person who played an important role for the stutterer. Male relatives were also mentioned. This was often the father or grandfather or an uncle or brother.

Two healers were interviewed in Doula. Their responses were sometimes difficult to understand. They revealed a syncretism between Christianity and animism, and that stuttering was considered a fate. They reported that they did not know the cause of the stuttering of their patients, although they assumed it has to do with the nutrition of the child when young or that of the mother during pregnancy. Treatment with plants seemed to be the only therapy they offered. One forbade his stuttering patients to use salt, nervousness, sexual love (*sic*) and alcoholic drinks. The healers were paid. Payment depended on severity of the client's stutter and included a goat, palm oil, some acajou nuts, two lizard eggs, a white waistcloth, 10 lumps of sugar.

4 Conclusion

The results from the questionnaire do not provide an exhaustive picture. What is striking is that diverse countries that are sometimes far away from each other have a common approach towards the disorder: These traditional practices seem to persist in most countries of the French speaking part of black Africa (at least). The treatments are all preceded by rituals, magic spells and formulae which even an African cannot possibly know as they have been transmitted from father to son and guarded jealously by all healers, godlike persons, wizards, medicine men or sorcerers.

If the mere report of some of these religious practices appears disappointing, knowledge about them could shed light on stuttering. Stuttering is certainly regarded in a different way from the way Westerners view it. For example, Dean Williams argued that animism pervaded approaches to stuttering in the West. Furthermore, he argued that this approach should be dismissed (which it largely has) in favor of ones based upon scientific collection and analysis of data about speakers who stutter. In some ways the practices described here have similarities with the underlying conviction in some members of our societies that adults who stutter have mental delay. Additionally, Jung's psychoanalytic approach suggesting deep-rooted animism that affects many aspects of behavior would support the possibility that an individual suffering from stuttering may need to establish a connection between his own world (expressed in his stuttering) and that of ancestors and gods.

The imagery proposed by and contained in animism practices allows an internal dialogue between oneself and the world of spirits, comparable to the dialogue that takes place for instance with representations proposed by the therapist; I am thinking of the work of Nicole Charpy with pictures that propose dreams of another world. If there is for an African child a lack of language, this might prevent the necessary symbolization to integrate the taboos of his lineage, his family or the adult that broke the rules of his tribe.

The relation between animism and the modern world is a topic that intrigues sociologists and ethnologists. With a concept of primitive religion at the start, some see at present animism as a return to solidarity, bringing peace or conflicts in a world where a great number of wars are justified on religious grounds.

For us simply, knowing that African culture relies essentially on the oral tradition (the spoken word), we should not be too surprised about the lot of children suffering from stuttering. The task at hand is to make these children, the deaf or cerebral palsied children understood to be speaking beings that need help. They should not be rejected or ignored (this is the task as seen by the international stuttering association, ISA, which seeks to send therapists to Africa to support the self-help groups and perhaps also train practitioners). We will still have to inform ourselves a lot before being able to match our knowledge with these cultures.

Finally, as far as the profession of communication therapist is concerned, it would be helpful to examine these traditional practices into stuttering and for other disorders too. Some patients in Western countries come from Africa and elsewhere and sit between two cultures. Acknowledging the differences and being aware of them is the best way to listen to the patients and to live up to their expectations.

Editors' note This chapter is based on a presentation by Anne-Marie Simon at an international meeting held in Toulouse, 18th March 2006.

It provides a unique perspective concerning traditional treatment practices in the developing world. Anne-Marie describes how treatments are based in animism (the idea that conscious spirits occurs in all objects, not just human beings).

References

Griaule, M. (1935a) *Burners of Men: Modern Ethiopia*. 1st US edition translated by Rich, E.G. Lippincott: Philadelphia (The story of an expedition into the interior of Abyssinia in the early 1930s; a time when Abyssinia was trying to fight off Mussolini.

Griaule, M. (1935b) *Abyssinian Journey*. John Miles: London (Travel account of an ethnographic and linguistic study on behalf of the French Government in the 1930s.).

Griaule, M. (1938a) *Masques dogons*. Paris: Institut d'Ethnologie.

Griaule, M. (1938b) *Jeux dogons*. Paris: Institut d'Ethnologie.

Griaule, M. and Dieterlen, G. (1950) Un système soudanais de sirius. *Journal de la Société des Africanistes* 20, 273–294.

Appendix: Survey on traditional practices against stuttering in Africa

Date:

Initials:

Age: **Sex:**

Country:

You are (tick)   **A person who stutters**

                            Parent of a person who stutters

Are there other persons in your family who stutter?   YES   NO

Age of these person(s)?

Rank in the family (e.g. 1st of three siblings = 1/3)?

Relationship with you?

How do you account for your stuttering yourself?

(1) When you were a child, did your parents consult a traditional practitioner or a healer?   YES   NO

If YES, what advice did they receive?

What measures did they take against your stuttering?

Do you remember these practices? Can you describe them? (IMPORTANT)

(2) As an adolescent or adult, who did you consult about your stuttering:

a traditional practitioner? a healer? another person?

What advice did you receive?

What practices or methods did you follow?

Did you observe any effect on your speech?

Is there in your immedite family, tribe or lineage a person who played a particular role with respect to you as a person who stutters?

Are there any feasts or rites that you attended to in order to dispel your disorder? If YES, please describe them?

(3) At the moment do you follow any traditional practices? If YES, please describe them?

(4) Are you bound to secrecy about these practices? YES NO

(5) Are you embarrased to answer this survey even though it is anonymous? YES NO

In a society where traditional practices, animistic or other, are common and adhered to by a great number of persons, how much credence do you give to these practices. Indicate by marking a cross on the following scale

No credence at all --
total credence

Remarks:

All remarks are welcome

Thanks again. A-M Simon

Part 3

Bilingual Language Diversity, Stuttering and Its Treatment

Chapter 11

Review of Research on the Relationship between Bilingualism and Stuttering

JOHN VAN BORSEL

Summary

This chapter gives an overview of the research on stuttering and bilingualism. Although the relationship between bilingualism and stuttering received clinical interest already in the 19th century, the review shows that much is still to be learned. It is still a matter of debate whether or not bilingualism can cause stuttering and many questions are still open with regard to prevalence and manifestation of stuttering in bilinguals, as well as with regard to the assessment and treatment of bilinguals who stutter. One reason why research in this area is making only slow progress is probably the diversity of the population of bilingual speakers but it is also this diversity that constitutes the challenge for both clinicians and researchers.

1 Introduction

The relationship between stuttering and bilingualism is a topic that has received clinical interest for more than two centuries. Already in the 19th century the French physician Jean Marc Itard, for instance, sometimes advised that stuttering children be placed in the care of a foreign governess who would compel the use of a foreign language in order to overcome stuttering (Eldridge, 1968). Apparently Itard assumed that it was possible to stutter in one language and be fluent in another one. It is not clear where Itard got this idea from, but it is highly unlikely that it was based on research findings. Research into the relationship between stuttering and bilingualism only dates back to recent times and systematic studies remain relatively scarce even today. This paucity of research on bilingualism and stuttering is quite remarkable as it has been estimated that over 50% of the world's population is bilingual. It has even been suggested that bilingualism is the norm worldwide (Grosjean, 1982) and that bilinguals outnumber unilinguals worldwide (De Bot & Kroll, 2002). It certainly is a fact that bilingualism is present in every country, in all classes of society and at all age levels.

A first glance at the literature that has been published on stuttering and bilingualism shows that the picture is quite diverse, in different respects. Studies on bilingualism differ as to the number and age of participants reported. Studies differ as to language combinations involved, as to the age of acquisition of the second language, as to proficiency and usage of the languages by the participants, as to the methodology in assessing stuttering and as to the methodology in assessing bilingualism. Studies on bilingualism and stuttering further differ as to what is considered bilingualism and what is considered stuttering. Actually, one finds the complete range of bilingualism as outlined by Siguan and MacKay (1987) going from 'the total, simultaneous and alternating mastery of two languages' to 'some degree of knowledge of a second language in addition to spontaneous skills which any individual possesses in his (her) first language' (p. 13). With regard to what is considered stuttering, the majority of studies deal with the well-known type of developmental dysfluency. But there are also a few reports on acquired stuttering, i.e. stuttering that manifested itself for the first time beyond the typical childhood period of stuttering onset. In the latter case the stuttering is often of neurogenic origin. Furthermore, research on stuttering and bilingualism reflect a diversity of types of studies ranging from almost anecdotal case studies to well-designed group studies.

The purpose of this chapter is to give an overview of the research on stuttering and bilingualism. It should be clear that given not just the diversity of studies available but the paucity as well, any conclusions drawn from this overview must be considered tentative. This chapter is organized around a number of recurrent topics in the literature: the prevalence of stuttering in bilinguals, the manifestation of stuttering in bilinguals, the diagnosis of stuttering in bilinguals and the treatment of stuttering in bilinguals.

2   The Prevalence of Stuttering in Bilinguals

One of the most under-researched aspects of stuttering and bilingualism is certainly prevalence. While for monolinguals there is a general consensus that prevalence of stuttering is about 1% worldwide (Bloodstein & Bernstein Ratner, 2008), there is no similar knowledge about the occurrence of stuttering in bilinguals. Only a few studies on stuttering prevalence in bilinguals have been reported and they all focused on whether stuttering is more prevalent in bilinguals than in monolinguals rather than on prevalence of stuttering in bilinguals per se.

A survey of the public schools of East Chicago involving 4827 children (2405 boys, 2422 girls) aged 4 to 17 (average 8.54) by Travis *et al.* (1937) reported an overall prevalence of stuttering of 2.61%. In children who spoke only English, prevalence was lower than in those speaking English and one or two foreign languages (1.80% versus 2.80% and 2.38% respectively). Similarly, Stern (1948) who studied 1861 children in four schools of Johannesburg, South Africa, found a prevalence of 1.66% in monolinguals and a prevalence of 2.16% in children who had been bilingual prior to age 6 years.

On the other hand, Au-Yeung *et al.* (2000) in an internet survey on bilingualism and stuttering found a similar prevalence of stuttering among their 656 bilingual and 138 monolingual respondents (respectively 21.65% and 21.74%). In that study any person interested could enter a website and respond to a series of questions regarding language usage and the occurrence of speech disorders.

The question of prevalence of stuttering in bilinguals is by no means purely of theoretical interest. It is not unusual for parents of a stuttering child to inquire if the dysfluency in their child is perhaps the result of exposure to two languages and whether they should give up the bilingualism (at least temporary) and elect for a monolingual education. In fact, the idea lives among some scholars that stuttering can originate from bilingualism and that therefore a bilingual education should be deferred until the child has acquired good control of a first language. This idea was put forward by, for instance, Karniol (1992) and more recently also by Howell *et al.* (2009). The latter found that in a group of 38 stuttering bilingual children aged 8–10 years, those who had spoken two languages during the preschool years outnumbered those who had spoken only one non-English language during the preschool years whereas in a cohort of age-matched non-stuttering bilingual children, the proportions were reversed. Based on these findings the authors concluded that bilingual children are more prone to starting to stutter and that if a child uses a language other than English in the home, deferring the time when they learn English may reduce the chance of stuttering onset.

Studies on the prevalence of stuttering in bilinguals should be interpreted with great caution. A weakness of surveys like that of Travis *et al.* (1937) and Stern (1948) is that the presence of stuttering in the participants is based on a single assessment. Given the well-known variability in symptoms of stuttering across time and situation (Ingham & Costello, 1984), a single assessment can hardly be considered a valid procedure. Moreover, assessing fluency in the bilingual participants in such surveys, almost certainly implies assessment in one or more languages that the investigator himself is not acquainted with. As shown in a study by Van Borsel and Britto Pereira (2005), identifying stuttering merely by reliance on the symptoms in a language one is not familiar with may be risky. The risk is even higher if the language to be judged is more remote from the investigator's native language (Van Borsel *et al.*, 2008) (see also Section 4. The diagnosis of stuttering in bilinguals). A possible solution would be to call upon the help of a native speaker. In the study of Travis *et al.* (1937), this is what was actually done. A variety of people helped as interpreters in that study including personnel directors of oil refineries and steel mills, priests, merchants, foreign school-masters, and interpreters for docks and unloading companies. However, apart from the fact that finding native speakers who can function as observers may be difficult, it is evident that such untrained, inexperienced interpreters may not provide useful or dependable information about stuttered speech (Finn & Cordes, 1997).

An internet survey like the one of Au-Yeung *et al.* (2000) also has its methodological flaws. One may wonder how reliable self-report is when it comes to distinguishing, for instance, between developmental stuttering and normal non-fluency or language formulation problems, or between stuttering and other fluency disorders such as cluttering. More-over, people are likely to seek out websites of their main interests or concerns. Perhaps this explains the unusually high ratio of respondents who stuttered in this study.

Whether the methodology adopted in the recent study by Howell *et al.* (2009) is a valid method to compare the prevalence of stuttering in mono-linguals and bilinguals is still a matter of debate. According to Packman *et al.* (2009), drawing conclusions about the general population of bilin-gual children from a clinical cohort is not appropriate. They suggest that the best way to establish if there is a relationship between stuttering and bilingualism is with an epidemiological study. On the other hand, epi-demiological studies are not without problems. An epidemiological study necessitates, for instance, grouping together bilinguals that may be quite heterogeneous.

In addition to the question of whether stuttering is more prevalent in bilinguals than in monolinguals, one may further wonder if there might be any prevalence differences among certain subgroup of bilinguals. A fac-tor that may play a role in this respect is age of acquisition of the two languages. It is interesting that in the study by Stern (1948) the bilingual participants with a higher stuttering rate than the monolingual partici-pants had been bilingual prior to the age of 6. In the study of Au-Yeung *et al.* (2000) participants who started second-language acquisition between the ages of 7 and 12 stuttered less often than those who started second language acquisition before the age of 7. And the bilingual children who stuttered in the study of Howell *et al.* (2009) all had used another language than English since birth. Taken together these data suggest that espe-cially younger children are vulnerable to stuttering if they are exposed to two languages. In agreement with this is the observation that adults who learn a second language appear to be 'immune' to developing stut-tering. To the best of our knowledge, stuttering onset in adults learning a second language has never been reported. Further research seems war-ranted comparing the prevalence of stuttering in children hearing two languages from birth and thus growing up in a so-called Bilingual First

Language Acquisition setting with that in children first growing up mono-lingually and coming in to regular contact with a second language only later, thus growing up in a so-called Early Second Language Acquisition setting (De Houwer, this volume). As pointed out by De Houwer, the dynamics, expectations and emotional demands are different in both settings. For instance, families of children growing up in a bilingual first-language acquisition will want children to learn to understand and speak two languages from the beginning. Perhaps demands like this make these children more vulnerable to stuttering.

Another factor that may be of influence on the stuttering prevalence in bilinguals is similarity of the languages involved. The prevalence of stuttering may be higher in bilinguals speaking two linguistically related languages than in those speaking two totally different languages. Closely related pairs of languages conceivably produce more confusion and hence may lead more often to stuttering. Conversely, however, it could also be that non-related language pairs demand more resources in learning two different lexical and syntactic systems and, for that reason causes stutter-ing to arise more often. Unfortunately, the data that are available at present do not allow the question whether the degree of similarity between the languages spoken is a factor in the prevalence of stuttering in bilinguals to be determined.

Further insight into the impact of bilingualism on stuttering might also be obtained from a systematic comparison of stuttering prevalence in countries with a high probability for its inhabitants to be bilingual with that of countries with a low such probability. Greenberg (1956) developed a diversity index which expresses the probability that any two randomly selected people from the same country have different mother tongues. This diversity index is computed based on the population of each lan-guage as a proportion of the total population and ranges from 1 (total diversity, no two people have the same mother tongue) to 0 (no diversity at all, everybody speaks the same mother tongue). It would seem logical that in countries with a higher diversity index, the number of people using more than one language is also higher. If bilingualism is a factor in stut-tering prevalence, then one would expect a higher stuttering prevalence overall in countries with a higher diversity index. As far as we are aware of, this type of study has not yet been undertaken so far.

3 The Manifestation of Stuttering in Bilinguals

A topic that received considerable attention in the literature on stut-tering and bilingualism is that of the manifestation of stuttering in bilinguals and in particular whether bilinguals stutter in one or both languages. Nwokah (1988) outlined three theoretical possibilities: (1) Stut-tering occurs in one language and not in the other; (2) Stuttering occurs in both languages with similar behavior in each language (the same-hypothesis) and (3) Stuttering occurs in both languages but varies from one language to the other (the difference-hypothesis).

3.1 Stuttering in one language and not in the other

Nwokah concluded that stuttering occurring in one language and not in the other is a highly unusual situation based on her research in Nigeria involving 16 people who stutter who spoke Igbo and English. None of her participants stuttered in one language only. She moreover hypothesized that if such a pattern exists, it must be in individuals who are far more dominant in one language than the other. A review of the literature of cases of stuttering in bilinguals that compare the occurrence of dysfluency in each language seems to support Nwokah's conclusion. Indeed, bilingual persons who stutter in one language and not in the other are rather exceptional. Dale (1977) reported four bilingual Cuban-American male adolescents (average age 13 years) who were born in the United States. They all spoke only Spanish at home and were all quite proficient in Spanish and English. Each reported that they began to stutter in Spanish. None of the participants exhibited dysfluent speech while speaking English. According to Deal the boys' stuttering probably originated when they started to forget some of their Spanish vocabulary, demonstrating normal dysfluencies, which then were identified as stuttering by the parents. Pressure to speak Spanish fluently conceivably induced fear in the boys, leading to more dysfluencies.

Stuttering in one language and not in the other was also observed in the study by Howell *et al.* (2009). Of 38 bilinguals who stuttered, all of whom spoke a second language in addition to English, two (i.e. 5.3%) stuttered in just one of their languages. Remarkably, they stuttered in their first language but not in English.

A few more references to stuttering in one language only can be found in Van Riper (1971). One is the case of an individual who lived on Southampton Island and according to an informant stuttered in English but not in Eskimo. The other is that of a Pakistani stutterer who himself reported not to stutter when he read his Holy Book written in a language he can read but not understand. Since these reports refer to uncontrolled second-hand information, the value of them is questionable.

3.2 Stuttering in both languages with similar behavior in each language

Equally unusual to stuttering in only one language is the apparent occurrence of a similar pattern of stuttering in both languages. Apart again from an anecdotal report in Van Riper (1971) (a Japanese stutterer who communicated that he feared the same sounds in English and German as in Japanese), examples of studies that conform to Nwokah's same hypothesis were reported by Roberts (2002), Woods and Wright (1998), and Lebrun *et al.* (1990). Of two male English-French bilinguals, Roberts (2002) mentions that, at least for a monologue task, they were 'equally disfluent in French and English' (p. 15). Woods and Wright (1998) described the case of a man who reported that his stuttering was equally severe while speaking Russian (his first language) as while speaking English (his second language). Lebrun *et al.* (1990) mention that in a French-Dutch speaking male who began to stutter following brain damage, the severity of the speech impediment fluctuated but never disappeared and 'affected his French and Dutch equally' (p. 255). It is important to note that in the latter case the dysfluency was of neurogenic origin. As Ringo and Dietrich (1995) pointed out, stuttering of neurogenic origin may be more pervasive than developmental stuttering and tends to occur across all speech tasks. Perhaps the case by Lebrun *et al.* (1990) must be interpreted in the light of this. It is also important to note that neither the study of Woods and Wright (1998) nor the study of Lebrun *et al.* (1990) present actual measurements to support the statement of equal influence of both languages. As illustrated by a study of Bernstein Ratner and Benitez (1985) in a Spanish-English-speaking bilingual, clinical impressions of degree of stuttering may be quite misleading. While both the clinicians and the participant in this study thought that fluency was equally compromised in English and Spanish, an analysis of spontaneous speech samples showed almost twice as many dysfluencies in English as in Spanish. The reports of the studies by Woods and Wright (1998) and Lebrun *et al.* (1990) thus should be treated with care.

3.3   Stuttering in both languages but varying from one language to the other

By far the most common pattern of dysfluency in bilinguals who stutter seems to be that stuttering occurs in both languages but varies from language to language. Several studies are available now that illustrate this pattern (see Table 11.1). In some of these studies participants demonstrated different degrees of stuttering severity but yet similar patterns and distributions of stuttering (for instance, in Jayaram, 1983; Scott Trautman & Keller, 2000; Lim *et al.*, 2008). In other studies different patterns and distributions of stuttering were seen, with or without different degrees of stuttering severity (Bernstein Ratner & Benitez, 1985; Cabrera & Bernstein Ratner, 2000; Jankelowitz & Bortz, 1996; Nwokah, 1988; Schäfer, 2008; Shenker *et al.*, 1998; Watt, 2000).

3.3.1   *Stuttering severity and language proficiency*

An intriguing question in cases of different severity of stuttering from one language to the other is what factors are behind this difference.

Table 11.1 Studies illustrating that stuttering in bilinguals may vary from language to language

Study	Languages	N	Age	Different Severity?	Different patterns/ distribution?
Jayaram (1983)	Kannada/English	10	19–32	Y	N
Bernstein Ratner and Benitez (1985)	Spanish/English	1	50	Y	Y
Nwokah (1988)	Igbo/English	16	16–40	Y	Y
Jankelowitz and Bortz (1996)	English/Afrikaans	1	63	Y	Y
Shenker et al. (1998)	English/French	1	2;8	Y	Y
Cabrera and Bernstein Ratner (2000)	Spanish/English	1	5	?	Y
Scott Trautman and Keller (2000)	Spanish/English		20	Y	N
Watt (2000)	Kinyarwanda/ French/Swahili/English	1	19	Y	Y
Reardon (2000)	Indian....	40		Y	
Meline et al. (2006)	Chinese/English	1		Y	
Carias and Ingram (2006)	Spanish/English	4	4–10	Y	Y
Lim et al. (2008)	English/Mandarin	14	12–33	Y	N
Schäfer (2008)	English/German	15	10–59	Y	Y
Van Borsel et al. (2009)	Dutch/English	1	39;9	Y	Y

A possible candidate is language proficiency. Indeed, a number of studies suggest that stuttering may be more severe in the less-proficient language. This pattern was observed for instance in Jankelowitz and Bortz (1996) and Scott Trautman and Keller (2000) and also confirmed in a few studies explicitly devoted to investigating the relationship between language proficiency and stuttering.

Schäfer (2008) analyzed stuttering characteristics in 15 German-English bilingual people who stuttered, ranging in age between 10 and 59 years (mean 25). In the majority of the participants (12/15) the severity of stuttering, determined according to the percentage of syllables and percentage of words stuttered, was found to be significantly more severe in English (the second language) compared to German (the first language). On the other hand, the degree of language proficiency in English, as determined from a cloze test and a post-conversational questionnaire, did not highly correlate with stuttering behavior.

Lim *et al.* (2008) examined the influence of language dominance on the manifestation of stuttering in 30 English-Mandarin bilinguals who stuttered (age 12–44 years, mean 21.7). Interestingly, the participants in this study did not only include individuals who, according to a self-report classification tool, were more proficient in one language than the other (15 English-dominant, 4 Mandarin-dominant) but also 11 so-called balanced bilinguals, i.e. bilinguals who used their two languages equally or with equal levels of proficiency. The English-dominant and Mandarin-dominant participants were found to exhibit greater stuttering in their less dominant language, whereas the balanced bilinguals evidenced similar levels of stuttering in both languages. Note that Lim *et al.* (2008) categorized their participants according to 'language dominance' rather than 'language proficiency'. Language dominance is partly determined by language proficiency but also by other aspects such as frequency and domain of language use (see also below).

The finding of equal stuttering severity in the case of balanced bilinguals was also reported previously by Roberts (2002). In this study, two participants began learning their second language between the ages of 6 and 10 (and therefore were considered balanced bilinguals). They exhibited equal amounts of stuttering in both languages. Two other participants began learning their second language between the ages of 11 and 15 (and therefore were considered unbalanced bilinguals) and they exhibited more stuttering in their second language.

The likelihood that language proficiency is a factor in the differential stuttering severity between languages in bilinguals is further supported by some experiments with normal speakers. It is well known that delaying auditory feedback in normal speakers produces speech disruptions that some authors consider to be reminiscent of stuttering (Fairbanks, 1955; Lee, 1950). As reported by MacKay and Bowman (1969) and confirmed by Van Borsel *et al.* (2005), the speech of fluent bilinguals or multilinguals is less disrupted when they speak the language(s) they are more familiar with.

While judging from the aforementioned studies, language proficiency would seem to be an important factor in the severity of stuttering across languages in bilinguals; it may not be the only factor involved. To begin with, a number of studies have observed exactly the opposite pattern than that found by Jankelowitz and Bortz (1996), Scott Trautman and Keller (2000), Schäfer (2008) and Lim *et al.* (2008).

Jayaram (1983) studied 10 bilingual stutterers (age 19–32; mean 25.6 years) speaking Kannada, a language from South India, as their primary language and English in addition. The participants were reported to stutter more in Kannada than in English, especially in spontaneous speech. It should be noted, though, that the difference may not have been statistically significant. In an English-French speaking pre-school girl with English as the dominant language, Shenker *et al.* (1998) observed more stutter-like dysfluencies in English than in French (respectively 13.51% versus 9.89%). The symptoms considered to be stutter-like dysfluencies were not specified (Shenker, this volume). Similarly, in a 11-year 9 month-old Spanish-English bilingual speaker, Howell *et al.* (2004) found higher stuttering rates in Spanish, the more developed language, than in English, both during monologue (38.5% versus 18.4%, respectively) and conversation (29.5% versus 19.7%, respectively). Carias and Ingram (2006) in four Spanish-English bilingual children (age 4–10 years) reported that in all four cases, the language with the most dysfluencies was also the more proficient language, as measured by mean length of utterance (MLU) that is a standard measure used in language development. Also Meline *et al.* (2006) found more stuttering in the more proficient language (Chinese) in a Chinese-English bilingual stutterer. It must be added, however, that in the latter study the participant had received recent treatment in English which may have influenced the results. Still another case with more stuttering in the more proficient language was reported by Van Borsel *et al.* (2009). In a bilingual (Dutch-English) speaking woman who started to stutter after a whiplash trauma, significantly more dysfluencies were observed in the patient's native language (Dutch) in conversation (23.5% versus 4.2%) and in picture description (16.1% versus 7.2%). Apparently also in acquired stuttering different degrees of severity can be observed with the more proficient language being affected most.

Further suggestion that language proficiency may not be the only factor involved in the severity of stuttering across languages in bilingual speakers comes from the studies by Bernstein Ratner and Benitez (1985) and Nwokah (1988). The 16 participants in Nwokah's study were said to be 'equally competent in English and Igbo and to use both languages daily'. The participant in Bernstein Ratner and Benitez (1985) 'had spoken

Spanish and English since learning to speak and he used both languages almost equally'. Thus, in both studies balanced bilinguals were examined. As such language proficiency in these cases cannot have been of influence. Yet the participants of these two studies stuttered more in one language than the other.

Another interesting study with regard to the role of language proficiency in stuttering severity is that of Watt (2000). She reported a 19-year-old severe stutterer who spoke four languages. The stuttering was not equally severe in all languages but varied from language to language. However, there appeared to be no correlation with self-reported level of oral proficiency or reported frequency of use. Rather stuttering severity varied from least to most severe in order of the age of acquisition of each language (Kinyarwanda < French < Swahili < English). Thus, age at which this individual started speaking his languages was a more important predictor of stuttering severity than language proficiency or frequency of use.

From the studies reviewed above it is clear that the role of language proficiency in the origin of different degrees of stuttering in different languages as seen in many bilinguals requires further investigation. The studies reviewed also raise some questions and draw attention to some methodological issues. One issue concerns the method for determining stuttering severity. It is obvious that reliance on clinical impression and self-evaluation only, as happened in a number of studies, is inadequate. At least there should be some formal measurement of stuttering severity. This could be a measurement not only in terms of percentage of stuttered syllables but also as percentage of stuttered words. As pointed out by Schäfer (2008), it is recommendable to perform both types of measurements. Languages may differ with respect to the amount of multisyllable words, potentially yielding different overall levels of dysfluency when examined according to percentage of stuttered syllables and percentage of stuttered words. In languages with higher proportions of multi-syllable words lower percentages of syllables stuttered will be calculated compared to languages with fewer proportions of multi-syllable words. In addition, studies that compare stuttering severity in different languages in bilinguals should reflect on the significance of any difference observed. When is a difference in stuttering severity (measured as percentage of stuttered syllables or percentage of stuttered words) between two languages in a bilingual person clinically significant? How large should the difference in stuttering severity be to call it a real difference?

Further aspects that need to be reckoned with when comparing the severity of stuttering across different languages are the language mode in which severity is assessed and the type of dysfluencies counted. Regarding language mode, it is quite common to find that stuttering rate varies depending on the task involved (reading, conversation, monologue, etc.).

Unfortunately studies often base comparison on a single mode. As to the symptoms that are considered, it must be remembered that certain types of dysfluency, though occurring in people who stutter, are not typical of stuttering. Examples of such symptoms are phrase repetitions, revisions and interjections. Including such dysfluencies in severity counts when comparing stuttering across languages, may blur the picture, with results reflecting dysfluency variation due to second-language influence rather than degree in stuttering severity. The inclusion of word repetitions is particularly problematic, as some consider them to be a stuttering symptom and others do not (see Howell and Rusbridge, this volume).

Similar to a formal assessment of stuttering severity, a formal assessment of language proficiency is necessary. And again the question arises as to what is the most appropriate method. Apart from clinical impression and self-evaluation the studies, reviewed above, used a variety of measures to determine language proficiency including length of exposure to a language (Nwokah (1988), mean length of utterance (Carias & Ingram, 2006), a cloze test (Jankelowitz & Bortz, 1996; Schäfer, 2008), questionnaires (Jankelowitz & Bortz, 1996; Schäfer, 2008), part of the Bilingual aphasia test by Paradis (http://www.mcgill.ca/linguistics/research/bat/) (Jankelowitz & Bortz, 1996), and a specially developed self-report classification tool (Lim *et al.*, 2008).

The concept of language proficiency is a complex one. As discussed by Lim *et al.* (2008) there is considerable overlap between 'language proficiency' and 'language dominance' and levels of proficiency and degrees of dominance tend to correlate. Yet the two should be distinguished. A speaker may have almost native-like proficiency in two languages but still consider one language to be better than the other. Alternatively, he may be dominant in one language but not be highly proficient in that language. Moreover, language proficiency is composed of several components (comprehension and expression, verbal and written) and the proficiency in each of these modalities can vary over time (Roberts & Shenker, 2007). In addition, next to 'language proficiency' and 'language dominance' investigators have used such terms as 'primary language' and 'native language' when comparing stuttering in the languages of bilinguals. It is advisable that whatever term is used, it is clearly defined and a clear description is given of how the aspect referred to was assessed or measured.

3.3.2 Different patterns and distributions of stuttering

As mentioned above, when a bilingual person stutters in both languages, the stuttering may not only differ in severity from language to language but different patterns and distributions of stuttering may be demonstrated also. A number of studies include examples of such differences. As one can see from Table 11.2 the differences may pertain to which

Table 11.2 Studies reporting different patterns and/or distributions of stuttering in the two languages of bilinguals

Study	*Participant(s)*	*Stuttering pattern/distribution*
Bernstein Ratner and Benitez (1985)	50-year-old Spanish-English bilingual	Had more difficulty initiating sentences and clauses in Spanish than in English and initial noun phrases attracted as much dysfluency as did verb phrases in English, but they were not a large source of dysfluency in Spanish. On the other hand, conjunctions and clause initial words seemed to attract twice as much dysfluency in Spanish as in English
Nwokah (1988)	16 Nigerian high-school-educated bilingual stutterers speaking Igbo and English, age 16 to 40	An overuse of fillers such as 'er' or 'mm' was common in English, whereas these did not occur in Igbo. In addition, English-initial consonants were more frequently stuttered than vowels, whereas the opposite pattern was observed in Igbo.
Jankelowitz and Bortz (1996)	63-year-old English-Afrikaans-speaking male	Tended to be more aware of his stuttering in Afrikaans than in English, and evidenced a greater adaptation effect in Afrikaans than in English but a greater consistency in English than in Afrikaans. In addition, his dysfluencies were predominantly more typical than atypical in Afrikaans than in English.
Shenker *et al.* (1998)	English-French speaking pre-school girl	No significant differences between English and French as to the loci of stuttering, classified according to type of dysfluency, placement of stuttered word in a sentence, and word length. However, more word repetitions were observed in French and more part-word repetitions in English (the dominant language).
Cabrera and Bernstein Ratner (2000)	5-year-old Spanish-English bilingual boy	Demonstrated higher proportions of dysfluencies on reflexives in Spanish, and higher proportions on adjectives in English.
Howell *et al.* (2004)	11-year 9-month-old Spanish-English bilingual boy	Stuttering occurred more on function words than on content word in the boy's second language (English). In the child's first language (Spanish) the opposite was seen, i.e. more stuttering on content words than on function words.

Table 11.2 (Continued)

Study	Participant(s)	Stuttering pattern/distribution
Schäfer (2008)	15 German-English bilinguals	In German, the predominant language, stuttering occurred significantly more often on content words. In English, the second language, no such significant difference between stuttering on function and content words was observed. Across languages significantly more stuttering occurred on content words in German and more stuttering on function words in English.
Van Borsel *et al.* (2009)	39;9-year-old Dutch/English woman	Part word repetitions and revisions in Dutch but not in English

phrases (noun phrases versus verb phrases), which types of words (reflexives, adjectives, conjunctions, function words versus content words) or which types of sounds (vowels versus consonants in a particular position) attract more dysfluencies. The difference may also pertain to which types of dysfluencies (interjections, part word repetitions, revisions, word repetitions versus part-word repetitions, typical versus atypical dysfluencies) occur most frequently in language. Furthermore, there can be a difference with respect to awareness of the dysfluency by the stuttering individual and with respect to such phenomena as the adaptation effect and consistency effect.

Explaining the observed differences is not always straightforward. Bernstein Ratner and Benitez (1985) and Cabrera and Bernstein Ratner (2000) assumed that in their cases the differences in the loci of dysfluencies across the two languages were associated mainly with differences between English and Spanish sentence structure. Cabrera and Bernstein Ratner (2000) pointed out, for instance, that Spanish reflexives are word-initial rather than word-final as in English, and English adjectives precede, rather than follow the nouns they modify whereas Spanish does the opposite. They used these observations to explain the higher proportion of dysfluencies on reflexives in Spanish, and the higher proportion on adjectives in English in their subject. Also Schäfer (2008) referred to language inherent characteristics to explain the differences observed in her participants. More stuttering occurs on content words in German due to longer words in German. This difference would, moreover, be closely related to overall language abilities. Participants were more proficient in German than in English and overall produced longer words in English.

Similarly, the English-French-speaking pre-school girl in Shenker *et al.* (1998) demonstrated more stutter-like dysfluencies in English than in French probably because French was still less developed and included more monosyllable words than English.

More detailed comparison of the stuttering distribution and patterns in different languages with attention to a greater number of variables in studies with more different language pairs is needed in order to better understand the possible factors that lead to differential stuttering in the languages of bilinguals.

4 The Diagnosis of Stuttering in Bilinguals

As already mentioned above, assessing fluency in bilingual individuals will often imply assessment in a language that the clinician himself is not (fully) acquainted with. If the client is a severe stutterer, identifying stuttering in a foreign language may not be so difficult (Watson & Kayser, 1994). In such cases, clinicians will often observe excessive tension and secondary behaviors without difficulty even though the language is unfamiliar. However, there is still a lack of empirical evidence concerning whether or how well clinicians are able to make reliable and valid judgments about the presence of stuttering in languages or dialects other than their own (Finn & Cordes, 1997).

Humphrey (2004) investigated whether bilingual English-Spanish-speaking judges are better at making dysfluency judgments in Spanish than monolingual English-speaking judges. He asked judges to view two videotaped narrative samples (one in English and one in Spanish) of a dysfluent bilingual English-Spanish speaker and to identify dysfluencies. Both the bilingual English-Spanish-speaking judges and the monolingual English-speaking judges judged the Spanish-language narrative to contain a greater percentage of dysfluencies than the English-language narrative. However, the two groups did not identify a significantly different percentage of dysfluencies in the English sample or in the Spanish sample. This seems to suggest that familiarity with Spanish made no significant difference when judging dysfluencies in Spanish. It must be remarked, however, that the study was conducted in South Florida. It is fairly likely, therefore, that the monolingual English-speaking judges had developed some familiarity with certain features of Spanish. As Humphrey (2004) acknowledged, the results might have been different in an area with different demographics.

By contrast, a study by Van Borsel and Britto Pereira (2005) showed that language familiarity does influence stuttering judgment. In a series of observer experiments 14 native speakers of Brazilian Portuguese identified and judged stuttering in Dutch speakers and in Portuguese speakers. Fourteen native speakers of Dutch identified and judged stuttering in

Brazilian Portuguese speakers and in Dutch speakers. Results showed that judges can make a similar level of judgment in a native and a foreign language, and that native and foreign judges can make a similar level of judgment irrespective of native/foreign differences. It was also found, however, that for the identification of non-stutterers, both panels performed better in their native language than in the foreign language, and in their native language they both performed better than the other panel. Moreover, the Dutch judges performed significantly better in identifying native stutterers than foreign stutterers. Both panels were generally also less confident, and found identification of stuttering more difficult in the foreign language than in the native language and when asked for the characteristics that helped them identify stutterers, they provided less detail in the foreign language than in the native language.

A further study (Van Borsel *et al.*, 2008) expanded on the findings of Van Borsel and Britto Pereira (2005) and explored the hypothesis that closeness to a person's native language is a determining factor in judgments of stuttering in an unfamiliar language. In that study it was found that a panel speaking Dutch and a panel speaking English (both West Germanic languages) performed better in identifying Dutch people who stutter and people who do not stutter than a panel speaking Brazilian Portuguese (a Romance language), thus confirming the existence of a closeness of language influence. Results further suggested that when the native language is more remote from the unfamiliar language there is a higher risk for false positive identification in particular.

It is of importance to note that in the latter study the closeness of the language hypothesis was tested by presenting video-recordings of one group of stuttering and non-stuttering people speaking a particular language to several panels who had various linguistic backgrounds. One of the problems with this approach is that the panels involved may not have exactly the same clinical training or previous experience with stuttering. A possible strategy to rule out clinical training as an eventual confounding variable would be to use naive listeners as judges. However, this approach too is not straightforward. To what extent are naive listeners capable of diagnosing stuttering and to what extent can one generalize findings from naive listeners to trained professionals? An alternative design for testing the closeness of language hypothesis might be to set up experiments in which one single panel makes fluency judgments of recordings in different languages with various levels of similarity to the native language. As such the possible influence of differences in clinical training or previous experience with stuttering would be ruled out. This approach requires, however, that the various recordings present stuttering and non-stuttering people that are equally difficult or equally easy to assess from language to language. Composing such samples is by no means easy, if possible at all. The best option then in future studies seems to adopt both strategies (one recording/multiple panels and multiple recordings/one panel) and reckon with the weakness of each type. From a clinical point of view, studies on judgment of languages that reflect linguistic situations as they occur in reality at some point in time would seem most valuable.

5   The Treatment of Stuttering in Bilinguals

5.1   One language or two languages?

One of the recurrent questions in the literature regarding the treatment of bilingual persons who stutter is if treatment should be given in one language or in both languages? Any discussion on this topic must anyhow consider, however, that therapy in both languages is very often not possible. It is estimated that currently over 6900 languages are spoken worldwide, some 347 (5%) of which have at least one million speakers (Lewis, 2009). Needless to say that this creates the possibility of a great many language pairs spoken by bilinguals. As such, the more important question is probably not, 'Should the treatment should be given in one or in both languages?' but rather, 'If therapy is given in one language, may one count on generalization to the other, untreated language?'

Theoretically speaking, when treating stuttering in one language, there may be no generalization to the untreated language, there may be a similar improvement in both languages, there may be less improvement in the untreated language than in the treated language and (less likely it would seem) there may be more improvement in the untreated language than in the treated language.

A number of studies have reported on generalization of treatment in bilinguals including Woods and Wright (1998), Humphrey *et al.* (2001), Humphrey (1999, 2004), Rousseau *et al.* (2005), and Lim (2007 and this volume) (Table 11.3). In these studies participants were of various ages, used various language combinations, which they learned at various ages and demonstrated stuttering to various degrees at the onset of therapy. Moreover, different types of therapy were used and duration of therapy varied from study to study. Also, in some studies treatment took place in the primary language, in others in the secondary language, mainly because of practical circumstances (i.e. depending on the language the therapist had mastered). Nonetheless, each of these studies reported that treatment in one language resulted in spontaneous improvement in the untreated language. The available studies also suggest, however, that the degree of fluency transfer from the treated to the untreated language may vary. In some cases improvement was larger in the treated language than in the untreated language, in others the degree of improvement in

Table 11.3 Studies have reported on generalization of treatment in bilinguals

Study	Participants	Languages	Therapy	
			Type	*Language*
Woods and Wright (1998)	adult male	Russian/English	simplified regulated breathing treatment	English
Humphrey *et al.* (2001)	11-year-old twin girls	Arabic/English	fluency shaping and stuttering modification	Arabic
Humphrey (2004)	3 males, 1 female*	English/Spanish or French	fluency shaping and stuttering modification	English
Rousseau *et al.* (2005)	7-year-old boy	French/English	Lidcombe program	French
Lim (2007)	14 males (12 to 33 y)	English/Mandarin	smooth speech intensive program	English

*also described in Humphrey (1999)

the untreated language was equal or even somewhat higher than that in the untreated language. There is also some suggestion that generalization does not always occur for all aspects. Humphrey (1999), for instance, noted that treatment in English in his participant brought about a clinically significant decrease of percentage of stuttered syllables in both English and Spanish. However, a decreased situational avoidance score observed in English was not accompanied by a similar significant decrease in Spanish. Overall, the factors that determine generalization in monolingual treatment of bilinguals are presently unclear and require further investigation.

While stuttering treatment in one language is probably the most viable option in most cases, treatment in both languages is of course not impossible. Some questions that arise then are: should both languages be treated simultaneously or not and if not, which language should be treated first and for what reason? Data on treatment in both languages almost exclusively come from studies with the Lidcombe program. Perhaps this is no coincidence. In contrast to other therapy approaches that rely mostly on direct intervention from the therapist, the Lidcombe program is conducted by the parents and not by the therapist. A detailed overview of studies with the Lidcombe program in bilinguals can be found in the chapter by Shenker in this volume. In some of these studies treatment was input simultaneously in two languages (Bakhtiar & Packman, 2009; Gutmann & Shenker, 2006; Harrison *et al.*, 2010; Roberts & Shenker, 2007). In other studies therapy started in one language and only after some time therapy was given in the other language too (Roberts & Shenker, 2007; Rousseau *et al.*, 2005; Shenker *et al.* 1999). The language chosen to start therapy first, time of introduction of the therapy in the other language, the individuals involved in the therapy (clinician, mother, father) and the language pairs spoken, all varied from study to study. In all studies of bilingual treatment conducted thus far, fluency increased in both languages, irrespective of whether the two languages were treated simultaneously or sequentially.

Apparently both monolingual and bilingual treatment seems to work in bilinguals who stutter. One further question then is why one would chose bilingual treatment if monolingual treatment is also effective? Indeed, one may wonder if, in the published cases of bilingual treatment, this treatment was necessary at all. It is of course possible that bilingual treatment reduces the treatment time compared to monolingual treatment, but as far as can be determined, this issue has not yet been investigated. In the same vein, in cases of sequential bilingual treatment, one may wonder if bilingual intervention from the start would not have reduced therapy time. Again, to the best of our knowledge, studies on this issue are nonexistent.

5.2 Therapy outcome?

Apart from some evidence that treatment in one language may generalize to the other untreated language, and that both monolingual and bilingual treatment work, there is also some evidence now that therapy outcome in bilingual speakers is not necessarily worse than in monolingual speakers.

Druce *et al.* (1997) in a study investigating an intensive behaviorally oriented treatment program for 6-to 8-year-old children who stutter found no significant difference between percentage of syllables stuttered for 6 bilingual and 9 monolingual participants either before treatment or after treatment and no significant association was seen between bilingualism and outcome 18 months post-program. The bilingual children in this study all started their bilingual education during the first 5 years of life and spoke Slovenian, German, Greek, Hindi or Italian in addition to English. Treatment and (unfortunately) also measures of treatment outcome were confined to English. Results confirmed those of an earlier, similar investigation (Debney & Druce, 1988) in 33 children, 55% of which had a bilingual background. Also in this group results did not show a significant effect of bilingualism on outcome.

Furthermore, the studies with the Lidcombe program showed that median treatment time to arrive at stage 2 of this therapy approach (i.e. when the child reaches zero or near-zero levels of stuttering for three consecutive clinic visits) was not significantly different between bilingual and unilingual children (see Shenker, 2004; Findlay *et al.*, 2008). Also, the gains achieved in therapy are maintained after discharge from treatment (see Shenker, this volume).

Yet, therapy in bilinguals may require some adaptation in order to yield the same outcome as in monolinguals as a study by Waheed-Khan (1998) showed. In that study two comparisons were presented of each 20 bilingual speakers and 20 monolingual English speakers who received fluency shaping therapy. The initial comparison revealed that bilingual children were less successful than monolingual children. The average number of therapy sessions attended and completion of homework assignments was lower among the bilingual children than monolingual children, and the bilingual children were less successful in achieving fluency and in consistently self-correcting their dysfluencies in conversation. It is only when a specialized therapy program was developed for bilingual speakers including the mandatory participation of a family member who functioned as a 'speech helper' that outcome in the bilinguals improved to a level comparable to that of monolingual speakers (second comparison).

The study of Waheed-Khan (1998) reminds us also of an important consideration pertaining to both assessment and treatment of bilingual stutterers, namely that bilingual stutterers are often bicultural as well. A number of recommendations for incorporating the cultural background of bilingual clients who stutter in assessment and treatment can be found in Finn and Cordes (1997) and Leith (1986). Much remains to be learned, however, and empirical data concerning the interactions between cultures and stuttering are still very scanty (Finn & Cordes, 1997; Shames, 1989).

6 Conclusions

Although the relationship between bilingualism and stuttering received clinical interest already in the 19th century, the present literature review shows that much is still to be learned. Several questions regarding bilingualism and stuttering are still a matter of debate, have only been answered partially or await further data to support our present assumptions. Among these are: Is stuttering more prevalent in bilinguals than in monolinguals? Does bilingualism cause stuttering? Does stuttering in bilinguals always manifest in both languages? Can one make reliable and valid judgments about the presence and severity of stuttering in a language that is not one's own? Is closeness to the mother tongue a determining factor in judgments of stuttering in an unfamiliar language?

Should treatment be given in both languages or in one language? And, is outcome of therapy in bilingual speakers worse than in monolingual speakers? One reason why research in this area is making only slow progress is probably the diversity of the population of bilingual speakers. No two bilinguals are alike, or as Haugen (1953) viewed it, the only common thing about bilinguals is that they are not monolingual. On the other hand, it is also this diversity that constitutes the challenge for both clinicians and researchers.

References

Au-Yeung, J., Howell, P., Davis, S., Charles, N. and Sackin, S. (2000) *UCL Survey on Bilingualism and Stuttering*. Paper presented at the 3rd World congress on Fluency Disorders, Nyborg, Denmark, 7–11 August 2000.

Bakhtiar, M. and Packman, A. (2009) Intervention with the Lidcombe program for a bilingual school-age child who stutters in Iran. *Folia Phoniatrica et Logopaedica* 61, 300–304.

Bernstein Ratner, N. and Benitez, M. (1985) Linguistic analysis of a bilingual stutterer. *Journal of Fluency Disorders* 10, 211–219.

Bloodstein, O. and Bernstein Ratner, N. (2008) *A Handbook on Stuttering* (6th edn). New York: Delmar.

Cabrera,V. and Bernstein Ratner, N. (2000) *Stuttering Patterns in the Two Languages of a Bilingual Child*. Paper presented at the ASHA annual convention, Washington DC, November 16–19.

Carias, S. and Ingram, D. (2006) Language and disfluency: Four case studies on Spanish-English bilingual children. *Journal of Multilingual Communication Disorders* 4, 149–157.

Dale, P. (1977) Factors related to dysfluent speech in bilingual Cuban–American adolescents. *Journal of Fluency Disorders* 2, 311–314.

Debney, S. and Druce, T. (1988) Intensive fluency program. Long-term follow-up study. *Australian Communication Quarterly* 4, 9–10.

De Bot, K. and Kroll, J.F. (2002) Psycholinguistics. In N. Schmitt (ed.) *Introduction to Applied Linguistics* (pp. 133–149). London: Arnold Publishers.

Druce, T., Debney, S. and Byrt, T. (1997) Evaluation of an intensive treatment program for stuttering in young children. *Journal of Fluency Disorders* 22, 169–186.

Eldridge, M. (1968) *A History of the Treatment of Speech Disorders*. Edinburgh: Livingstone.

Fairbanks, G. (1955) Selective vocal effects of delayed auditory feedback. *Journal of Speech and Hearing Disorders* 20, 333–346.

Findlay, K., Shenker, R.C. and Matthews, S. (2008) *Treatment Time with the Lidcombe Program for Bilingual Children*. Poster presented at the American Speech Language and Hearing Association. Chicago, Ill.

Finn, P. and Cordes, A.K. (1997) Multicultural identification and treatment of stuttering: A continuing need for research. *Journal of Fluency Disorders* 22, 219–236.

Greenberg, J.H. (1956) The measure of linguistic diversity. *Language* 32, 109–115.

Grosjean, F. (1982) *Life with Two Languages: An Introduction to Bilingualism.* Cambridge, MA: Harvard University Press.

Gutmann, V. and Shenker, R.C. (2006) *Achieving Fluency in Bilingual Children with the Lidcombe Program.* Poster Presented at the American Speech Language and Hearing Association, Miami, Florida.

Harrison, E., Kingston, M. and Shenker, R.C. (2010) Case studies in evidence-based management of stuttering preschoolers. Manuscript submitted for publication.

Haugen, E. (1953) *The Norwegian Language in American: A Study in Bilingual Behavior.* Philadelphia: University of Pennsylvania Press.

Howell, P., Davis, S. and Williams, R. (2009) The effects of bilingualism on stuttering during late childhood. *Archives of Disease in Childhood* 94, 42–46.

Howell, P., Ruffle, L., Fernández-Zúñiga, A., Gutiérrez, R., Fernández, A.H., O'Brien, M.L., Tarasco, M., Vallejo-Gomez, I. and Au-Yeung, J. (2004) Comparison of exchange patterns of stuttering in Spanish and English monolingual speakers and a bilingual Spanish-English speaker. In A. Packman, A. Meltzer and H.F.M. Peters (eds) *Theory, Research and Therapy in Fluency Disorders. Proceedings of the 4th World Congress on Fluency Disorders, Montreal, Canada* (pp. 415–422). Nijmegen: Nijmegen University Press.

Humphrey, B. (1999) *Bilingual Stuttering: Can Treating One Language Improve Fluency in Both?* Poster session presented at the annual convention of the American Speech-Language-Hearing Association, San Francisco, CA.

Humphrey, B.D. (2004) Judgements of disfluency in a familiar vs. an unfamiliar language. In A. Packman, A. Meltzer and H.F.M. Peters (eds) *Theory, Research and Therapy in Fluency Disorders. Proceedings of the 4th World Congress on Fluency Disorders, Montreal, Canada* (pp. 423–427). Nijmegen: Nijmegen University Press.

Humphrey, B., Natour, Y. and Amayreh, M. (2001) *Bilingual Stuttering: Comparing Treatment Studies of Children vs. Adults.* Paper presented at the annual convention of the Florida Association of Speech-Language Pathologists and Audiologists, Orlando FL.

Ingham, R.J. and Costello, J.M. (1984) Stuttering treatment outcome evaluation. In J. Costello (ed.) *Speech Disorders in Children* (pp. 313–346). San Diego, CA: College-Hill.

Jankelowitz, D.L. and Bortz, M.A. (1996) The interaction of bilingualism and stuttering in an adult. *Journal of Communication Disorders* 29, 223–234.

Jayaram, M. (1983) Phonetic influences on stuttering in monolingual and bilingual stutterers. *Journal of Communication Disorders* 16, 278–297.

Karniol, R. (1992) Stuttering out of bilingualism. *First Language* 12, 255–283.

Lebrun, Y., Bijleveld, H. and Rousseau, J.J. (1990) A case of persistent neurogenic stuttering following a missile wound. *Journal of Fluency Disorders* 15, 251–258.

Lee, B.S. (1950) Some effects of sidetone delay. *Journal of the Acoustical Society of America* 22, 639–640.

Leith, W.R. (1986) Treating the stutterer with atypical cultural differences. In K. St. Louis (ed.) *The Atypical Stutterer* (pp. 9–34). San Diego, CA: Academic.

Lewis, M.P. (ed.) (2009) *Ethnologue: Languages of the World* (16th edn). Dallas, TX: SIL International. Online version: http://www.ethnologue.com/.

Lim, V.P.C. (2007) *A Comparison of Stuttering Behavior and Fluency Improvement in English-Mandarin Bilinguals Who Stutter.* A thesis submitted in fulfillment of the requirements for the degree of Doctor of Philosophy. Australian Stuttering Research Centre. The University of Sydney.

Lim, V.P.C., Lincoln, M., Chan, Y.H. and. Onslow, M. (2008) Stuttering in English–Mandarin bilingual speakers: The influence of language dominance on stuttering severity. *Journal of Speech, Language, and Hearing Research* 51, 1522–1537.

MacKay, D.G. and Bowman, R.W. (1969) On producing the meaning in sentences. *American Journal of Psychology* 82, 23–39.

Meline, T., Stoehr, R.W., Cranfield, C. and Elliot, A. (2006) *Stuttering and Late Bilinguals: What is the Evidence to Date?* Paper presented at the American Speech-Language-Hearing Association Annual Convention, Miami, FL.

Nwokah, E.E. (1988) The imbalance of stuttering behavior in bilingual speakers. *Journal of Fluency Disorders* 13, 357–373.

Packman, A., Onslow, M., Reilly, S., Attanasio, J. and Shenker, R. (2009) Stuttering and bilingualism. *Archives of Disease in Childhood* 94, 248.

Paradis, M. Bilingual Aphasia Test (BAT). http://www.mcgill.ca/linguistics/research/bat/.

Ringo, C.C. and Dietrich, S. (1995) Neurogenic stuttering: An analysis and critique. *Journal of Medical Speech–Language Pathology* 3, 111–122.

Roberts, P.M. (2002) Disfluency patterns in four bilingual adults who stutter. *Journal of Speech-Language Pathology and Audiology/Revue d'orthophonie et d'audiologie* 26, 5–19.

Roberts, P.M. and Shenker, R.C. (2007) Assessment and treatment of stuttering in bilingual speakers. In E. Conture and R.F. Curlee (eds) *Stuttering and Related Disorders of Fluency* (3rd edn) (pp. 183–209) New York: Thieme Medical Publishers, Inc.

Rousseau, I., Packman, A. and Onslow, M. (2005, June) *A Trial of the Lidcombe Program with School Age Stuttering Children*. Paper presented at the Speech Pathology National Conference, Canberra, Australia.

Schäfer, S.M.C.M. (2008) *Stuttering Characteristics of German-English Bilingual Speakers*. A thesis submitted in partial fulfillment of the requirements for the Degree of Masters of Science in Speech-language-therapy in the University of Canterbury. University of Canterbury.

Scott Trautman, L. and Keller, K. (2000) *Bilingual Intervention for Stuttering: A Case in Point*. Paper presented and the ASHA annual convention,Washington, DC, November 16–19.

Shames, G.H. (1989) Stuttering: An RFP for a cultural perspective. *Journal of Fluency Disorders* 14, 67–77.

Shenker, R.C. (2004) Bilingualism in early stuttering: Empirical issues and clinical implications. In A.K. Bothe (ed.) *Evidence-based Treatment of Stuttering: Empirical Bases and Clinical Application* (pp. 81–96). Mahwah, NJ: Lawrence Erlbaum Associates.

Shenker, R.C., Conte, A., Gingras, A., Courcey, A. and Polomeno, L. (1998) The impact of bilingualism on developing fluency in a preschool child. In E.C. Healey and H.F.M. Peters (eds) *Second World Congress on Fluency Disorders Proceedings, San Francisco, August 18–22* (pp. 200–204). Nijmegen: Nijmegen University Press.

Siguan, M. and Mackay, W.F. (1987) *Education and Bilingualism*. London: Kagan Page in association with UNESCO.

Stern, E. (1948) A preliminary study of bilingualism and stuttering in four Johannesburg schools. *Journal of Logopaedics* 1, 15–25.

Travis, L.E., Johnson, W. and Shover, J. (1937) The relation of bilingualism to stuttering. *Journal of Speech Disorders* 2, 185–189.

Van Borsel, J. and Britto Pereira, M. M. (2005) Assessment of stuttering in a familiar versus an unfamiliar language. *Journal of Fluency Disorders* 30, 109–124.

Van Borsel, J., Leahy, M.M. and Britto Pereira, M.M. (2008) Judging stuttering in an unfamiliar language: The importance of closeness to the native language. *Clinical Linguistics and Phonetics* 22, 59–67.

Van Borsel, J., Sunaert, R. and Engelen, S. (2005) Speech disruption under delayed auditory feedback in multilingual speakers. *Journal of Fluency Disorders* 30, 201–217.

Van Borsel, J., Meirlaen, A., Achten, R., Vingerhoets, G. and Santens, P. (2009) Acquired stuttering with differential manifestation in different languages: A case study. *Journal of Neurolinguistics* 22, 187–195.

Van Riper, C. (1971) *The Nature of Stuttering*. Englewood Cliffs, NJ: Prentice-Hall.

Waheed-Khan, N. (1997) Fluency therapy with multilingual clients. In E.C. Healey and H.F.M. Peters (eds) *Proceedings of the Second World Congress on Fluency Disorders, San Francisco. August 18–22* (pp. 195–199). Nijmegen: Nijmegen University Press.

Watson, J.B. and Kayser, H. (1994) Assessment of bilingual/bicultural children and adults who stutter. *Seminars in Speech and Language* 15, 149–164.

Watt, N. (2000) Analysis of language factors in a multilingual stutterer. *South African Journal of Communication Disorders* 47, 5–12.

Woods, D.W. and Wright, L.W. (1998) Dismantling simplified regulated breathing: A case of a bilingual stutterer. *Journal of Behavior Therapy and Experimental Psychiatry* 29 (2), 179–186.

Chapter 12

Stuttering in English-Mandarin Bilinguals in Singapore

VALERIE P.C. LIM AND MICHELLE LINCOLN

Summary

English and Mandarin are the two most spoken languages in the world, yet there is little information about how stuttering manifests in Mandarin, or in bilinguals who speak both English and Mandarin. This chapter outlines our clinical and research experience with stuttering in Singapore, and in particular, with English-Mandarin bilinguals who stutter.

1   Introduction

We start the chapter with a brief overview of the demographics and language background of the population of Singapore. We next describe the differences between English and Mandarin languages so that the reader has a better understanding of the structural differences between them. This is followed by a discussion of our clinical experience with the assessment and treatment of preschoolers, school-age children, adolescent and adult bilinguals who stutter (BWS) in Singapore. We then provide some local research data on adolescent and adult BWS. Specifically, we report on how stuttering manifests in English-Mandarin BWS, and how such individuals respond to treatment. We end the chapter with a proposed model of bilingual stuttering that attempts to explain our research findings, and highlight some areas for future research.

2   Background Information about Singapore

Singapore is a city-state in which multilingualism is the norm at all levels of society (Gupta, 1994). The Singapore resident population is approximately 3.6 million, and comprises four main ethnic groups namely Chinese (74.7%), Malay (13.6%), Indian (8.9%), and Others (2.8%) ('Singapore in Figures, 2009'). There are four official languages spoken in Singapore – English, Mandarin, Malay, Tamil – but there are also many dialectal variations of Chinese that are used (e.g. Cantonese, Hokkien, Teochew etc.). The main language used for instruction in schools is English.

271

Depending on their ethnic background, children in Singapore are usually exposed to at least two of the four languages in the home through local television and radio broadcasts and other public services (e.g., transport, shopping centers). They are expected to become bilingual and literate in English, and in either Mandarin, Malay or Tamil during their primary education which occurs from 6 to 12 years of age. Even though bilingualism in this form continues through secondary education and into adulthood, the use and level of proficiency in each language varies across Singaporean children. In general, Singaporeans function at the bilingual end of the monolingual-bilingual mode continuum described by Grosjean (2001). According to Grosjean, bilinguals can be in a totally monolingual language mode, where one language is thought to be active while the other is deactivated, to the bilingual end of the continuum, where both languages are thought to be active. At the bilingual end of the continuum, bilinguals communicate with other bilinguals in their two (or more) languages, and can frequently language mix and code-switch. While some Singaporean children develop balanced abilities in both languages, others maintain a dominant language, or are dominant in particular language modalities (i.e. speaking or understanding). For example, it is common for many bilingual Singaporeans to use Mandarin, Malay and Tamil for everyday speaking but to read and write mainly in English. Hence, they would develop better written proficiency in English than for their other languages.

The literacy rate in Singapore is relatively high (96%) ('Singapore in Figures, 2009') with many Singaporeans literate in two languages. For example, a recent report from the Department of Statistics showed that more than half of the Chinese population above the age of 15 are literate in English and Mandarin ('Population Trends, 2006'). As the majority of the population comes from an ethnic Chinese background, this bilingual cohort is the largest ethnic group presenting at stuttering clinics in Singapore. Consequently, the focus of our research has been on stuttering in English-Mandarin bilinguals. In the following section we introduce the main similarities and differences between the English and Chinese languages that are relevant to multilingualism and stuttering in Singapore (for a comprehensive discussion, see Lin, 2001).

3 Differences between English and Mandarin-Chinese

3.1 Background information

English and Chinese originate from separate language families: Indo-European and Sino-Tibetan. There is a vast difference between the two languages in terms of their respective written forms, syntax, morphology, phonology and syllable structure. There are many variants of English (e.g. Cockney, American English, Scottish English) and Chinese (e.g.

Mandarin, Cantonese, Hokkien), and their respective spoken forms vary according to the dialect, or the region or country in which the language is spoken.

3.2 Linguistic differences

Unlike in English syntax and morphology, inflections are not used in Chinese. In particular, there are no plural markings on the verb, no case or agreement markings, and no tense suffixes. Additionally, English and Chinese contrast with respect to word order and word order cues (Li *et al.*, 1993). English and Chinese also have distinct segmental phonemic inventories and their phonotactic constraints are distinct from each other. Syllabic structure in English can be very complex; syllables may begin with up to three consonants (as in *straight* or *splash*), and occasionally end with as many as four (as in *prompts*). See Howell and Rusbridge (this volume) for further details. Conversely, the phonotactic system of Chinese languages is relatively simple. For instance, the Mandarin-Chinese syllable structure has three elements: syllable initials, syllable finals and tones. Syllable initials can consist of either vowels (vowel initials) or consonants (consonantal beginnings). There are no consonant clusters in Mandarin, hence, the consonantal beginning of a syllable can only be a single consonant (Li & Thompson, 1981). Syllable finals are the part of the syllable that excludes the initial. There are only two syllable final consonants in standard Mandarin: /n/ and /ŋ/ (Tseng, 1988). However, unlike the syllable structure of English, the Chinese syllable must be affiliated with a lexical tone (see next section) in order for any syllable to become lexically meaningful.

Chinese words are formed using either one or more Chinese characters. Each Chinese character is a logograph, or a monosyllabic morpheme. As such, the meaning of each word is easily apparent. For example, the word 'car' in Mandarin is represented by the single character 车 [che[1]][1]. On the other hand, the word 'bicycle' in Mandarin is made up of three Chinese characters 脚踏车 [jiao[3] da[4] che[1]] all of which are individually meaningful (i.e. 'leg', 'step', and 'car'). Conversely, English words are made up of one or more letters. Although letter-to-sound correspondence may be weak in some instances, it is possible to read many unknown English words by decoding their constituent parts. Thus, in contrast with English, one must know the pronunciation that is associated with the Chinese character in order to read it correctly (for details, see Weekes *et al.*, 1998).

3.2.1 Tone, pitch and stress differences

Chinese languages are tonal languages. Lexical tones are described as contrastive variations in pitch or fundamental frequency (F_0) at the syllable level (Keung & Hoosain, 1979; Packard, 1992; Yiu & Fok, 1995).

Table 12.1 Illustration of lexical tones for Mandarin and Cantonese

Tone/Description	Syllable	Word meaning
Mandarin		
Tone 1 – high-level	ma^1	mother
Tone 2 – high-rising	ma^2	plant
Tone 3 – low-falling-rising	ma^3	horse
Tone 4 – high-falling	ma^4	to scold
Cantonese		
Tone 1 – high-falling	yi^1	clothes
Tone 2 – mid-rising	yi^2	chair
Tone 3 – mid-level	yi^3	opinion
Tone 4 – low-falling	yi^4	son
Tone 5 – low-rising	yi^5	ear
Tone 6 – low-level	yi^6	two

They minimally distinguish individual Chinese words that are not differentiated by segmental (consonant or vowel phonemes) information (Baudoin-Chial, 1986; Gandour, 1987) (see Table 12.1). Thus, lexical tones alter the meaning of Chinese words in the same way that phonemes minimally differentiate words in English (e.g. bat vs. pat). The number and type of lexical tones are known to vary across the different Chinese languages. For example, Mandarin has four lexical tones whereas Cantonese has six (see Table 12.1).

Although each Chinese character or syllable is associated with a lexical tone when it stands alone, the same syllable may take on a different tone when it is followed by another syllable without any change in its meaning. Such phonological rules are called *tone sandhi* (Li & Thompson, 1981; Matthews & Yip, 1994). Tone sandhi are described as the change of tones when syllables are juxtaposed (Li & Thompson, 1981). Application of these tone sandhi rules modifies the original production of lexical tones at the phonetic level (i.e. spoken level) only. For instance, the Mandarin word for 'fruit' is represented by two syllables, 水 [$shui^3$] and 果 [guo^3]. Each of the two characters is originally associated with the Mandarin third tone. A tone sandhi rule stipulates that when two third tone syllables are articulated in succession (e.g. tone 3-tone 3), the former syllable is always pronounced as a second tone (i.e. 水果 or $shui^2$ guo^3). As the application of this tone sandhi rule only affects its spoken form, the written character and meaning of the word do not change.

In English, differences in pitch are not related to the lexicon in the same way (Cruttenden, 1986). English is considered a stress-timed language (see Abercrombie, 1967; Grabe & Low, 2002 for full discussion) where stress patterns are used to influence the timing and rhythm of speech. However, there is still debate as to whether the English spoken in different countries can be similarly classified[2]. Syllable stress refers to the relative emphasis that may be given to certain syllables in a word, and is produced by changes in the pitch, duration and loudness of sounds. The production of syllable stress may vary according to the length and context of the utterance produced. Moreover, English utterances also use intonation – variations in time, amplitude and voice pitch that are superimposed over phrases or sentences – to convey syntactic, pragmatic and affective information and to minimally distinguish sentence types (Blumstein & Cooper, 1974; Cooper & Klouda, 1987). Intonation and stress-like patterns have been observed in Chinese, but generally with fewer possibilities than in English (Cruttenden, 1986). For example, the statement 'this is my pen' in English can also be produced as a question form by using a rising intonation on the last word. In Mandarin, however, the same statement 这是我的笔 can only turn into a question form by adding a grammatical particle 吗 at the end of the sentence: 这是我的笔吗?

4   Models of Speech Processing in English and Mandarin

There are several models of speech production available in the literature which describe the speech planning process for English (e.g. Dell, 1986; Dell & Oseaghdha, 1992; Garrett, 1982; Levelt, 1989; Levelt *et al.*, 1999; Roelofs, 2000). Since lexical tones are an integral part of the Chinese language, the speech planning process for Chinese languages also needs to incorporate modifications for lexical tone production. As the WEAVER++ model developed by Levelt and his colleagues (1989, 1999) has been adapted to accommodate the production of words in Chinese (see Chen, 1999; Chen *et al.*, 2002, 2003) we chose to explore this model in some depth to see if it can account for stuttering in both English and Mandarin.

There is similar conceptual preparation, parallel retrieval of segmental and prosodic features, sequential linking of segments in the syllable structure and the activation of motor programs for syllables for both English and Mandarin. However, to produce a two-syllable Chinese word, the lemma (representation of the syntactic properties of the word that is extracted from memory) connects to the two morpheme units, and specifies their order of appearance (Chen *et al.*, 2002). In the case of the Chinese word 电话 (meaning telephone), the two morphemes [dian^4] and [hua^4] are activated, and a syllable and a tone are also retrieved. At this stage, the syllable has phonological segments but lacks tone representation. There is neurolinguistic evidence for independent phonological tiers for segments and lexical tones in the constitution of a word in tone languages (Gandour *et al.*, 1994; Snider and van der Hulst, 1992). Studies of aphasic individuals have shown that the production of phonological segments (e.g. consonants and vowels) and tones can be independently disrupted following brain damage (Gandour *et al.*, 1994; Liang & Heuven, 2004; Lim, 1998a, 1998b; Naeser & Chan, 1980; Packard, 1992).

It is postulated that the retrieved lexical tones are represented and processed in a manner similar to linguistic stress in English (Chen, 1999). Hence they are encoded as part of the phonological frame. Once the tonal frame is created and the syllable unit is accessible, the content of the syllable is linked with the tonal frame (Chen *et al.*, 2002). Chen and colleagues also suggest that full preparation of each syllable occurs before stress patterns and tone sandhi rules (where applicable) are applied. The integrated phonological word representation [dian^{4}hua^4] is then passed down to the phonetic level where the tone is translated into the vowel that carries it and is configured as a pitch contour. The appropriate articulatory programs are then activated. As the in case for English, it is assumed that a syllable inventory exists so that articulatory programs do not have to be generated from scratch each time a word is produced. In comparison with English, however, the number of syllables stored in the Chinese syllabary is believed to be smaller. Moreover, whereas online changes in syllable structure and word stress patterns occur frequently in English speech, such resyllabification between syllables in Mandarin is less likely (Chen *et al.*, 2003).

4.1.1   Relation to stuttering

Levelt *et al.*'s WEAVER++ model was developed within Levelt's general theoretical framework for speech production, and is discussed in this chapter for two reasons. First, it is one of the models that has been used by researchers to discuss how language factors affect stuttering (Bernstein Ratner & Wijnen, 2007; Kolk & Postma, 1997). Second and more importantly, it has been previously used to accommodate the production of words in Chinese (see Chen, 1999; Chen *et al.*, 2002, 2003). We discuss the Leveltian model in this chapter *not* with the purpose of identifying the origin of stuttering within the speech production process. Rather, we use it to explore the potential differences that may be expected in the manifestation of stuttering between Chinese and English. Notwithstanding, we are aware that the Levelt model has been critiqued (see, for example, Howell, 2010), and that alternative models of language processing (e.g. Dell, 1986; Dell & Oseaghdha, 1992) have also been used to explain how stuttering arises in monolinguals and bilinguals (see, for example, Howell & Dworzynski, 2005; Howell *et al.*, 2004). Models are useful only in as much as they facilitate the generation of research questions that test the elements of the model and it is with this in mind that we are exploring the Levelt model. The elements that Howell (2004) identifies as controversial about this model (those involving perceptual monitoring) are not employed in our work.

To summarize so far, we have introduced the inherent differences in language structure and linguistic processing between the English and Chinese languages. English is stress-timed while Chinese is tonal. While the syllable and segmental structure of Chinese is simpler than English, the processing of the Chinese word needs to incorporate an additional important feature – lexical tone. Since it has been proposed that stuttering can be influenced by factors such as linguistic stress (Natke *et al.*, 2004; Wingate, 1984) and phonetic structure (cf. Bernstein Ratner, 2005b; Dworzynski & Howell, 2004; Howell *et al.*, 2000), it was of interest to study whether the degree and pattern of stuttering across English and Chinese differ. For instance, would the frequency of stuttering in Mandarin be lower than that in English because of its simpler phonetic structure? This notion provided the impetus for an investigation of stuttering in Mandarin-Chinese, and more specifically, in bilinguals who stutter who speak both English and Mandarin. Before we present our data on English-Mandarin BWS, we felt that it would benefit the reader to first be acquainted with the stuttering services in Singapore.

5 Assessment of Stuttering in Singapore

There are currently no prevalence or incidence data for stuttering in Singapore. Nonetheless, clinicians in Singapore have been managing preschoolers, school-aged children, adolescents and adults who stutter for more than two decades. Although most Singaporeans are bilingual, clinicians in Singapore (the first author included) have for the longest time been assessing BWS in the language that the clinicians themselves are most comfortable with. More often than not, this language is English. There are several reasons as to why this monolingual practice was, and probably still is, the principal approach that is adopted.

Compared to other countries, the speech language pathology profession in Singapore is in its infancy. At present, there are approximately 180 speech language pathologists serving a total population of 4.8 million. Services for stuttering are available in a limited number of government hospitals and private clinics, and to date only a small number of Speech Language Pathologists (SLPs) have experience in managing individuals who stutter ('SHAS Directory of Services', 2009). Before 2007, all clinicians in Singapore were trained overseas (e.g. in the US, UK, or Australia), and received their academic and clinical training in the English language. It is possible that the overseas trained clinicians may not have adequate technical knowledge of the local languages to handle the linguistic complexity of the clients in Singapore. Additionally, as there are four official languages and numerous dialects spoken in Singapore, bilingual clinicians may still not always understand or speak the languages of their clients. As such, clinicians may not feel comfortable, or may not be able to accurately assess or treat stuttering in the languages that they are not familiar with, or speak less proficiently in (see Van Borsel & Medeiros de Britto Pereira, 2005). Therefore, even though clinicians in Singapore recognize the advantages of assessing all the languages in their bilingual clients' repertoire (see, for example, Kohnert, 2009; Roberts, 2001), they may not possess adequate skills, resources or time to assess stuttering in two (or more) languages. Furthermore, up until recently, local stuttering research data were non-existent, and there was no information on which to base assessment and treatment decisions for people who stutter.

In the more recent years, SLPs at the Singapore General Hospital (SGH) Stuttering Clinic have started to adopt a bilingual approach when assessing BWS. In order to diagnose stuttering in BWS, we take comprehensive language and stuttering case histories, and, whenever possible, conduct speech assessments and analyses in the client's two languages. Observed stuttering behaviors are interpreted with consideration of the client's level of proficiency in one language relative to the other, the domain and frequency of language use, and the topic of conversation to which the client is accustomed. This is because slower speech rate, pauses, revisions, interjections or shorter sentences may reflect bilingual coping strategies, or normal disfluencies that may be related to limited language proficiency rather than stuttering per se (Roberts & Shenker, 2007; Watson & Kayser, 1994). In the absence of specific diagnostic guidelines for BWS, SLPs at the SGH Stuttering Clinic generally take into consideration the presence or absence of the following factors when making a differential diagnosis of stuttering, especially in young children: (a) stuttering behaviors in both languages, (b) secondary behaviors in both languages, (c) negative reactions towards communication in both languages, and (d) familial history of stuttering (see Howell *et al.*, 2009; Mattes & Omark, 1991; Roberts & Shenker, 2007; Van Borsel *et al.*, 2001; Watson & Kayser, 1994). Such factors may also apply to older children and adults who stutter.

6   Management of Stuttering in Singapore

Clinicians in Singapore use different types of treatment approaches in their management of preschoolers, school-aged children, adolescents and adults who stutter (see Table 12.2). Although there are a relatively wide variety of treatments practiced in Singapore, their usage is dependent on the SLP's clinical training background and personal experience. It is not uncommon for clinicians to use a hybrid approach or a combination of treatments for different groups of people who stutter.

Table 12.2 Therapeutic approaches available for people who stutter in Singapore

Preschoolers	*School-aged children*	*Adolescents/adults*
Lidcombe Program	Lidcombe Program	Prolonged Speech
	GILCU /ELU	Time Out
	Prolonged Speech	Altered Auditory Feedback (AAF)
	Time Out	Cognitive Behavioural Therapy[1]

[1] Mainly conducted by Psychologists/Psychiatrists

A logical question when treating stuttering in bilinguals is whether BWS should receive treatment in one or both languages. Monolingual and bilingual treatment approaches have been trialed previously, both with positive outcomes (see, for example, Roberts & Shenker, 2007; Shenker, 2004; Shenker *et al.*, 1998; Waheed-Khan, 1998). However, we agree with Roberts and Shenker (2007) that BWS may not necessarily need treatment in both languages. This issue of whether monolingual or bilingual treatment is superior remains unclear since there is currently insufficient data to draw conclusions.

6.1 Preschoolers who stutter

There are numerous treatment approaches that are available for early stuttering intervention (see Bloodstein & Bernstein Ratner, 2008; Conture & Curlee, 2007; Guitar, 2006), but the approach that has been most extensively researched is the Lidcombe Program of Early Stuttering Intervention (LP; see Onslow *et al.*, 2003). There are at least 13 clinical trials of the LP with preschoolers (see Jones *et al.*, 2008), three of which are randomized control trials (Jones *et al.*, 2005; Lattermann *et al.*, 2008; Lewis *et al.*, 2008). All of these studies show that LP is efficacious in reducing stuttering in preschool-aged children. Even though the empirical data for the LP is striking, other researchers have raised issues regarding this treatment approach (Bernstein Ratner, 2005a; Bloodstein & Bernstein Ratner, 2008). Moreover, the LP may not work for all children and it is still uncertain which treatment option best fits individual families (Franken *et al.*, 2005). Alternative treatment approaches have also yielded positive outcomes similar to that of the LP (see, for example, Franken *et al.*, 2005; Trajkovski *et al.*, 2006, 2009).

Nonetheless, the LP is the main treatment approach that is used in Singapore. At the time of writing, there are only a handful of Singaporean

SLPs who have had formal training in the LP. Our collective clinical experience at the SGH Stuttering Clinic is that preschool-aged children who stutter in Singapore generally respond well to the LP. For reasons described previously (see Section 5 of this chapter), the majority of preschool children seen at our clinic receive monolingual treatment in English. Although Singaporean children who attend daycare facilities or preschool may start some bilingual language exposure between 2 and 6 years of age, few develop sufficient proficiency levels in both languages to allow for bilingual stuttering intervention. Thus, for all of these reasons, only a small number of children in our clinic are treated in both languages.

Irrespective of whether the LP is delivered in one or both languages, our collective clinical observation is that the children at our clinic show stuttering reductions in both languages (see also Roberts & Shenker, 2007; Shenker, 2004; Shenker *et al.*, 1998). However, we are yet to perform any formal audit of our clinical files of children who have been treated with the LP in our clinic, or collect any formal efficacy data for the use of the LP with bilingual Singaporean preschool children to empirically support this observation. This topic remains a high priority for future research.

The implementation of the LP in our clinic is not problem-free. We do encounter hurdles which are not uncommon to our colleagues outside of Singapore. For example, possibly due to the Asian culture, we have found that some parents can be very reserved and uncomfortable with overt praise, and/or feel overly self conscious about being observed in action with their children. As the LP is essentially a behavioral program where parental training is key, these issues affect the degree of parental participation in the program. The other common challenge that we face is that parents/caregivers have difficulty maintaining weekly therapy sessions in view of their own work schedules or their child's other co-curricular activities. We try to overcome these issues by approaching the concept of parent training sensitively, and to be as flexible and accessible to parents as we possibly can.

6.2 School-aged children

As children who attend primary school in Singapore receive bilingual education, they would usually have two languages in their repertoire. While some children have somewhat balanced abilities in both languages, the majority of children referred to our clinic have one language that is more dominant than the other. Similar to our approach with preschool children, most school-aged children at our clinic receive treatment mainly in English. Table 12.2 shows the different types of treatment approaches that are used in Singapore. Although our clinical records and our clients' self-report indicate that stuttering reduces in both languages post-treatment (see also Roberts & Shenker, 2007), we currently have not systematically collected or analyzed any efficacy data to support these observations. As is the case with preschool children, research on how school-aged children in Singapore respond to stuttering treatment is highly warranted.

Nonetheless, our clinical experience is that school-aged children who stutter, compared to preschool-aged children and adolescents and adults who stutter, are 'more difficult' to treat, and may often take a longer time to respond to treatment. Apart from stuttering being less tractable with age and time, another plausible reason for this observation in Singapore is that school-aged children are engaged in a myriad of activities (e.g. school, co-curricular activities, private tuition, music classes etc.) and it is often difficult for them to receive consistent weekly therapy, or to have time for daily speech practice.

6.3   Adolescents and adults who stutter

Adolescent and adult BWS in Singapore usually have different language dominance profiles, and varying levels of proficiency in both languages. For this group, frequency and domain of language use become more important determiners of language dominance than factors such as age of language acquisition since bilinguals tend to lose dominance in a language when it is not used, or is used less frequently (Grosjean, 1998; White & Genesee, 1996). As adolescent and adult BWS need to use different languages for various social conversations or specific tasks (e.g. sitting for an oral exam in Mandarin, giving a presentation or talking to peers in English), they generally desire to be able to speak fluently in more than one language.

In spite of their bilingual profile, adolescent and adult BWS in Singapore have also traditionally received treatment in English only. There are numerous treatment approaches available for treating adolescent and adults who stutter (see Bloodstein & Bernstein Ratner, 2008; Conture & Curlee, 2007; Guitar, 2006; Hewat *et al.*, 2006). In Singapore, clinicians mainly use speech restructuring techniques such as prolonged speech or smooth speech as the main treatment approach for advanced stuttering (see Table 12.2). Speech restructuring has been repeatedly shown to successfully alleviate stuttering in adolescents and adults who stutter (e.g. Andrews *et al.*, 1980; Block *et al.*, 2005; Harrison *et al.*, 1998; Ingham, 1987; O'Brian *et al.*, 2001; Venkatagiri, 2005). However, the techniques can have a negative impact on speech naturalness (cf. O'Brian *et al.*, 2003), and can affect one's desire to continue using the restructured speech in the long term (Cream *et al.*, 2003). Relapse is therefore quite common.

Previous research on speech restructuring techniques has primarily been conducted on non-Asian populations. Unlike the case for preschool and school-aged children, we do have systematic data about adolescent and adults BWS in Singapore. Specifically, our data suggest that:

(a) stuttering frequency can be manifested differently across languages, (b) the use of speech restructuring techniques can effectively reduce stuttering in English-Mandarin adolescent and adult BWS in Singapore, and, (c) positive treatment effects in one language can generalize to the other language.

Stuttering treatment for adolescent and adult BWS is usually offered on a weekly basis or via non-residential, intensive treatment programs. Similar to individuals with advanced stuttering in the West (Guitar, 2006), our clinical experience in Singapore is that such individuals have typically developed negative feelings associated with speaking situations (see Iverach, Jones *et al.*, 2009; Iverach, O'Brian *et al.*, 2009; Kraaimaat *et al.*, 1991; Kraaimaat, Vanryckeghem, & Van Dam-Baggen, 2002; Mahr & Torosian, 1999; Menzies *et al.*, 1999; Messenger *et al.*, 2004; Schneier *et al.*, 1997; Stein *et al.*, 1996). Accordingly, we have found that both their stuttering and their psychological well-being need attention in the treatment process. Thus, whenever necessary, our adolescent and adult clientele are referred to psychologists or psychiatrists for assessment and management of their anxiety.

7 Singapore Stuttering Data

In the first author's clinical experience, adolescent and adult BWS seen at our facility varied in their self-report of, and in their formal assessment results with respect to (a) the language they stuttered more in pretreatment, and (b) the language that they were more fluent in following treatment. This clinical experience sparked off a series of investigations regarding the manifestation and treatment of stuttering in BWS. Since our largest clientele of BWS were English-Mandarin bilinguals, we began and are currently engaged in ongoing research to investigate stuttering in English-Mandarin BWS with a view to developing better guidelines for our own clinical practice, and to develop a deeper understanding of the disorder itself and how it is affected by language structure and use (see Sections 3 and 4 of this chapter).

7.1 Manifestation of stuttering in English-Mandarin BWS in Singapore

In 2008, we investigated the severity and type of stuttering in a group of English-Mandarin BWS to determine whether stuttering was different across the two languages, and whether the differences were influenced by language dominance (see Lim *et al.*, 2008a). Details of the study are found in Lim *et al.* (2008a); however, we provide a synopsis below.

7.1.1 Assessment of language dominance

For the purpose of the study, language dominance was defined as that which reflected the differences in processing each of the two languages

(Birdsong, 2006) and indicated the relative ability levels of the two languages *within* the same individual (for full discussion on language dominance, see Chen & Leung, 1989; Kotz & Elston-Guttler, 2004; McElree *et al.*, 2000). To determine language dominance, we developed and validated a self-report classification tool (Lim *et al.*, 2008b).

It has been argued that self-report ratings are subjective, and may either over or underestimate relative proficiency in the two languages (see Tsai and colleagues, this volume). Hence, self-report ratings may not be considered ideal for assessing language dominance. Notwithstanding, there is a growing body of research which shows that self-assessments of proficiency are valid and reliable measures of language skills, and are correlated highly with ratings by experienced judges and standardized test (Grosjean, 1982; Langdon *et al.*, 2005; Oscarson, 1989). Further, objective assessments of language dominance have their own limitations. There is little consensus about which objective test is best: standardized or non-standardized assessments of language ability (e.g., Bialystok & Miller, 1999; Jared & Kroll, 2001), scores from a standardized examination such as TOEFL (e.g. Golestania, Alario, Meriaux, *et al.*, 2006), or various laboratory tests of speed, fluency and automaticity (e.g. Flege *et al.*, 2002). Thus, it has been argued that a more acceptable approach might be to first determine language dominance using self-report ratings (Langdon *et al.*, 2005), and then use the results of objective tests to substantiate rather than determine language dominance (Grosjean, 1998).

7.1.2 Self-report classification tool (Lim et al., 2008a)

The self-report classification tool is a questionnaire which gathered information on all languages in the participants' repertoire across the four language modalities: understanding, speaking, reading and writing. The criteria used to determine language dominance were based on the participants' self-ratings of language proficiency using a seven-point rating scale (Kohnert *et al.*, 1998), ranking of the language they use most often at home, work, and socially, and quantification of how frequently they use each language. A language was considered dominant if: (a) it consistently received a higher language proficiency rating across the language modalities, (b) was spoken and heard daily and used for either reading or writing at least weekly, and (c) was used in at least two out of the three possible language environments: home, work/school and social. A participant had to fulfill all three self-report criteria in order to be classified as Mandarin-dominant or English-dominant, while failure to satisfy the three criteria was taken to imply balanced bilingualism (for details, see Lim *et al.*, 2008b).

The self-report classification described above was validated on a group of 168 English-Mandarin bilingual University undergraduates in Singapore (Lim *et al.*, 2008b). The accuracy of this classification tool in determining language dominance was then tested using a discriminant analysis (DA; Garson, 2006). In this analysis, the grouping variable was language dominance (English-dominant, Mandarin-dominant, balanced) while the independent variables were the *raw scores* for language proficiency, frequency of language use and domain of language use in both languages. The discriminant analysis performed on the self-report data revealed an overall correct classification rate of 88%. Based on the large sample size in that study, this accuracy rate was high and significant when compared to the random probability of 33% ($p < 0.001$). The categorization of bilingual groups was also supported by the scores obtained on objective vocabulary tests conducted in English and Mandarin as well as their language history data (e.g. age of acquisition, years of language exposure). Together, these results indicated that the self-report tool achieved a reliable three-way classification into English-dominant, Mandarin-dominant and balanced bilinguals.

7.1.3 Participants

Thirty English-Mandarin bilinguals who stutter (BWS) aged 12–44 years were recruited for the study. Using the self-report classification tool, 15 BWS were classified as English-dominant, 4 as Mandarin-dominant and 11 as balanced bilinguals. A discriminant analysis (Garson, 2006) was again performed on the data for the 30 BWS. This yielded a 100% (95% CI 90.5%–100%) accuracy rate for group membership and was found to be significant when compared with the random probability of 33% ($p < 0.001$). Participant characteristics and performance on a receptive vocabulary test also supported this classification result.

7.1.4 Method

Speech samples from each participant were collected in English and in Mandarin. The samples in each language consisted of two beyond clinic audio-recorded conversations (i.e. a telephone call with an unfamiliar person and a home recording with a familiar person), and one within clinic video recording of a conversation with the clinician. All speech samples were on familiar topics (e.g. family, occupation, hobbies etc.) and lasted approximately 10 minutes in duration. The speech samples were analyzed by two Singaporean English-Mandarin bilingual clinicians for percent syllables stuttered (%SS), perceived stuttering severity (SEV) and types of stuttering behaviors using the Lidcombe Behavioral Data Language (LBDL; Packman & Onslow, 1998; Teesson *et al.*, 2003) in each language.

The LBDL classifies stuttering behaviors according to three categories: repeated movements (RM), fixed postures (FP) and superfluous behaviors (SB). These are further sub-categorized into seven descriptors: syllable repetition (SR), incomplete syllable repetition (ISR), multisyllabic unit repetition (MSUR), fixed postures with audible airflow (FPWAA), fixed postures without audible airflow (FPWOAA) and verbal superfluous behaviors (VSB) or nonverbal superfluous behaviors (NVSB) (see Packman & Onslow, 1998). Intra-judge and inter-judge agreement for the LBDL have been investigated previously, with higher agreement reported for experienced than non-experienced judges (LBDL; Packman & Onslow, 1998; Teesson *et al.*, 2003).

Packman and Onslow claim that this taxonomy of stuttering better reflects the kinematics of the speech mechanism, and hence can be used reliably to describe stuttering behaviors across all ages and languages. The LBDL taxonomy may indeed be useful for comparing the types of stutters across languages. This is especially the case when word and syllable boundaries are less distinct in one language (i.e. Mandarin) than the other (i.e. English). Taking the example of the word 'bicycle' again, a repetition of the first character/syllable 脚 in the word 脚踏车 (directly translated as 'leg', 'step', and 'car' in Mandarin) could either be classified as a word or syllable repetition.

Using the LBDL in our study, single-syllable whole-word repetitions were included under the category of syllable repetition. The Pearson correlation coefficient was used to analyze intra- and inter-judge reliability. Intra-judge reliability for the number of repeated movements, fixed postures and superfluous behaviors identified by the first judge across the two ratings was 0.98, 0.96 and 0.96 respectively. Inter-judge reliability for the total number of the stutters that were identified as repeated movements, fixed postures and superfluous behaviors between the first and second judge was 0.91, 0.74 and 0.79 respectively.

7.1.5 Results

Our results showed that the English-dominant and Mandarin-dominant BWS exhibited higher %SS scores in their less-dominant language (see reference for full results). The scores for the balanced bilinguals, on the other hand, were similar across languages (see Figure 12.1). Our results also showed that the bilingual groups did not differ with respect to the percentage of stutters per LBDL category between English and Mandarin (see Figure 12.2). As there were no significant differences for each LBDL descriptor across languages, the type of stutters according to bilingual groups were analyzed in terms of their broader categories: repeated movements, fixed postures and superfluous behaviors. Although the small sample size within each group precluded the use of statistical analyses, the number of repeated movements, fixed postures and superfluous behaviors did not appear to be markedly different between English and Mandarin for either English-dominant, Mandarin-dominant, or balanced bilinguals. Taken together, this suggested that the same types of stutters were found to manifest in both languages

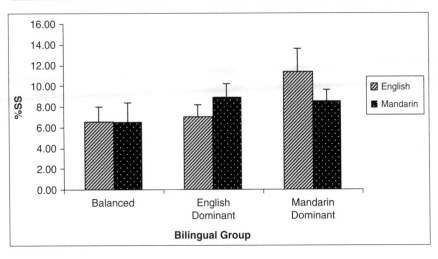

Figure 12.1 Mean percent syllables stuttered (%SS) and severity rating (SEV) scores for English and Mandarin according to bilingual group
Source: Reprinted from JSLHR (with permission)

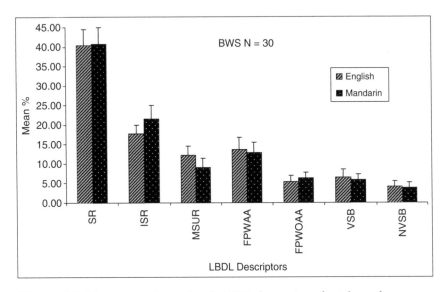

Figure 12.2 Mean percentage of each LBDL descriptor of total number stutters for English and Mandarin
Note: Lidcombe Behavioural Data Language (LBDL), syllable repetition (SR), incomplete syllable repetition (ISR), multisyllabic unit repetition (MSUR), fixed postures with audible airflow (FPWAA), fixed postures without audible airflow (FPWOAA), verbal superfluous behaviors (VSB), and nonverbal superfluous behaviors (NVSB).
Source: Reprinted from JSLHR (with permission)

irrespective of language dominance. We will discuss these results in subsequent sections of this chapter.

7.2 Treatment of English-Mandarin BWS in Singapore

In a second study, we evaluated whether stuttering reductions in English generalized to Mandarin following treatment in English only, and whether treatment generalization was influenced by language dominance. Our data analysis is still ongoing at the time of writing, but we present data from two case studies in this chapter.

7.2.1 Participants

Both participants were male, aged between 27 and 28 years, bilingual in English and Mandarin, and had previously participated in our 2008 study. Using the self-report classification tool described and validated by Lim *et al.* (2008b), one participant was classified as an English-dominant bilingual while the other was categorized as a Mandarin-dominant bilingual. Their bilingual profiles are displayed in Table 12.3. The English-dominant bilingual acquired English earlier than Mandarin, had longer exposure and formal education in English compared to Mandarin, and obtained higher scores on the English version of the Mulitlingual British Picture Vocabulary Scales (see Lim *et al.*, 2008b; Rickard Liow *et al.*, 1992) and on the self-rated language proficiency scale in English than in Mandarin. With the exception of having a longer formal education in English than in Mandarin, the profile for the Mandarin-dominant bilingual showed the reverse pattern. It is not unusual for Singaporean students to have more years formal education in English than Mandarin because the latter is discontinued once students enter the polytechnics or tertiary education.

7.2.2 Treatment program and method

Both participants underwent a speech restructuring intensive program (IP) in English which was adapted from that used by Block and her colleagues (2003, 2005). Our IP involved a three-day, non-residential program which was delivered by experienced clinicians. The first 2 days of the program comprised fluency instatement where participants learnt *Smooth Speech*. They were taught to speak at 60 syllables per minute (SPM), then slowly advancing to a comfort rate of about 180 to 200 SPM. Participants were also taught to focus on achieving natural sounding speech when they acquired speech rates of 120 SPM or higher. Midway through the third day of the IP, participants practiced the transfer of fluent speech to every day speaking situations. This was followed by six, two-hour follow-up sessions that were conducted once a week. During these sessions, the clinician reviewed participants' home practice recordings and use of Smooth Speech, allowed the participants to practice the technique at specified speech rates, and reinforced self-management strategies to facilitate generalization and maintenance of stutter-free speech beyond the clinic.

Table 12.3 Profile of the two English-Mandarin BWS

	English-dominant	*Mandarin-dominant*
Variables		
Age	28	27
Age of language exposure		
English	2	2
Mandarin	6	5
Years of formal instruction		
English	15	14
Mandarin	12	10
Years of language exposure		
English	26	25
Mandarin	22	22
MBPVS Percentage score		
English	92.0	80.0
Mandarin	66.7	66.7
English proficiency (1–7 scale)		
Understanding	7	5
Speaking	7	4
Reading	7	4
Writing	7	4
Mandarin proficiency (1–7 scale)		
Understanding	4	6
Speaking	3	6
Reading	3	6
Writing	3	5

Note: MBPVS = Multilingual British Picture Vocabulary Scale

Treatment was conducted in English only for the entire program. No other specific advice about using the technique in Mandarin was given.

Three 10-minute conversations in English and Mandarin, sampled at pretreatment, immediately post-IP, 4 weeks and 12 weeks post-IP, were analyzed by two English-Mandarin bilingual clinicians for %SS. The %SS scores results for the two participants are displayed in Figure 12.3.

7.2.3 Results

The BWS in both case studies stuttered more in their less-dominant language pretreatment (Table 12.4). The English-dominant BWS stuttered

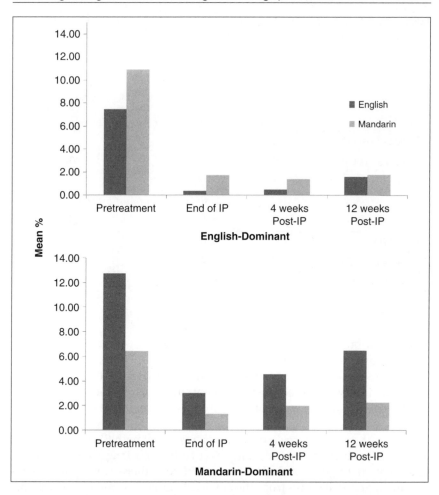

Figure 12.3 Mean Percent Syllables Stuttered (%SS) Scores for English and Mandarin at pretreatment, end of IP, 4-weeks post-IP and 12 weeks post-IP for the English-dominant and Mandarin-dominant bilingual

more in Mandarin (10.93 %SS) than in English (7.47 %SS) while the Mandarin-dominant BWS stuttered more in English (12.7 %SS) compared to Mandarin (6.43 %SS). Both BWS showed stuttering reductions in English and in Mandarin following treatment; however, the pattern of fluency improvement was found to be different for each individual. The mean %SS scores in English for the English-dominant BWS decreased to 0.37 %SS, 0.47 %SS and 1.6 %SS at the end of IP, 4 weeks post-IP and 12 weeks post-IP respectively while his scores for Mandarin were 1.77 %SS, 1.37 %SS and 1.80 %SS at the end of IP, 4 weeks post-IP and 12 weeks post-IP respectively. Conversely, the Mandarin-dominant BWS was found to have English mean %SS scores of 3.0 %SS at the end of IP, 4.57 %SS

Table 12.4 Mean Percent Syllables Stuttered (%SS)) Scores according to language across the four assessment occasions

Assessment occasion	English	Mandarin
	English-dominant bilingual	
Pretreatment	7.47	10.93
End of IP	0.37	1.77
4 weeks Post-IP	0.47	1.37
12 weeks Post-IP	1.60	1.80
	Mandarin-dominant bilingual	
Pretreatment	12.7	6.43
End of IP	3.0	1.33
4 weeks Post-IP	4.57	2.00
12 weeks Post-IP	6.45	2.27

at 4 weeks post-IP and 6.45 %SS at 12 weeks post-IP while his scores for Mandarin were lower: 1.33 %SS, 2 %SS and 2.27 %SS at the end of IP, 4 weeks post-IP and 12 weeks post-IP respectively. Although stuttering reductions were noted post treatment, these results indicated a small but progressive increase in stuttering from one assessment occasion to the other.

The results for our two case studies showed that both BWS experienced an overall reduction in stuttering severity in both languages following treatment in English only. This indicated that there was spontaneous treatment generalization from the treated language to the untreated language. Even though the English-dominant bilingual exhibited a mild increase in residual stuttering at 12 months post-IP, the treatment generalization effect was observed to be fairly stable over time. For the Mandarin-dominant bilingual, however, residual stuttering in Mandarin – the untreated language – appeared to be more stable than that observed for English. Perhaps the more interesting observation was that the extent of treatment generalization was noted to be disproportionate across the two languages. Albeit more prominent in the case of the Mandarin-dominant BWS, both participants had higher residual stuttering in the less-dominant language compared to the dominant language despite being treated in the same language (i.e. English).

While the above results are noteworthy, we acknowledge it only provides data for a small part of larger puzzle that needs further unraveling. Unlike our previous study (Lim *et al.*, 2008a), we did not conduct any

LBDL analyses to determine whether there were any differences in the type of stutters pre- and post-treatment. One could wonder if the same results would be obtained if other symptom counts had been measured before and after treatment. Further, we also did not measure whether there were any improvements in participants' well-being, or report on changes in their speech naturalness following treatment. We hope to report such information when more of our data is analyzed. Until then, we provide a general discussion of our findings to date.

8 General Discussion

The study of stuttering manifestations in English-Mandarin BWS (discussed earlier) produced some interesting findings. First, our data provides evidence which casts doubt on the notion that stuttering patterns in Chinese languages, Mandarin in this case, are different from the patterns observed in English because of the apparent differences in linguistic processing between the two languages. Rather, as we did not find any differences in the type using LBDL and frequency of stuttering using symptoms that include whole monosyllable word repetitions between Mandarin and English, we suggested that language dominance and not language dissimilarity affected the way in which stuttering was displayed in BWS. Second, although the frequency of stuttering in each language was found to be related to language dominance, the result of no significant difference in the topography of stuttering between the two languages may imply that stuttering in English and in Mandarin reflects a similar manner of breakdown during the process of speech production.

Our findings are inconsistent with those of Howell *et al.* (2004),who found quantitative differences in the type of stutters across languages in a Spanish-English BWS. Specifically, Howell *et al.* reported that the BWS produced more non-stalling disfluencies (e.g. incomplete syllable repetitions, fixed postures with and without audible airflow) than stalling disfluencies (e.g. syllable repetitions, multisyllable unit repetitions) in Spanish compared to English. One possible reason for the conflicting results could be that Howell *et al.* used a different analysis procedure in their study. They examined stuttering rates according to content words (CW) and function words (FW) and found that their Spanish-English BWS stuttered more on CW than on FW, in the dominant than the non-dominant language. In a more recent study of five English-Mandarin BWS, Tsai and colleagues (this volume) found no consistent pattern in the distribution of stutters on CW and FW across the English and Mandarin. It is not clear whether the inconsistent findings across the studies are related to the different languages examined (i.e. Mandarin-English vs. Spanish-English), or the types of stuttering symptoms analyzed. What is notable, however, is that we found no difference in the topography of stuttering despite English and Mandarin being more structurally dissimilar than Spanish and English. Indeed, the relationship between the type and frequency of stuttering and language dominance warrants further investigation.

The treatment data from our two case studies of adult BWS provide preliminary data to show that stuttering reductions in English spontaneously generalized to Mandarin following treatment in English only. Our results are consistent with the small number of studies and conference papers cited in Roberts and Shenker (2007) and Van Borsel, Maes, and Foulon (2001) which also show that fluency improvements from the treated language spontaneously transfer to the untreated language. Further, in our two case studies, stuttering remained lower than pretreatment levels for up to 12 weeks post-IP. However, the English-dominant and Mandarin-dominant BWS displayed greater fluency improvements in their dominant language whether or not this language received direct intervention. Such findings allow us to speculate that the extent of treatment generalization may also be associated with language dominance. That is, it is possible that language dominance influences the successful transfer of fluency improvements to the less-dominant language, particularly if treatment is conducted in the dominant language. However, when the less-dominant language is treated, it may be that the effects of stuttering treatment in this language may be obscured by relative language dominance.

The finding of more residual stuttering in the less-dominant language pretreatment, and less fluency improvement in the less-dominant language after treatment coupled with the finding that fluency in this language may dissipate over time may suggest that BWS have greater difficulty in achieving and maintaining fluency in the less-dominant language. Whether this trend is apparent in all BWS or whether it is qualitatively or quantitatively different in bilingual and monolingual people who stutter remains unclear. As it is known that advanced stuttering is intractable and prone to relapse, even monolinguals who stutter may find maintaining fluency after treatment challenging. Recently, Howell *et al.* (2009) reported that a group of children in the United Kingdom who were bilingual from birth had an increased risk of stuttering and a lower likelihood for recovery from stuttering than children who are late bilinguals or who are monolingual speakers. In our study, however, both participants acquired their dominant language first, but still stuttered into adulthood. Based on our own experiences, we believe that bilingualism does not pose an added risk for stuttering (see Bloodstein and Bernstein Ratner, 2008 for discussion). Although our data collection is still ongoing, we attempt to explain the results of both of our studies by exploring the existing information about stuttering and bilingual language processing.

9 A Potential Bilingual Stuttering Model – Our Preliminary Thoughts

We think that our findings of greater stuttering in the less-dominant language pre- and post-treatment might potentially be explained by factors which affect the processing of two languages, and of a less familiar language (see also Roberts, 2002). To illustrate this, Figure 12.4 portrays the scenario of an English-dominant BWS who stutters more in Mandarin. We first discuss the processes of the bilingual model before we explore the potential reasons for the stuttering results reported here.

As discussed earlier we have used Levelt's (1989) distinct stage model of spoken word production and the adaptations of several researchers (e.g. De Bot, 1992; De Bot & Schreuder, 1993; Green, 1986) to incorporate a framework for bilingual speakers. Adjustments to the model were necessary to account for the fact that bilinguals have two languages at their disposal, and are able to separate and mix their languages during speech.

It has been previously suggested that the presence of more than one active language can impose problems of cognitive control (Abutalebi & Green, 2007). Competition between languages can affect performance on various linguistic and cognitive tasks (see Hernandez *et al.*, 2005 for further discussion). Thus, when speaking in one language, there is a need to inhibit the activity of the other. Such language suppression can occur internally within the language itself or externally from the other language, although it has been postulated that the latter is more likely during spontaneous use (Green, 1986, 1993). Green (1986) also asserted that the activation and control of languages consumes limited resources. If such resources are insufficient, control becomes imperfect and speech errors result. This may account for the presence of involuntary intrusions and interference in the speech of bilinguals with or without brain damage. For example, bilinguals with aphasia make semantic, phonemic and even tonal paraphasic errors in their speech, and healthy bilingual individuals frequently demonstrate slip-of-the-tongue phenomena during speech production. These behaviors, together with evidence from studies employing lexical decision, translation tasks and priming paradigms, indicate that there is interaction between the bilingual's two languages at the level of semantic, orthographic, phonological and phonetic processing between the two linguistic systems and is denoted by the dotted arrows in Figure 12.4.

The interaction between the two languages in a bilingual has support in the brain imaging literature. To date, there is still disagreement over whether the brain regions activated by a bilinguals' two languages overlap (e.g. Chee *et al.*, 1999a; Chee *et al.*, 1999b), or are partially different (e.g. Dehaene *et al.*, 1997; Kim *et al.*, 1997; Tham *et al.*, 2005). The inconsistent results could very well be attributable to the different tasks

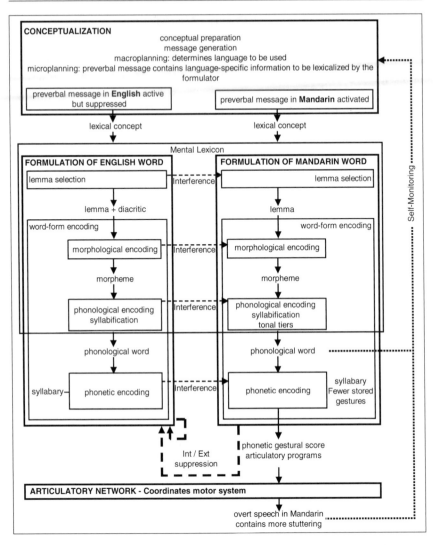

Figure 12.4 Sketch of model of an English-dominant adult BWS speaking in Mandarin, the less-dominant language

Source: Adapted from Green (1989), De Bot (1992), De Bot and Schreuder (1993)

and languages investigated across studies. However, it is noteworthy that three of the studies were conducted on Singaporean participants, and showed both overlapping and distinct areas of activation, even for structurally dissimilar languages such as English and Mandarin (Chee *et al.*, 1999a; Chee *et al.*, 1999b; Tham *et al.*, 2005).

Some researchers have linked the differences in cortical representation across languages with the age at which the second language is acquired. For instance, Kim *et al.* (1997) found that brain activation in bilinguals was overlapping for early bilinguals, while late bilinguals showed separate centers of activation. However, there are several reasons why this opinion is problematic. The cut off age used to separate early and late bilinguals often differs across the published studies and continues to be a contentious topic. In addition, even early English-Mandarin bilinguals who acquired both languages by five years of age have been found to show distinct areas of brain activation for both languages (e.g. Tham *et al.*, 2005). It has also been reported that attained proficiency is more important than age of acquisition in determining cortical representation of a second language (Perani *et al.*, 1998). It is not uncommon to find bilinguals who are more proficient in their second language even though it was acquired later in life because they were using the second language more frequently. Indeed, recent investigations indicate that the interaction between a bilingual's languages is complex, and that other factors may play a greater role in the representation of languages in a bilingual. These include language proficiency, computational demands of each language, the level of exposure to each language, and amount of daily language exposure or usage (see Chee *et al.*, 2002; Hernandez, 2009; Perani & Abutalebi, 2005; van Heuven & Dijkstra, 2010; Vingerhoets *et al.*, 2003).

It has been demonstrated repeatedly that interference and bilingual performance during language switching and translation show directional asymmetry associated with language proficiency (Goral *et al.*, 2006). More specifically, bilinguals tend to suffer more interference from the dominant language when speaking in the less-dominant language than vice versa. Evidence is also available which shows that bilinguals are slower in translating from the more-proficient language to the less-proficient language than vice versa., and that these latency differences decrease with increasing L2 proficiency (e.g. de Groot & Poot, 1997; Kroll & Stewart, 1994). The levels of accuracy, automaticity and speed in identifying and retrieving lexical items have also been found to correlate with the level of proficiency in each language (e.g. Chen & Leung, 1989; Kotz & Elston-Guttler, 2004; McElree *et al.*, 2000), and with factors such as the amount of similarity between languages and patterns of language use (e.g. Goral *et al.*, 2006).

To explain why language proficiency affects bilingual performance, Green (1986, 1993) argued that greater energy is expended when bilinguals speak in the weaker language because the production of this language is less automatized and requires greater cognitive control. Hence, there may be fewer resources left to suppress the activation of the dominant language (Costa *et al.*, 1999). This theory finds some support from neuroimaging data (e.g. Chee *et al.*, 2002; Green *et al.*, 2006; Hernandez & Meschyan, 2006; Perani *et al.*, 1998).

In relation to stuttering, it has been suggested that increased linguistic demands on the speech planning and production system can lead to increased stuttering (Bernstein Ratner & Benitez, 1985; Bernstein Ratner & Sih, 1987; Kleinow & Smith, 2000; Melnick & Conture, 2000; Silverman & Ratner, 1997; Smith & Kleinow, 2000; Yaruss, 1999). However, it is recognized that stuttering frequency at any one point in time is likely to be influenced by an interplay of linguistic, motoric and emotional factors (Guitar, 2006; Packman *et al.*, 1996). Although research data are still emerging, vulnerability of the speech motor system to higher processing demands has also been reported in some groups of people who stutter (PWS) who were subjected to dual task paradigms (Bosshardt, 1997, 1999, 2002; Bosshardt *et al.*, 2002; Bosshardt & Fransen, 1996; Smits-Bandstra & De Nil, 2007; Smits-Bandstra *et al.*, 2006). For example, Smits-Bandstra and colleagues found that the performance of PWS on practiced dual tasks was comparatively slower, less accurate and more attention-demanding than that of those who do not stutter. Such data may imply that PWS may perhaps be affected by higher computational load and may have difficulty with the automatization of sequence skill learning even after practice.

In our previous study (Lim *et al.*, 2008a), we suggested that bilinguals may stutter more in their less-dominant language because of the need to perform concurrent attention-demanding processes in that language (Bosshardt, 1999, 2002, 2006; Bosshardt *et al.*, 2002). For example, to speak in the less-dominant language, bilinguals not only need to plan and assimilate the different features of the word and sentence (e.g. semantic, syntactic, phonological and phonetic) but at the same time also need to repress the activation of and interference from the dominant language. The accuracy, speed and automaticity of processing two languages has been found to be influenced by language dominance (e.g. Chen & Leung, 1989; de Groot & Poot, 1997; Kotz & Elston-Guttler, 2004; Kroll & Stewart, 1994; McElree *et al.*, 2000). De Houwer (this volume) provided an overview of research which indicated that bilinguals may have a cognitive and linguistic advantage over monolinguals. However, this data is for infants and children. What we allude to here is that bilingual adults appear to have decreased processing ability in their less-dominant language compared to their dominant language. So, although there may be some advantages to being bilingual, perhaps increased stuttering in the less-dominant language is one of the drawbacks to being bilingual.

Our opinion is that such simultaneous, incremental and competing processes may create a cascading effect which may drain the resources of an already unstable motor speech system. This can perhaps reduce one's ability for speech control (Green, 1986, 1993), and hence, more stuttering can result. This might account for findings that BWS stutter in both languages, but more so in the language that is less dominant and which requires greater control. Along the same line, it is plausible that BWS continue to have higher residual stuttering in their less-dominant language even after treatment since (a) language proficiency remains unchanged after stuttering treatment, and (b) there are still ongoing processing demands placed on the speech planning and production system in this language. The idea that language planning may affect stuttering levels across the different languages spoken by BWS has also been raised previously by Roberts (2002).

At this juncture, however, our data are still preliminary. As such, our proposals regarding the bilingual stuttering model remain purely speculative. We await the full analyses of the results of our larger group study as we hope that the data will help us to better understand the influence of language dominance on stuttering severity and treatment generalization. In particular, it would be interesting to know if our group of balanced bilinguals will also exhibit uneven fluency gains across English and Mandarin despite having more equal proficiency across the two languages.

Due to the limitations in our data to date, our bilingual stuttering model also needs to undergo further testing. For example, we need to examine stuttering frequency in unbalanced bilinguals with a range of dominant and less-dominant languages. Since the structural distance between two languages may influence the degree of interference from one language to the other, it would be of value to compare within the same study, pre- and post-treatment stuttering levels in language pairs that are more structurally dissimilar (i.e. English-Mandarin), with languages that are less dissimilar (e.g. English-Malay or Mandarin-Cantonese). Additionally, since we suggest that language interference and processing is also associated with language dominance, it may also be beneficial to assess whether stuttering frequency would vary across groups of BWS with a range of differences in the degree of dominance. Take for example the case of a bilingual who is proficient in their dominant language but only able to produce short utterances in their less-dominant language. It would be surprising to find that stuttering in this case was more frequent in the less-dominant language. In this example linguistic and motoric complexity is reduced in the less-dominant language which may offset the effect of the cognitive load on stuttering. Further, based on Nwokah's (1988) proposal that BWS could stutter more in the language that they had negative experiences with, the issue of anxiety or other sociopsychological factors related to speaking a second language needs further examination. A study examining whether healthy bilinguals and BWS experience different levels of anxiety or fears when speaking in their less-dominant language would thus be relevant. Other studies of BWS which examine and compare the loci of stuttering and/or code switching events pretreatment and post treatment, and laboratory studies which examine BWS under dual tasking procedures may also shed more light on the impact of concurrent language processing on the degree of fluency improvements in the less-dominant language. We also need to assess if our model will apply to bilingual children who stutter. All the above information will no doubt help us to fully test the bilingual stuttering model presented in this chapter.

10   Implications for Assessment and Treatment of BWS

The results of our research have provided us with some initial guidelines for the assessment and treatment of BWS. Since our results suggest that language dominance may be an important factor in the interpretation of the results for both stuttering manifestation and treatment generalization effects in BWS, SLPs and researchers who work with bilinguals in Singapore (and perhaps elsewhere) will need to interpret bilingual behavioral data in the light of the bilinguals' language dominance profile. This has implications not only for stuttering or other speech and language disorders in bilinguals, but also for normal bilingual behavioral data as well.

If the results of our larger group study indicate that language dominance does in fact affect treatment generalization, then speech language pathologists who deliver treatment in only one language will also need to consider their clients' language dominance profile in deciding which language to provide treatment in. Clinicians may continue to deliver treatment in one language only as stuttering reductions in the treated language may spontaneously and simultaneously generalize to the untreated language. However, since our data suggest that some BWS may still have higher residual stuttering in one language compared to the other, clinicians may need to base treatment options according to their clients' requirements. For instance, they may need to extend stuttering treatment to the untreated language, particularly if fluent communication in that language is an important goal of the client after treatment.

11   Conclusion

Singapore is still in its infancy as far as stuttering research is concerned. There is still much to learn about bilingual stuttering, and in particular BWS who speak Asian languages. Nonetheless, with continued research with our current and future international collaborators, we hope that we will continue to build upon the existing data on BWS so that clinicians who work with BWS around the world will have clearer best practice guidelines for bilingual stuttering assessment and treatment.

Notes

1. Chinese word for 'car' written in Pinyin. Pinyin is the standard romanization system for modern Chinese (ISO 7098:1982, superseded by ISO 7098:1991). The number in superscript reflects the tone number; a numeral used in a notational system for marking the different lexical tones in Standard Mandarin.
2. British English has been classified as a stress-timed language (Abercrombie, 1967) whereas Singapore Colloquial English has been described more as a syllable-timed language (Low *et al.*, 2000; Platt and Weber, 1980; Tongue, 1974).

References

Abercrombie, D. (1967) *Elements of General Phonetics*. Edinburgh: Edinburgh University Press.

Abutalebi, J. and Green, D.W. (2007). Bilingual language production: The neurocognition of language representation and control. *Journal of Neurolinguistics* 20(3), 242–275.

Andrews, G., Guitar, B. and Howie, P. (1980) Meta-analysis of the effects of stuttering treatment. *Journal of Speech and Hearing Disorders* 45, 287–307.

Baudoin-Chial, S. (1986) Hemispheric lateralization of Modern Standard Chinese tone processing. *Journal of Neurolinguistics* 2(1–2), 189–199.

Bernstein Ratner, N. (2005a) Evidence-based practice in stuttering: Some questions to consider. *Journal of Fluency Disorders* 30(3), 163–188.

Bernstein Ratner, N. (2005b). Is phonetic complexity a useful construct in understanding stuttering? *Journal of Fluency Disorders* 30(4), 337–341.

Bernstein Ratner, N. and Benitez, M. (1985) Linguistic analysis of a bilingual stutterer. *Journal of Fluency Disorders* 10(3), 211–219.

Bernstein Ratner, N. and Sih, C.C. (1987) Effects of gradual increases in sentence length and complexity on children's disfluency. *Journal of Speech and Hearing Disorders* 52, 278–287.

Bernstein Ratner, N. and Wijnen, F. (2007) The vicious cycle: Linguistic encoding, self-monitoring and stuttering. In J. Au-Yeung and M.M. Leahy (eds) *Research, Treatment and Self Help in Fluency Disorders: New Horizons. Proceedings of the Fifth World Congress on Fluency Disorders* (pp. 84–90). Dublin: The International Fluency Association.

Bialystok, E. and Miller, B. (1999) The problem of age in second-language acquisition: Influences from language, structure, and task. *Bilingualism: Language and Cognition* 2, 127–145.

Birdsong, D. (2006) Dominance, proficiency, and second language grammatical processing. *Applied Psycholinguistics* 27(1), 46–49.

Block, S. and Dacakis, G. (2003) *La Trobe Fluency Clinic: Student Manual*. Melbourne: La Trobe University.

Block, S., Onslow, M., Packman, A., Gray, B. and Dacakis, G. (2005) Treatment of chronic stuttering: Outcomes from a student training clinic. *International Journal of Language & Communication Disorders* 40(4), 455–466.

Bloodstein, O. and Bernstein Ratner, N. (2008) *The Handbook of Stuttering* (6th edn). Clifton Park, NY: Delmar Learning.

Blumstein, S. and Cooper, W. (1974) Hemispheric processing of intonation contours. *Cortex* 10(2), 146–158.

Bosshardt, H-G. (1997) Mental effort and speech fluency. In W. Hulstijn, H.F.M. Peters and P.H.H.M. Van Lieshout (eds) *Speech Production: Motor Control,*

Brain Research and Fluency Disorders (pp. 503–514). The Netherlands: Elsevier Science.

Bosshardt, H-G. (1999) Effects of concurrent mental calculation on stuttering, inhalation and speech timing. *Journal of Fluency Disorders*, 24(1), 43–72.

Bosshardt, H-G. (2002) Effects of concurrent cognitive processing on the fluency of word repetition: Comparison between persons who do and do not stutter. *Journal of Fluency Disorders* 27(2), 93–114.

Bosshardt, H-G. (2006) Cognitive processing load as a determinant of stuttering: Summary of a research programme. *Clinical Linguistics & Phonetics* 20(5), 371–385.

Bosshardt, H-G., Ballmer, W. and De Nil, L.F. (2002) Effects of category and rhyme decisions on sentence production. *Journal of Speech Language and Hearing Research* 45(5), 844–857.

Bosshardt, H-G. and Fransen, H. (1996) Online sentence processing in adults who stutter and adults who do not stutter. *Journal of Speech and Hearing Research* 39(4), 785–797.

Chee, M.W., Tan, E.W. and Thiel, T. (1999a) Mandarin and English single word processing studied with functional magnetic resonance imaging. *Journal of Neuroscience* 19(8), 3050–3056.

Chee, M.W.L., Caplan, D., Soon, C.S., Sriram, N., Tan, E.W.L., Thiel, T., *et al.* (1999b) Processing of visually presented sentences in Mandarin and English studied with fMRI. *Neuron* 23(1), 127–137.

Chee, M.W.L., Hon, N., Lee, H.L., and Soon, C.S. (2002) Relative language proficiency modulates BOLD signal change when bilinguals perform semantic judgments. *NeuroImage* 13(6), 1155–1163.

Chen, H.-C. and Leung, Y.-S. (1989). Patterns of lexical processing in a nonnative language. *Journal of Experimental Psychology: Learning, Memory, and Cognition* 15(2), 316–325.

Chen, J.-Y. (1999) The representation and processing of tone in Mandarin Chinese: Evidence from slips of the tongue. *Applied Psycholinguistics* 20, 289–301.

Chen, J.-Y., Chen, T.-M. and Dell, G.S. (2002) Word-form encoding in Mandarin Chinese as assessed by the implicit priming task. *Journal of Memory and Language* 46(4), 751–781.

Chen, J.-Y., Lin, W.-C. and Ferrand, L. (2003) Masked priming of the syllable in Mandarin Chinese speech production. *Chinese Journal of Psychology* 45(1), 107–120.

Conture, E.G. and Curlee, R.F. (eds) (2007) *Stuttering and Related Disorders of Fluency* (3rd edn) New York: Thieme Medical Publishers Inc.

Cooper, W.E. and Klouda, G.V. (1987) Intonation in aphasic and right-hemisphere-damaged patients. In J.H. Ryalls (ed.) *Phonetic Approaches to Speech Production in Aphasia and Related Disorders* (pp. 59–77). Boston: College-Hill Press.

Costa, A., Miozzo, M. and Caramazza, A. (1999) Lexical selection in bilinguals: Do words in the bilingual's two lexicons compete for selection? *Journal of Memory and Language* 41(3), 365–397.

Cream, A., Onslow, M., Packman, A. and Llewellyn, G. (2003) Protection from harm: The experience of adults after therapy with prolonged speech. *International Journal of Language & Communication Disorders* 38(4), 379–395.

Cruttenden, A. (1986) *Intonation*. New York: Cambridge University Press.

De Bot, K. (1992) A bilingual production model: Levelt's 'speaking' model adapted. *Applied Linguistics* 13, 1–24.

De Bot, K. and Schreuder, R. (1993) Word production and the biligual lexicon. In R. Schreuder and B. Weltens (eds) *The Bilingual Lexicon* (pp. 191–214). Amsterdam: John Benjamins.

de Groot, A.M.B. and Poot, R. (1997) Word translation at three levels of proficiency in a second language: The ubiquitous involvement of conceptual memory. *Language Learning* 47(2), 215–264.

Dehaene, S., Dupoux, E., Mehler, J., Cohen, L., Paulesu, E., Perani, D., *et al.* (1997) Anatomical variability in the cortical representation of first and second language. *Neuroreport* 8(17), 3809–3815.

Dell, G.S. (1986) A spreading-activation theory of retrieval in sentence production. *Psychological Review* 93(3), 283–321.

Dell, G.S. and Oseaghdha, P.G. (1992) Stages of lexical access in language production. *Cognition* 42(1–3), 287–314.

Dworzynski, K. and Howell, P. (2004). Predicting stuttering from phonetic complexity in German. *Journal of Fluency Disorders* 29(2), 149–173.

Flege, J.E., Mackay, I.R.A. and Piske, T. (2002) Assessing bilingual dominance. *Applied Psycholinguistics* 23(4), 567–598.

Franken, M.C.J., Kielstra-Van der Schalka, C.J. and Boelens, H. (2005) Experimental treatment of early stuttering: A preliminary study. *Journal of Fluency Disorders* 30(3), 189–199.

Gandour, J. (1987) Tone production in aphasia. In J. Ryalls (ed.) *Phonetic Approaches to Speech Production in Aphasia and Related Disorders* (pp. 45–57). Boston, MA: College-Hill.

Gandour, J., Akamanon, C., Dechongkit, S., Khunadorn, F. and Boonklam, R. (1994) Sequences of phonemic approximations in a Thai conduction aphasic. *Brain and Language* 46(1), 69–95.

Garrett, M.F. (1982) Production of speech: Observations from normal and pathological use. In A.W. Ellis (ed.) *Normality and Pathology in Cognitive Functions* (pp. 19–76). London: Academic Press.

Garson, D.G. (2006) Discriminant Function Analysis, http://www2.chass.ncsu.edu/garson/pa765/discrim.htm. Retrieved 12 September 2006.

Golestania, N., Alario, F.-X., Meriaux, S., Bihan, D.L., Dehaene, S., and Pallier, C. (2006) Syntax production in bilinguals. *Neuropsychologia* 44(7), 1029–1040.

Goral, M., Levy, E.S., Obler, L.K. and Cohen, E. (2006) Cross-language lexical connections in the mental lexicon: Evidence from a case of trilingual aphasia. *Brain and Language* 98(2), 235–247.

Grabe, E., and Low, E.L. (2002) Durational variability in speech and the rhythm class hypothesis. In N. Warner and C. Gussenhoven (eds) *Papers in Laboratory Phonology* (Vol. 7, pp. 515–546). Cambridge: CUP.

Green, D.W. (1986) Control, activation, and resource: A framework and a model for the control of speech in bilinguals. *Brain and Language* 27(2), 210–223.

Green, D.W. (1993) Towards a model of L2 comprehension and production. In R. Schreuder and B. Weltens (eds) *The Bilingual Lexicon* (pp. 249–278). Amsterdam: John Benjamins.

Green, D.W., Crinion, J. and Price, C.J. (2006) Convergence, degeneracy, and control. *Language Learning* 56, 99–125.

Grosjean, F. (1982) Life with two languages: An introduction to bilingualism. *Bilingualism: Language and Cognition* 1(2), 131–149.

Grosjean, F. (1998) Studying bilinguals: Methodological and conceptual issues. *Bilingualism* 1(2), 131–149.

Grosjean, F. (2001) The bilingual's language modes. In J.L. Nicol (ed.) *One Mind, Two Languages: Bilingual Language Processing* (pp. 1–22). Malden, MA: Blackwell Publishers Ltd.

Guitar, B. (2006) *Stuttering: An Integrated Approach to Its Nature and Treatment* (3rd edn). Baltimore: Lippincott Williams & Wilkins.

Gupta, A.F. (1994) *The Step-Tongue: Children's English in Singapore*: Clevedon: Multilingual Matters.

Harrison, E., Onslow, M., Andrews, C., Packman, A. and Webber, M. (1998) Control of stuttering with prolonged speech: Development of a one-day instatement program. In A. Cordes and R.J. Ingham (eds) *Treatment Efficacy in Stuttering: A Search for Empirical Bases*. San Diego, CA: Singular Publishing Group.

Hernandez, A.E. (2009) Language switching in the bilingual brain: What's next? *Brain and Language* 109(2–3), 133–140.

Hernandez, A.E., Li, P. and MacWhinney, B. (2005) The emergence of competing modules in bilingualism. *Trends in Cognitive Sciences* 9(5), 220–225.

Hernandez, A.E. and Meschyan, G. (2006) Executive function is necessary to enhance lexical processing in a less proficient L2: Evidence from fMR1 during picture naming. *Bilingualism: Language and Cognition* 9(2), 177–188.

Hewat, S., Onslow, M., Packman, A. and O'Brian, S. (2006) A Phase II clinical trial of self-imposed time-out treatment for stuttering in adults and adolescents. *Disability and Rehabilitation* 28(1), 33–42.

Howell, P. (2010) Language processing in fluency disorders. In J. Guendouzi, F. Loncke and M. Williams (eds) *The Handbook on Psycholinguistics and Cognitive Processes: Perspectives on Communication Disorders*. London: Taylor & Francis.

Howell, P., Au-Yeung, J. and Sackin, S. (2000) Internal structure of content words leading to lifespan differences in phonological difficulty in stuttering. *Journal of Fluency Disorders* 25(1), 1–20.

Howell, P., Davis, S. and Williams, R. (2009) The effects of bilingualism on stuttering during late childhood. *Archives of Disorders of Children* 94, 42–46.

Howell, P. and Dworzynski, K. (2005) Planning and execution processes in speech control by fluent speakers and speakers who stutter. *Journal of Fluency Disorders* 30(4), 343–354.

Howell, P., Ruffle, L., Fernandez-Zuniga, A., Gutierrez, R., Fernandez, A.H., O'Brian, M.L., *et al.* (eds) (2004) *Comparison of Exchange Patterns of Stuttering in Spanish and English Monolingual Speakers and a Bilingual Spanish-English Speaker*. Nijmegen: Nijmegen University Press.

Ingham, R.J. (1987) *Residential Prolonged Speech Stuttering Therapy Manual*. Santa Barbara: Department of speech and hearing sciences, University of California.

Iverach, L., Jones, M., O'Brian, S., Block, S., Lincoln, M., Harrison, E., *et al.* (2009) The relationship between mental health disorders and treatment outcomes among adults who stutter. *Journal of Fluency Disorders* 34(1), 29–43.

Iverach, L., O'Brian, S., Jones, M., Block, S., Lincoln, M., Harrison, E., *et al.* (2009) Prevalence of anxiety disorders among adults seeking speech therapy for stuttering. *Journal of Anxiety Disorders* 23(7), 928–934.

Jared, D. and Kroll, J.F. (2001) Do bilinguals activate phonological representations in one or both of their languages when naming words? *Journal of Memory and Language* 44(1), 2–31.

Jones, M., Onslow, M., Packman, A., O'Brian, S., Hearne, A., Williams, S., *et al.* (2008) Extended follow-up of a randomized controlled trial of the Lidcombe program of early stuttering intervention. *International Journal of Language & Communication Disorders* 43(6), 649–661.

Jones, M., Onslow, M., Packman, A., Williams, S., Ormond, T., Schwarz, I., *et al.* (2005) Randomised controlled trial of the Lidcombe programme of early stuttering intervention. *British Medical Journal* 331(7518), 659–661.

Keung, T. and Hoosain, R. (1979) Segmental phonemes and tonal phonemes in comprehension of Cantonese. *Psychologia: An International Journal of Psychology in the Orient* 22(4), 222–224.

Kim, K.H., Relkin, N.R., Lee, K.M. and Hirsch, J. (1997) Distinct cortical areas associated with native and second languages. *Nature* 388, 171–174.

Kleinow, J. and Smith, A. (2000) Influences of length and syntactic complexity on the speech motor stability of the fluent speech of adults who stutter. *Journal of Speech Language and Hearing Research* 43(2), 548–559.

Kohnert, K. (2009) Cross-language generalization following treatment in bilingual speakers with aphasia: A review. *Seminars in Speech and Language* 30(03), 174–186.

Kohnert, K.J., Hernandez, A.E. and Bates, E. (1998) Bilingual performance on the Boston Naming Test: Preliminary norms in Spanish and English. *Brain and Language* 65(3), 422–440.

Kolk, H. and Postma, A. (1997) Stuttering as a covert repair phenomenon. In R.F. Curlee and G.M. Siegel (eds) *Nature and Treatments of Stuttering: New Directions* (pp. 182–203). Needham Heights, MA: Allyn & Bacon.

Kotz, S.A. and Elston-Guttler, K. (2004) The role of proficiency on processing categorical and associative information in the L2 as revealed by reaction times and event-related brain potentials. *Journal of Neurolinguistics* 17(2–3), 215–235.

Kraaimaat, F.W., Janssen, P. and Van Dam-Baggen, R. (1991) Social anxiety and stuttering. *Perceptual and Motor Skills* 72(3), 766–766.

Kraaimaat, F.W., Vanryckeghem, M. and Van Dam-Baggen, R. (2002) Stuttering and social anxiety. *Journal of Fluency Disorders* 27(4), 319–331.

Kroll, J.F. and Stewart, E. (1994) Category interference in translation and picture naming – Evidence for asymmetric connections between bilingual memory representations. *Journal of Memory and Language* 33(2), 149–174.

Langdon, H.W., Wiig, E.H. and Nielsen, N.P. (2005) Dual-dimension naming speed and language-dominance ratings by bilingual Hispanic adults. *Bilingual Research Journal* 29(2), 319.

Lattermann, C., Euler, H.A. and Neumann, K. (2008) A randomized control trial to investigate the impact of the Lidcombe Program on early stuttering in German-speaking preschoolers. *Journal of Fluency Disorders* 33(1), 52–65.

Levelt, W.J.M. (1989) *Speaking: From Intention to Articulation.* Cambridge, MA: MIT Press.

Levelt, W.J.M., Roelofs, A. and Meyer, A.S. (1999) A theory of lexical access in speech production. *Behavioral and Brain Sciences* 22(1), 1–38.

Lewis, C., Packman, A., Onslow, M., Simpson, J.M. and Jones, M. (2008) A Phase II Trial of Telehealth Delivery of the Lidcombe Program of early stuttering intervention. *American Journal of Speech Language Pathology* 17(2), 139–149.

Li, C.N. and Thompson, S.A. (1981) *Mandarin Chinese: A Functional Reference Grammar.* Berkeley, CA: University of California Press.

Li, P., Bates, E. and Macwhinney, B. (1993) Processing a language without inflections: A reaction time study of sentence interpretation in Chinese. *Journal of Memory and Language* 32(2), 169–192.

Liang, J. and Heuven, V.J.V. (2004) Evidence for separate tonal and segmental tiers in the lexical specification of words: A case study of a brain-damaged Chinese speaker. *Brain and Language* 91(3), 282–293.

Lim, V. (1998a) *Impairment of Lexical Tone Production in Stroke Patients with Bilingual Aphasia.* Unpublished Masters Thesis, La Trobe University, Melbourne.

Lim, V.P.C. (1998b) *Impairment of Lexical Tone Production in Stroke Patients with Bilingual Aphasia.* Unpublished Masters Thesis, La Trobe University, Victoria, Australia.

Lim, V.P.C., Lincoln, M., Chan, Y.H. and Onslow, M. (2008a) Stuttering in English-Mandarin bilingual speakers: The influence of language dominance on stuttering severity. *Journal of Speech, Language and Hearing Research* 51, 1522–1537.

Lim, V.P.C., Rickard Liow, S.J., Lincoln, M., Chan, Y.H. and Onslow, M. (2008b) Determining language dominance in English-Mandarin bilinguals: A self-report classification tool for clinical use. *Applied Psycholinguistics* 29(3), 389–412.

Lin, H. (2001) *A Grammar of Mandarin Chinese.* Muenchen: LINCOM Europa.

Low, E.L., Grabe, E. and Nolan, F. (2000) Quantitative characterizations of speech rhythm syllable-timing in Singapore English. *Language & Speech* 43(4), 377.

Mahr, G.C. and Torosian, T. (1999) Anxiety and social phobia in stuttering. *Journal of Fluency Disorders* 24(2), 119–126.

Mattes, L.J. and Omark, D.R. (1991) *Speech and Language Assessment for the Bilingual Handicapped.* San Diego: College-Hill Press.

Matthews, S. and Yip, V. (1994) *Cantonese: A Comprehensive Grammar.* London: Routledge.

McElree, B., Jia, G. and Litvak, A. (2000) The time course of conceptual processing in three bilingual populations. *Journal of Memory and Language* 42(2), 229–254.

Melnick, K.S. and Conture, E.G. (2000) Relationship of length and grammatical complexity to the systematic and nonsystematic speech errors and stuttering of children who stutter. *Journal of Fluency Disorders* 25(1), 21–45.

Menzies, R.G., Onslow, M. and Packman, A. (1999) Anxiety and stuttering: Exploring a complex relationship. *American Journal of Speech Language Pathology* 8(1), 3–10.

Messenger, M., Onslow, M., Packman, A. and Menzies, R. (2004) Social anxiety in stuttering: Measuring negative social expectancies. *Journal of Fluency Disorders* 29(3), 201–212.

Naeser, M.A. and Chan, S.W.C. (1980) Case-Study of a Chinese Aphasic with the Boston Diagnostic Aphasia Exam. *Neuropsychologia* 18(4–5), 389.

Natke, U., Sandrieser, P., van Ark, M., Pietrowsky, R. and Kalveram, K.T. (2004) Linguistic stress, within-word position, and grammatical class in relation to early childhood stuttering. *Journal of Fluency Disorders* 29(2), 109–122.

Nwokah, E.E. (1988). The imbalance of stuttering behavior in bilingual speakers. *Journal of Fluency Disorders* 13(5), 357–373.

O'Brian, S., Cream, A., Onslow, M. and Packman, A. (2001) A replicable, nonprogrammed, instrument-free method for the control of stuttering with prolonged speech. *Asia Pacific Journal of Speech, Language, and Hearing* 6, 91–96.

O'Brian, S., Onslow, M., Cream, A. and Packman, A. (2003) The Camperdown Program: Outcomes of a new prolonged-speech treatment model. *Journal of Speech, Language and Hearing Research* 46(4), 933–946.

Onslow, M., Packman, A. and Harrison, E. (2003) *The Lidcombe Programme for Early Stuttering Intervention: A Clinician's Guide.* Austin, TX: Pro-ed.

Oscarson, M. (1989) Self-assessment of language proficiency: Rationale and applications. *Language Testing* 6, 1–13.

Packard, J. (1992) *A Linguistic Investigation of Aphasic Chinese Speech.* Amsterdam: Kluwer Academic.

Packman, A. and Onslow, M. (1998) The behavioral data language of stuttering. In A. Cordes and R.J. Ingham (eds)*Treatment Efficacy in Stuttering: A Search for Empirical Bases.* San Diego, CA: Singular Publishing Group.

Packman, A., Onslow, M., Richard, F. and VanDoorn, J. (1996) Syllabic stress and variability: A model of stuttering. *Clinical Linguistics & Phonetics* 10(3), 235–263.

Perani, D. and Abutalebi, J. (2005) The neural basis of first and second language processing. *Current Opinion in Neurobiology* 15(2), 202–206.

Perani, D., Eraldo, P., Galles, N.S., Dupoux, E., Dehaene, S., Bettinardi, V., *et al.* (1998) The bilingual brain: Proficiency and age of acquisition of the second language. *Brain* 121, 1841–1852.

Platt, J.T. and Weber, H. (1980) *English in Singapore and Malaysia: Status, Features and Functions.* Kuala Lumpur: Oxford University Press.

Population Trends (2006) Singapore Department of Statistics, Department of Statistics, Ministry of Trade and Industry, http://www.singstat.gov.sg/pubn/popn/population2006.pdf.

Rickard Liow, S.J., Hong, E.L. and Tng, S.K. (1992) *Singapore Primary School Norms for the Multilingual British Picture Vocabulary Scale: English, Mandarin and Malay. Working Paper No. 43*: Department of social work & psychology, National University of Singapore.

Roberts, P.M. (2002) Disfluency patterns in four bilingual adults who stutter. *Revue d'orthophonie et d'audiologie* 26(1), 5–19.

Roberts, P.M. (ed.) (2001) *Aphasia Assessment and Treatment for Bilingual and Culturally Diverse Patients.* Philadelphia: Lippincott, Williams & Wilkins.

Roberts, P.M. and Shenker, R.C. (2007) Assessment and treatment of stuttering in bilingual speakers. In E.G. Conture and R.F. Curlee (eds) *Stuttering and Related Disorders of Fluency* (3rd edn), pp. 183–209. New York: Thieme Medical Publishers.

Roelofs, A. (2000) WEAVER++ and other computational models of lemma retrieval and word-form encoding. In L. Wheeldon (ed.) *Aspects of Language Production.* Hove, East Sussex: Psychological Press.

Schneier, F., Wexler, K.B.P. and Liebowitz, M.R. (1997) Social phobia and stuttering. *American Journal of Psychiatry* 154(1), 131.

SHAS Directory of Services. (2009) Singapore: Speech-Language and Hearing Association Singapore.

Shenker, R.C. (2004) Bilingualism in early stuttering: Empirical issues and clinical implications. In A.K. Bothe (ed.) *Evidence-based Treatment of Stuttering: Empirical Bases and Clinical Applications* (pp. 81–96). Mahwah, NJ: Lawrence Erlbaum Associates.

Shenker, R.C., Conte, A., Gingras, A., Courcy, A. and Polomeno, A. (1998) *The Impact of Bilingualism on Developing Fluency in a Preschool Child.* Paper presented at the Second World Congress on Fluency Disorders Proceedings, 18–22 August.

Silverman, S.W. and Ratner, N.B. (1997) Syntactic complexity, fluency, and accuracy of sentence imitation in adolescents. *Journal of Speech Language and Hearing Research* 40(1), 95–106.

Singapore in Figures 2009 (Publication. Retrieved 3 August 2009, from Singapore Department of Statistics: http://www.singstat.gov.sg/pubn/reference/sif2009.pdf

Smith, A. and Kleinow, J. (2000) Kinematic correlates of speaking rate changes in stuttering and normally fluent adults. *Journal of Speech Language and Hearing Research* 43(2), 521–536.

Smits-Bandstra, S. and De Nil, L.F. (2007) Sequence skill learning in persons who stutter: Implications for cortico-striato-thalamo-cortical dysfunction. *Journal of Fluency Disorders*, doi:10.1016/j.jfludis.2007.1006.1001.

Smits-Bandstra, S., De Nil, L.F. and Rochon, E. (2006) The transition to increased automaticity during finger sequence learning in adult males who stutter. *Journal of Fluency Disorders* 31(1), 22–42.

Snider, K. and van der Hulst, H. (eds) (1992) *The Phonology of Tone: The Representation of Tonal Register*. Berlin: Mouton de Gruyter.

Stein, M.B., Baird, A.M.A. and Walker, J.R. (1996) Social phobia in adults with stuttering. *American Journal of Psychiatry* 153(2), 278–280.

Teesson, K., Packman, A. and Onslow, M. (2003) The Lidcombe behavioral data language of stuttering. *Journal of Speech, Language, and Hearing Research* 46, 1009–1015.

Tham, W.W.P., Rickard Liow, S.J., Rajapakse, J.C., Tan, C.L., Ng, S.E.S., Lim, W.E.H., *et al.* (2005) Phonological processing in Chinese-English bilingual biscriptals: An fMRI study. *NeuroImage* 28(3), 579–587.

Tongue, R.K. (1974) *The English of Singapore and Malaysia*. Singapore: Eastern Universities Press.

Trajkovski, N., Andrews, C., O'Brian, S., Onslow, M. and Packman, A. (2006) Treating stuttering in a preschool child with syllable timed speech: A case report. *Behaviour Change* 23(4), 270–277.

Trajkovski, N., Andrews, C., Onslow, M., Packman, A., O'Brian, S. and Menzies, R. (2009) Using syllable-timed speech to treat preschool children who stutter: A multiple baseline experiment. *Journal of Fluency Disorders, January 14, 2009 Electronic Publication Ahead of Print*.

Tseng, T.F. (1988) *Colloquial Cantonese and Putonghua Equivalents*. New York: Hippocrene Books.

Van Borsel, J., Maes, E. and Foulon, S. (2001) Stuttering and bilingualism: A review. *Journal of Fluency Disorders* 26(3), 179–205.

Van Borsel, J. and Medeiros de Britto Pereira, M. (2005) Assessment of stuttering in a familiar versus an unfamiliar language. *Journal of Fluency Disorders* 30(2), 109–124.

van Heuven, W.J.B. and Dijkstra, T. (2010) Language comprehension in the bilingual brain: fMRI and ERP support for psycholinguistic models. *Brain Research Reviews* 64(1), 104–122.

Venkatagiri, H.S. (2005) Recent advances in the treatment of stuttering: A theoretical perspective. *Journal of Communication Disorders* 38(5), 375–393.

Vingerhoets, G., Borsel, J.V., Tesink, C., van den Noort, M., Deblaere, K., Seurinck, R., *et al.* (2003) Multilingualism: An fMRI study. *NeuroImage* 20(4), 2181–2196.

Waheed-Khan, N. (1997) Fluency therapy with multilingual clients. In E.C. Healey, and H.F.M.Peters (eds) *Proceedings of the Second World Congress on Fluency Disorders*, San Francisco, 18–22 August (pp. 195–199). Nijmegen: Nijmegen University Press.

Watson, J.B. and Kayser, H. (1994) Assessment of bilingual/bicultural children and adults who stutter. *Seminars in Speech and Language* 15, 149–164.

Weekes, B., Chen, M.J., Qun, H.C., Lin, Y.B., Yao, C. and Xiao, X.Y. (1998) Anomia and dyslexia in Chinese: A familiar story. *Aphasiology* 12(1), 77–98.

White, L. and Genesee, F. (1996) How native is near-native? The issue of ultimate attainment in adult second language acquisition. *Second Language Research* 12, 233–265.

Wingate, M.E. (1984) Stutter events and linguistic stress. *Journal of Fluency Disorders* 9(4), 295–300.

Yaruss, J.S. (1999) Utterance length, syntactic complexity, and childhood stuttering. *Journal of Speech Language and Hearing Research* 42(2), 329–344.

Yiu, E.M.L. and Fok, A.Y.Y. (1995) Lexical tone disruption in Cantonese aphasic speakers. *Clinical Linguistics and Phonetics* 9(1), 79–92.

Chapter 13

Linguistic Analysis of Stuttering in Bilinguals: Methodological Challenges and Solutions

PEI-TZU TSAI, VALERIE P.C. LIM, SHELLEY B. BRUNDAGE AND NAN BERNSTEIN RATNER

Summary

This chapter uses new computational tools to examine the content/function word distribution of stutters in adult bilingual stutterers' conversational language. We chose to examine Mandarin-English and Spanish-English people who stutter because of the contrasting typologies of all three languages. For example, Spanish has more function word members and both content and function words are highly affixed. In contrast, Mandarin has fewer free grammatical morphemes as well as some not seen in English.

When viewed on a detailed level that divides both classes of words into their component grammatical categories, most speakers did not show very consistent patterns of stuttering across classes of speech in their two languages. This could be because learning and pragmatic factors begin to shape linguistic features of stuttered speech after the teen years. Such a proposal suggests that examination of child bilingual stutterers would be a reasonable next step in understanding how linguistic features affect stuttering across the lifespan and across languages in bilingual speakers.

1   Introduction: Linguistic Factors and Stuttering

This chapter will explore our efforts to conduct linguistically based analyses of fluency patterns in bilinguals. To ground this discussion, it is first necessary to provide a rationale for performing linguistic analyses of the stuttering patterns of any speaker, whether bilingual or monolingual. Thus, we will begin by reviewing what has been learned about linguistic regularities in children and adults' stuttering, as well as some language-based factors that have been identified as influential in characterizing the overall profiles of people who stutter (PWS) across the age span.

A recent comprehensive overview of language factors in stuttering is provided in Hall, Wagovich and Bernstein Ratner (2007; hereafter

HW&BR), as well as in a chapter of the most recent revision of the *Handbook on Stuttering* (Bloodstein & Bernstein Ratner, 2008); we follow the HW& BR chapter's organization in laying out some of the primary concerns in relating linguistic factors to the understanding of stuttering before offering some case study profiles of bilingual stuttering.

1.1 Language skills in PWS

At this point in time, so much information is accumulating to suggest a certain level of language 'weakness' in individuals who stutter that the major findings in HW& BR had to be summarized in chart form; the charts spanned four entire pages.[1] More recently, a meta-analysis (Ntourou *et al.*, 2009) has combined a large number of these studies to reach the conclusion that there is substantive evidence of non-clinical levels of language impairment in broadly selected populations of people who stutter. By this, we mean that these individuals do not demonstrate concomitant clinically-significant language disorder that merits clinical intervention, but rather that an array of naturalistic, standardized test and experimental analyses has rather consistently shown lowered performance on the part of the stuttering participants when contrasted with typically fluent peers. These relative deficiencies are most robustly evident in the areas of overall performance on expressive and receptive language 'batteries', expressive and receptive vocabulary, length of spontaneous utterances in morphemes (MLU) and morphological completion. More general measures of syntactic production and comprehension appear less deficited.

The major lesson relevant to bilingual stuttering that we find most evident in this body of literature is that PWS as a group tend not to be as linguistically proficient in the use of one language; there is no reason to believe that proficiency of subsequent languages that are acquired would be superior. This, in turn, leads to another well-known phenomenon, in which level of linguistic challenge or demand impacts the likelihood of fluency breakdown.

1.2 Linguistic demand and stuttering

There are a number of ways to demonstrate that language demand affects stuttering frequency as well as other more general features of the disorder.

First, onset patterns are extremely consistent with the belief that stuttering emerges most often when children appear to be at the most dynamic stages of developing their first language (typically at ages 2;6–4 years) (Bloodstein & Bernstein Ratner, 2008). Next, naturalistic data amply associates more advanced language targets (e.g. longer, more syntactically complex language) with a higher frequency of stuttering and stuttered utterances (e.g. Buhr & Zebrowski, 2009; Melnick & Conture, 2000). Finally, experimental studies (for instance, those in which children or adults are asked to repeat or create modeled versions of stimulus utterances) also show that targets that can be characterized as being linguistically more complex tend to elicit greater amounts of stuttering (e.g. Bernstein Ratner & Sih, 1987). Critically, because we will return to this issue later in this chapter, such effects are largely confined to ages below eight years in monolingual children who stutter; above this age, typical language users who stutter are fairly immune to measures of language complexity (e.g. Silverman & Bernstein Ratner, 1997); rather, adults may be more vulnerable to precipitators that have been learned over time, such as feared words, addressees or contexts (e.g. Bloodstein & Bernstein Ratner, 2008; Manning, 2009; but see Howell (2010) for an alternative view).

1.3 Language proficiency: Impacts on stuttering recovery and therapeutic generalization

Two separate bodies of work independently suggest that language proficiency is a potent factor in stuttering. First, the work of the Illinois project suggests that those children who stutter (CWS) and possess relatively stronger language skills are more likely to experience spontaneous recovery (Yairi et al., 1996). Second, work done by Lim and colleagues (elsewhere in this volume) suggest that language dominance in bilinguals can be predictive of severity of stuttering symptoms (see also Jankelowitz & Bortz, 1996; Lim et al., 2008; Roberts, 2002), with the stronger language stuttered less (we recognize, however, that other studies have reported the opposite: Jayaram, 1983; Howell et al., 2004; Meline et al., 2006; see Van Borsel et al., 2001 for discussion). It is widely recognized that proficiency in the languages of a bilingual speaker vary along a substantive continuum (e.g. Perani et al., 1998), and that even listener judgment of 'native-like' proficiency or self-report may under- or over-estimate relative proficiency in the two languages, as well as proficiency when contrasted to a typical native speaker (Abrahamsson & Hyltenstam, 2009). Only recently has the literature on 'typical' bilingualism considered 'fluency' in the context considered by this text; some note that using speech disfluencies to track language competence may in fact be a useful construct in measuring language mastery (Hilton, 2008). Thus, in any speaker who is not a true 'balanced' bilingual, we might expect some elevated processing demands on one language spoken by a bilingual PWS. We personally find it more likely, given the merged psycholinguistic and second-language acquisition literatures, that stuttering would be somewhat worse in the weaker language of a bilingual speaker.

1.3.1　A note about concomitant disorders

We would be remiss in this chapter if we did not remind readers that a number of PWS actually demonstrate clinically relevant concomitant speech and language disorders (see Bloodstein & Bernstein Ratner, 2008). Particularly in the context of the bilingual speaker, where one component language might be more easily evaluated than the other, it should be noted that all PWS should receive as complete a diagnostic evaluation as is logistically possible given the clinical environment.

1.3.2　A note about differential diagnosis

We would also be remiss if we did not also note that individuals with relatively poorer language skills demonstrate higher levels of disfluency than more typical speakers; in some cases, these disfluencies can appear to be stutter-like in nature, even when someone more versed in stuttering would not label them as such (Boscolo *et al.*, 2002; Hall, 1996; Hall *et al.*, 1993). The literature on second-language or bilingual 'fluency' in this broadest sense is still in its infancy, but we would suggest that a high standard should be used in labeling disfluencies as stuttering, including some attention to qualitative features (such as tension) and self-concept as a person concerned about his or her speech fluency (cf. Bloodstein & Bernstein Ratner, 2008; Manning, 2009).

1.4　Broader linguistic impacts on fluency

Conversational demands related to the propositionality of speech (Eisenson & Horowitz, 1945; Young, 1980), the size of the audience being spoken to (Siegel & Haugen, 1964), and the nature of one's conversational partner (Sheehan *et al.*, 1967) all influence amount of stuttering. We will return to this concept later in discussion of our case study analyses, so we will introduce this concern here. It is indisputable that language in context is not language on paper being analyzed by a researcher. The literature amply demonstrates that affective and cognitive features of stuttering, particularly in older children, adolescents and adults can be very potent in precipitating fluency breakdown. These include broad issues involving conversational demand (how complex is the concept under discussion, as in academic or vocational environments), who is being spoken to (including past associations, the number and nature of the addressee(s)), and other contextual factors. It is widely recognized that the contexts in which bilinguals use their two or more languages may vary considerably in all these regards. Thus, issues such as the linguistic profile of a PWS in one or the other language may reflect things well beyond structural features of the language in question, and may reflect the contexts and past associations of the speaker's relative language practice and use.

2   Why is it Interesting to Compare Fluency Patterns in the Languages of Bilinguals?

Many studies early in the history of our field examined whether or not individual languages or cultures posed unequal risks of stuttering for speakers, or whether the presence of 'competing' languages in an individual might pose a risk factor for stuttering or recovery from stuttering. Given this, it is not surprising that many studies, even to this day, are concerned with whether or not stuttering is more frequent in some languages, or in bilinguals as opposed to monolinguals. We believe this issue is addressed in other chapters, but will voice our personal opinion that stuttering does not favor or disfavor any particular language(s), nor that bilingualism is a risk factor for beginning or continuing to stutter (see Bloodstein & Bernstein Ratner, 2008 for discussion).

In contrast, the authors of this chapter believe that we better understand how linguistic factors impact stuttering if we can closely examine patterns of dysfluency in a single speaker who knows and uses two different language systems. In this regard, we have relatively few studies to answer the question of whether or not linguistic factors that appear to characterize a speaker's fluency in one language 'carry over' to a second language. A few studies suggest some patterns in individuals (e.g. Bernstein Ratner & Benitez, 1985; see work by Howell and colleagues), while others suggest that motor planning issues are more important than linguistic factors in comparing fluency breakdown in bilingual stutterers (see, for example, Jayaram, 1984). Disagreements among studies may result, in part, from how the language samples are analyzed, as discussed below, in reference to our case studies.

3   What We Know to Date (and Its Limits)

3.1   Methodological issues

3.1.1   Children vs adults

It may be necessary to consider 'language age' as well as chronological age in analyzing language features in the speech of bilinguals. Adult-like language proficiency is normally achieved at around 8–10 years of age (in particular, for syntactic skill, as opposed to vocabulary use, which grows continuously over the lifespan (cf. Berko Gleason & Bernstein Ratner, 2008, but see Howell and Rusbridge, this volume for a contrasting view). Before this point, children's language skills are both variable and dynamic, suggesting that even children should be matched or sub-divided into smaller subgroups for linguistic analysis. In contrast, adults with a lifetime of experience that may shape language use may present with very different profiles of language-fluency interactions. We will return to this in discussion of our case studies because we believe that they suggest the importance of more studies of bilingual children (rare in the literature) as opposed to adults (the bulk of the literature).

3.1.2 Locus of disfluency and planning demand

When we try to associate disfluencies with language demand, we make an assumption that can be questioned. In so-called 'locus' analyses, we pinpoint the point in the utterance where fluency breakdown occurs and tend to presume that it was that spot in the utterance that provoked the disfluency. This is not necessarily a valid assumption, and alternate types of analyses may be more useful. In general, phrases and clauses are considered to be the larger planning units, rather than words (cf. Allum & Wheeldon, 2007; Ford & Holmes, 1978; Levelt & Maassen, 1981; Smith & Wheeldon, 1999, 2001); that is one reason why utterance and clause initiations robustly attract disfluencies (Bernstein, 1981). Given clause-level pre-planning, it is as likely that a disfluency signals relative difficulty in planning a subportion of the clause or constituent yet to come, rather than its initiating word (MacWhinney & Osser, 1977; Rispoli, 2003; Roll *et al.*, 2007). This is in fact how many researchers have characterized the likelihood of stuttering on function words in children – children stutter, not because the function words are difficult, but because they initiate larger planning units that are being pre-planned for production (see discussion relevant to stuttering in Chapters 8 and 12 of Bloodstein & Bernstein Ratner, 2008; and recent discussion relevant to disfluency patterns across the lifespan in McKee *et al.*, 2006).

3.1.3 What are the linguistic units of interest?

If one is to conduct a linguistic analysis, it is important to decide what aspect of language is of interest. One might divide into large word classes, such as the ubiquitous content-function word distinction. Such units have a measure of psycholinguistic validity reflected in patterns of language learning and language loss due to aphasia. Importantly, in virtually all languages, grammatical formulation exceeds that which is limited to free-standing function words and involves processes of lexical inflection that meld the 'open' and 'closed' classes of morphemes. The processes that integrate combinations of open and closed elements are also robustly evident in psycholinguistic research (e.g. Taft, 1984), even in very young children (cf. Silva-Pereyra *et al.*, 2007), which vexes the task of determining how to classify individual words. However, the research on this topic has been more focused on comprehension than production. In a rare test of morphological productivity in speech production, Janssen *et al.* (2002) supported the notion that, 'generating an inflectional frame costs time, and therefore it should be possible to measure it in appropriately designed chronometric experiments', implying an intermediate 'slot-and-filler' stage in language production that operates across word classes, and blurs the distinction between content and function words in the speech production process. A study by Marshall (2005) bears on this problem. She examined word-final grammatical morphology as a factor in stuttering, and found that some children and a small number of adults who stutter were more likely to stutter on morphologically complex words. To our knowledge, this is the only study that has taken such an approach to investigating stuttering loci and it would be valuable to both replicate the approach and extend such analyses to larger groups of younger children as well as speakers of other languages, particularly those with richer grammatical morphology than is seen in English.

In our preliminary analyses reported below, we report profiles that are organized in two different ways. The first is to collapse loci of stutters into those that affect the large classes of content and function words. The second is to perform a more 'microlinguistic' analysis of the specific parts of speech that are disfluently produced in the bilingual speakers' samples. A third approach has been utilized by some studies, particularly those conducted by Howell and colleagues, which is to sort utterances into phonological words (see Au-Yeung *et al.*, 2003), and then analyze the fluency characteristics of their initiating constituents. We have chosen not to do this for the samples reported here. One reason is that validating phonological words is difficult when using orthographically transcribed corpora, as we will illustrate below. In many phonological words, actual word boundaries are moved (e.g. defend it → defen dit; Levelt, 1989), which makes determining the locus of disfluency in relation to part of speech more difficult). Thus, we have decided to concentrate on the speakers' *target* output, rather than its phonological spell-out, in seeing whether or not grammatical factors appear to systematically guide the locus of stuttering in bilingual adults' speech.

To add to analytical complexity, most bilinguals use languages that do not bear close similarity to each other in terms of word formation, inflection and sentence types. This poses problems for comparisons. We provide an example below in considering how to treat Mandarin classifiers when drawing parallels between speakers' stuttering on this type of word and on other types of words in English.

3.2 One approach to analysis (CLAN MOR)

We have been gratified to see the development of a utility for research and clinical use that permits accurate and relatively easy 'parsing' of language targets and disfluency loci across a number of major languages. The utilities we will demonstrate here via case studies are available through the Child Language Data Exchange System (CHILDES; http://childes.

psy.cmu.edu/); they include an audio- or video-linking transcription utility that facilitates reliable coding of moments of fluency breakdown in a language sample, as well as a morphological parsing utility for use with a number of languages (MOR/POST), and frequency-searching routines (FREQ) that allow a full description of the data set and proportional accounts of fluency breakdown given the full characteristics of the language sample.

4 Case Studies

By way of background for our method of analysis, we note that the distribution of stutters has been analyzed extensively in relation to word class. Most studies made a broad distinction between content words (CW) and function words (FW), while only a few early studies specified the distinction among parts of speech (POS; e.g. noun, verb, pronoun, etc.).

Children who stutter, in general, stutter mainly on FW (e.g. Au-Yeung *et al.*, 2003; Bloodstein & Grossman, 1981; Howell *et al.*, 1999; Natke *et al.*, 2004) and AWS on CW (e.g. Brown, 1937; Dayalu *et al.*, 2002; Hahn, 1942; but see Soderberg, 1967). The difference in stuttering rates between CW and FW appears to be greater in young preschoolers than older children/adults who stutter, and that stuttering rate decreases on FW and increases on CW with age. These patterns have been observed in cross-sectional studies in English, German and Spanish, suggesting that the two word classes might affect stuttering differentially across age (Au-Yeung *et al.*, 2003; Dworzynski *et al.*, 2004; Howell *et al.*, 1999).

Grammatical class, or POS, also appears to be relevant to stuttering distribution. The few studies on POS showed some group tendencies in the ranking of difficulty among POS in English speakers who stutter, even though the specific order differed from study to study (Bloodstein & Gantwerk, 1967; Brown, 1937; Hahn, 1942; Quarrington *et al.*, 1962). Despite the inconsistency in specific findings across studies, word class appears to be a linguistic factor independent from other variables, such as initial phoneme, position and word length (e.g. Brown, 1937; Quarrington *et al.*, 1962).

Current research in typical adult language processing specifies processes involved in *specific* grammatical classes, rather than broad word class (e.g., the noun-verb distinction). Research evidence strongly suggests that grammatical class plays an important role in language processing, such as in sentence comprehension (Neville *et al.*, 1991), sentence production (Pechmann & Zerbst, 2002), phrase production (Pechmann *et al.*, 2004) and word production (Shapiro *et al.*, 2001). Although both classified in the content word class, nouns and verbs differ greatly in many respects. For example, in development, noun acquisition is generally earlier than verbs (Brown, 1957); in neuro-physiological studies, nouns and verbs appear to correspond to differential neural substrates (Kellenbach *et al.*, 2002; Shapiro *et al.*, 2005).

Since POS appears to play a role in language processing in people who do and do not stutter, it should also be the case in bilingual speakers who stutter (BWS). Studies previously discussed are mostly group studies, looking for group trends in monolingual speakers who stutter. That different studies found different patterns of stuttering between CW and FW and different rank orders among POS is consistent with the well-known observation that people who stutter are a heterogeneous population. Bilingual speakers provide a unique test case to analyze stuttering patterns across languages within individuals, which bypasses individual variability when examining linguistic factors in stuttering, although language dominance and language typology should be considered in conducting bilingual research. In the cases described below, we examined the distribution of stutters by grammatical class in both languages of each speaker. If stuttering distribution is related to grammatical class, we predicted that it should be fairly consistent in both languages within each BWS.

4.1 English-Mandarin analyses

4.1.1 Participants and method

Five adult English-Mandarin BWS, four male and one female, were included in the analyses, including two participants reported by Lim *et al.* (2008). Four BWS were judged as relatively balanced in both languages, whereas one was English-dominant, based on a survey of their language background with demographic information, including self-rating of language competencies across all modalities, report of age of language acquisition (AOA), exposure and daily use, etc.

All participants provided spontaneous language samples in both English and Mandarin on selected topics, yielding approximately 100 utterances per sample. Each sample was transcribed in 'Sonic' CHAT with linked audio/video recordings of the samples. All words in the transcripts were automatically tagged with their POS by running analyses using MOR and POST, both CHILDES utilities available for English and Mandarin. The POS output was inspected manually for all samples, and corrected for sparse categorization errors. All stuttering incidences in the samples were then coded as part-word repetition, whole-word repetition, block or prolongation; revisions, phrase repetitions and interjections were not included in the analyses, which focused on stutter-like dysfluencies (SLDs). Code switching, fillers, repetitions and revisions prior to the final forms were excluded from the analyses described below.

We obtained occurrence frequency and stuttering frequency in all samples by POS, using the CLAN programs (e.g. FREQ command).

Frequency by CW and FW was obtained by combining across the corresponding POS (these were manually corrected). In analyzing stuttering rates among POS and across languages within each BWS, we need to take into consideration the potential differences in occurrence rate across POS and the differences in overall stuttering rate across languages. Therefore, for each POS in each language sample, we calculated the stuttering ratio between the percent of the POS stuttered to the percent of total words stuttered (i.e., the stuttering frequency of each POS divided by the occurrence frequency of each POS, in relation to the total stuttering frequency divided by the total word frequency). It is worth noting that this ratio is consistent with the ratio between the percent of stuttering by POS to the percent of occurrence by POS (i.e. the stuttering frequency of each POS divided by the total stuttering frequency, in relation to the occurrence frequency of each POS divided by the total word frequency).

In brief, we will refer to this index as the stuttering ratio between the observed stuttering rate and the expected stuttering rate, reflecting stuttering tendency. A stuttering ratio of '1' reflects that the speaker is not stuttering disproportionately more or less on that particular word class, when compared to the speaker's overall stuttering rate. We obtained stuttering ratios by grammatical class (specific POS) and by the general word class (CW-FW distinction) for all language samples. Given that certain POS categories are not common to both English and Mandarin (such as classifiers in Mandarin and infinitive-*to* in English), only common POS across the two languages were included for POS analyses, while all words were included for CW-FW analyses. We compared the stuttering ratios by grammatical class and by word class across languages within individuals. We chose not to perform any statistical analyses on our data, given the small number of subjects (n = 5), and the obviously high level of variability we observed in the profiles, which was likely to produce null findings for the group as a whole. Descriptions of individual profiles are presented below.

4.1.2 Findings

The overall stuttering profiles of each BWS show that each of the four balanced BWS were similar in stuttering rates in both languages, whereas the unbalanced BWS stuttered more in the non-dominant language. There was a 5% difference in stuttering rates between two languages of the unbalanced BWS, while differences in the balanced BWS were below 2.5%. These individual profiles are consistent with prior findings that more stuttering is associated with the non-dominant language, suggestive of a relationship between language proficiency/dominance and stuttering (Jankelowitz & Bortz, 1996; Lim *et al.*, 2008; Schäfer & Robb, 2008; but see Jayaram, 1983).

4.1.2.1 Stuttering on CW and FW

Cross-linguistic comparisons of stuttering patterns between CW and FW showed two consistent profiles (BWS#1 and #2) and three inconsistent profiles (BWS#3, #4 and #5). As shown in Figure 13.1, the balanced BWS#1 stuttered consistently across languages, and stuttered fairly equivalently on both CW and FW, while the English-dominant BWS#2 stuttered consistently across languages, but disproportionately less on CW than FW. The other three BWS were balanced bilinguals, but all showed inconsistent cross-linguistic patterns with three very different individual profiles. BWS#3 stuttered fairly equivalently on both CW and FW in English, but stuttered disproportionately less on CW and more on FW in Mandarin. BWS#4 stuttered disproportionately less on CW and more on FW in English, but stuttered equivalently on both CW and FW in Mandarin. BWS#5 stuttered fairly equivalently on both CW and FW in English, but stuttered disproportionately more on CW and less on FW in Mandarin. Overall, stuttering tendency appeared to be either similar between CW and FW or greater on FW than CW.

These observations are inconsistent with the notion that AWS mainly stutter on CW, as mentioned earlier. Only one BWS showed this pattern and in one language only (BWS#5 in Mandarin). There are cross-linguistic differences in word class by the CW-FW distinction. For example, while all the English and Mandarin samples in our study included the same grammatical classes in the CW category (i.e. noun, verb, adverb and adjective) with similar positions in phrase structures between the two languages, Mandarin has several more grammatical classes in the FW

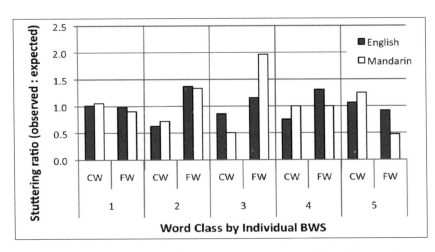

Figure 13.1 The distribution of stuttering on content and function words across English and Mandarin

category that are not present in English, such as sentence-final particles (e.g. *ma1* for questions), classifiers (e.g. *ben3* for 'book') and particle *de* (e.g. genitive marker, attributive marker and nominalization marker; Li & Thompson, 2003). The Mandarin-specific FW word classes are mostly particles that co-reference left (back) towards their modifiers or syntactic units (e.g. *san1-ben3 shu1* 'three-CLASSIFIER books'). These structure-final FW contributed to around 30% of the total FW in the Mandarin samples but only 1% of the total stuttering on FW in Mandarin; that is, stuttering rarely occurred on these language-specific FW. When these FW were excluded from analyses, stuttering distribution on CW and FW within individual BWS became more consistent across languages than originally observed, yet high individual variability among BWS was still present.

Despite the within- and between- individual differences, no BWS in our study showed opposite patterns of stuttering distribution on CW and FW across the two languages, including the unbalanced BWS (#2), who consistently stuttered more on FW than CW in both languages. Further, separate inspections of individual word class showed that the three BWS with greater tendency to stutter on one word class in one language and the opposite in the other (e.g. more stuttering on CW in English than Mandarin, and more stuttering on FW in Mandarin than English) were all balanced BWS. These observations differ from an earlier report of an unbalanced Spanish-English BWS, who stuttered more on CW, than FW, in the dominant than the non-dominant language (Howell *et al.*, 2004). The differences between the two studies might relate to the different languages examined and possibly in the types of disfluencies analyzed. Both studies reported a single case of unbalanced BWS, and thus more research is necessary to clarify the relationship among stuttering, word class and language dominance, if any. Our observations that stuttering distribution by CW-FW distinction showed cross-linguistic consistency in some balanced BWS but not all, and that the relative stuttering patterns on CW and FW differ widely across BWS. These findings suggest that the dichotomous, binary CW-FW distinction is not particularly useful in describing loci of stuttering in our adult BWS.

4.1.2.2 *Stuttering on parts of speech*

Cross-linguistic comparisons of stuttering in relation to specific grammatical class, POS, also showed very little consistency across languages within individual BWS. The POS common to both languages were first divided into two groups, those corresponding to content words (content POS), including noun, verb, adjective and adverb, and those corresponding to function words (function POS), including pronoun, conjunction, preposition, auxiliary, negation and quantifier. Ranking among content

POS based on stuttering distribution was consistent across languages only in one BWS (#4), who stuttered more on adverbs and nouns than on verbs and adjectives in both languages; all other BWS showed different rankings across languages. With such inconsistency in gross ranking among POS, it is not surprising that a closer examination of stuttering distributions by POS revealed little cross-linguistic consistency: BWS#1 showed similar stuttering tendency on verbs only, BWS#2 on nouns, adjectives and verbs, BWS#3 and #4 on adjectives only, and BWS#5 on nouns and verbs (Figure 13.2).

Analyses of function POS showed even less consistency within individual BWS. Rankings among function POS based on stuttering rates showed no similarity across languages in any BWS, and close examinations of stuttering distribution showed large cross-linguistic variability. For example, BWS#1 stuttered disproportionately more on quantifiers only in English and on prepositions only in Mandarin. BWS#2 stuttered disproportionately more on prepositions only in English and on negative forms only in Mandarin. BWS#3 stuttered on quantifiers, conjunctions and prepositions only in English and on negative forms only in Mandarin. BWS#4 stuttered disproportionately more on prepositions and pronouns only in English and on conjunctions and auxiliaries only in Mandarin. BWS#5 stuttered disproportionately more on conjunctions only in English and on quantifiers only in Mandarin (Figure 13.3).

These patterns are taken to suggest that specific part of speech is not useful in describing stuttering distributions in our adult BWS, which was the case with the binary CW-FW distinction discussed earlier. However, stuttering patterns by combining CW-FW and POS distinctions showed slightly more consistent cross-linguistic patterns of stuttering in content POS than function POS. Stuttering patterns were mostly less than or near the speaker's overall stuttering rate among content POS, whereas

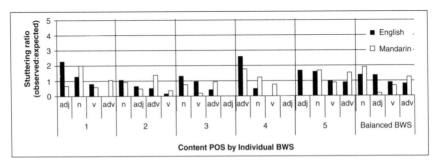

Figure 13.2 The distribution of stuttering on POS that corresponds to content words within individual BWS. POS are ordered by ranking in English, which is based on stuttering ratio from high to low

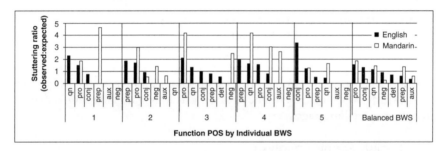

Figure 13.3 The distribution of stuttering on POS that corresponds to function words within individual BWS. POS are ordered by ranking in English, which is based on stuttering ratio from high to low

stuttering on function POS was much more variable and more categories were stuttered on greater than the overall stuttering rate.

4.1.3 Summary of English-Mandarin analysis

We obtained stuttering patterns that are consistent with the notion that stuttering could be related to language proficiency, as the balanced BWS all showed similar stuttering rates across languages while the unbalanced BWS showed higher stuttering rate in the non-dominant language. The poor cross-linguistic consistency in stuttering patterns by word class suggest that neither the dichotic CW-FW distinction nor the specific POS are reliable factors in describing stuttering patterns in adult BWS. The study does not support the notion that AWS stutter mainly on CW because of particular difficulty with CW retrieval/processing, compared to FW. No adult BWS in this study stuttered mainly on CW across languages. Yet, because this study examined only adult BWS, it does not provide support for or against any proposed developmental changes in stuttering between word classes. Previous cross-sectional studies on monolinguals who stutter have observed relatively smaller difference in stuttering between CW and FW in AWS than in young CWS, suggestive of a reduction in the CW-FW gap with age. This overall pattern does not preclude the possibility that word class no longer play a major role in the distribution of stuttering in AWS, and thus, it becomes a less useful variable for describing stuttering patterns. This corresponds to the overall finding of our study; that is, stuttering distributions in adult BWS do not reflect a direct or strong relationship between adult stuttering and grammatical factor. Future research on stuttering distribution and linguistic factors should be directed towards child BWS, whose stuttering patterns should be less affected by learned behaviors and/or coping strategies.

Cross-linguistic consistency of stuttering patterns by linguistic factors would provide strong support for the role of linguistic precipitators in the early stage of stuttering. The relationship between stuttering and linguistic factors might become less transparent with age, as learned behaviors become more influential on stuttering; thus, we propose that experimental studies of online linguistic processing will better capture the influence of linguistic factors, if any, on stuttering in AWS than does conversational corpus analysis. Corpus analysis may, however, be of greater use in studying children's fluency patterns as they gain language mastery in one or more languages.

4.2 English-Spanish analysis

4.2.1 Participant and method

Our English-Spanish bilingual person who stutters (hereafter 'ES') was a 28-year-old male. Speaking samples were obtained in Chile by a certified SLP. ES performed a variety of speaking tasks, including spontaneous speech, picture description and oral reading in each language. Using Roberts and Shenker's (2007) bilingual assessment protocol, ES judged himself to be a relatively balanced bilingual speaker, rating himself similarly in both languages for *understanding what people say, understanding what is read* and in the ability to *write*. He rated himself somewhat better at *expressing ideas* in Spanish than in English. ES self-rated his frequency of stuttering as similar in both English and Spanish. Although he reported relatively balanced proficiency in both languages, he spoke Spanish the majority of the time to family, friends and colleagues.

Speaking data presented here are from the reading tasks. During these tasks he read different portions of the book *The Little Prince* in both English and Spanish; these samples were an average of 239 words long. Reading samples were transcribed in Sonic CHAT mode and analyzed using MOR and POST, using the methods described above for the English-Mandarin samples. In order to compare across languages, we calculated a stuttering ratio as described above.

4.2.2 Findings

In terms of overall stuttering rate, ES stuttered more in English than in Spanish. In fact, he stuttered over twice as frequently in English (11.6% stuttered words) than in Spanish (5.93% stuttered words). Thus he does not follow the pattern of the balanced English-Mandarin speakers described above, who had relatively similar stuttering frequency across languages. Perhaps this is due not to his level of proficiency with each language but rather his frequency of use of each language in everyday conversations, which may lead to differing levels of automaticity for word retrieval and grammatical encoding in each language.

4.2.2.1 Stuttering on CW and FW

Stuttering ratios for content and function words for ES are in Figure 13.4.

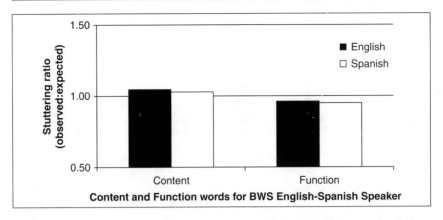

Figure 13.4 Stuttering ratio for content and function words across English and Spanish

ES stutters on CW and FW to similar degrees in both English and Spanish. In this respect his pattern is similar to that of BWS#1 above. This profile is different from that described by Howell *et al.* (1999) for an unbalanced Spanish-English bilingual who found more stuttering on CW than FW in the dominant (Spanish) language, and is inconsistent with the notion that AWS stutter more on CW than FW. It appears that proficiency level might matter; one possible hypothesis is that for ES, our balanced bilingual, we might expect similar patterns of stuttering across CW and FW in both languages if he is indeed equally proficient in both. Clearly more research is needed to describe what variables are influencing the loci of stuttering on CW versus FW, or perhaps this distinction is too 'coarse' to be of much explanatory use when it comes to cross-linguistic comparisons.

4.2.2.2 Stuttering on content parts of speech

Stuttering ratios for POS for content words are in Figure 13.5, ordered by stuttering ratios from high to low in English. Perhaps the most striking part of ES's POS profile is that despite being a relatively balanced bilingual speaker, certain parts of speech (nouns and adjectives) are stuttered more in English, whereas other parts of speech (verbs, adverbs) are stuttered more in Spanish. These inconsistencies in loci across languages suggest that the language being spoken 'frames' where stuttering occurs. Thus, in a language such as Spanish, where verbs can mark both person and tense and sentence-initial pronouns may be dropped, we see more stuttering on verbs than on nouns. It is extremely plausible that this pattern is caused by the primarily utterance-initial position of these items in Spanish, where processing load is universally regarded as highest. In contrast, stuttering is more frequent on English nouns and noun phrase

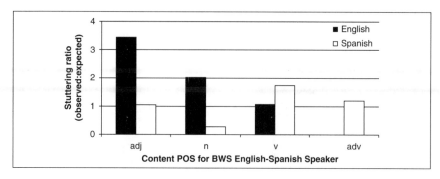

Figure 13.5 The distribution of stuttering on POS that corresponds to content words for a bilingual English-Spanish PWS. POS are ordered by ranking in English, from high to low stuttering ratio

constituents, which are utterance-initial, as required by the grammar of that language. Simply put, ES stutters on utterance-initial words, but the grammatical characteristics of these words differ greatly across his two languages.

4.2.2.3　*Stuttering on function parts of speech*

Stuttering ratios for POS for function words are in Figure 13.6. Prepositions and determiners were stuttered with relatively similar frequency in both languages; this pattern is not seen in any of the English-Mandarin speakers. For the ES speaker pronouns and conjunctions were stuttered more frequently in Spanish. This pattern matches BWS 1, 2 and 3, who all stuttered more on pronouns in Mandarin than in English. His profile for conjunctions is similar to other English-Spanish BWS reported in the literature (Bernstein Ratner & Benitez, 1985). For conjunctions, his profile matches that of BWS4 only, who stuttered on conjunctions in Mandarin far more frequently than in English.

4.2.3　*Summary of English-Spanish analysis*

ES stuttered more in Spanish than in English, despite his self-rating of similar frequencies of stuttering in both languages. Amount of stuttering on CW and FW was similar across languages. In terms of content POS, we observed more stuttering on nouns and adjectives in English, and more stuttering on verbs and adverbs in Spanish. For function POS, we saw approximately equal amounts of stuttering in both languages for prepositions and determiners, and more stuttering in Spanish for pronouns and conjunctions. For this adult Spanish-English speaker, there do not appear to be any consistent patterns across languages in terms of stuttering loci.

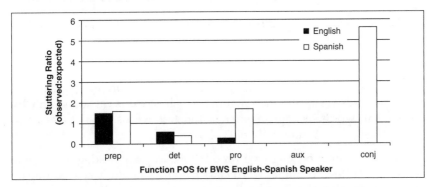

Figure 13.6 The distribution of stuttering on POS that corresponds to function words for a bilingual English-Spanish PWS. POS are ordered by ranking in English, from high to low stuttering ratio

5 Conclusions

We will begin discussion with comments about methods in analyzing linguistic properties of stuttered events in conversational speech. To do a linguistic analysis properly, one need to know how many opportunities a speaker has produced a given POS. This essentially requires either hand- or computer-assisted grammatical tagging of elements in complex spontaneous utterances. To do this on a large corpus of data, whether from one speaker or many, takes a fairly powerful parser, not available until recently, even for English. In this chapter, we essentially demonstrate the feasibility of using emerging analytical tools to a fairly old question of interest in stuttering research. The parsers that we used from the Childes Project ran fairly smoothly on our spontaneous data, requiring relatively little post-parser decision-making about word-level grammatical descriptions. These grammatical tags, in turn, were relatively easy input to frequency analyses of potential and observed loci of stuttering events. Thus, we hope these case studies will enable other researchers to pursue linguistic analyses of stuttering in other age-groups and languages.

In terms of our actual findings regarding the grammatical loci of stutters in bilingual speakers, analysis of our small sample does not suggest systematic effects of grammar across the languages and speakers we studied. This was particularly true when we attempt to 'drill down' to do a within-category analysis of the types of content and function words that were stuttered. In some respects, this should not be surprising. Currently we do not have the data to determine where we agree or not with Howell's notion that these should be similar across languages, leaving primarily phonological and prosodic differences across content words as languages vary:

> Content words in English and Spanish appear to operate equivalently insofar as they give an exchange relation. Some properties of content words remain roughly constant between the two languages (e.g., word frequency differences, their role in syntactic constructions). Other properties differ (e.g., phonological structure of Spanish content words is simpler than that in English, stress is carried mainly by content words in English whereas function words can be stressed in Spanish). (Au-Yeung *et al.*, 2003: 764)

During the course of language production, we would suggest that the ordering of utterance-initial word class members might very well impact stuttering profiles, as seen most dramatically in our Spanish speaker.

Dividing stutter loci into a dichotomous CW and FW split will make profiles of stuttering across languages and even developmental stages somewhat 'neater', but on closer examination, this level of analysis obscures quite a bit of real 'messiness' in describing what kinds of words our speakers are actually stuttering on in each of their languages. We would also suggest that it limits what we can learn about grammatical formulation and stuttering, and does not capitalize on emerging models of language production, which do not have a level at which retrieving or realizing these dichotomous classes are clearly distinguished. In fact, particularly as we move from a language such as English, where function words such as articles and verbal auxiliaries have little morphological relationship to content words, many languages (such as Spanish) greatly blur how such items mix in the encoding process, with rich systems of gender and number marking, and extensive person-marking on verbs. We note, however, that even for our Mandarin speakers, whose language is morphologically sparse, without function affixation on most content words, we didn't see many uniform patterns either across speakers or within their dual language profiles.

The content-function word contrast has been of long-standing and long-lasting interest to researchers in stuttering. But the original distinction is only part of a four-way distinction typically made in morphology, which also includes grammatical and lexical affixes, which are known to participate in utterance assembly as well as language comprehension. It may be valuable to explore alternative ways of describing the loci of stuttered events, in terms of incremental constituent phrase building, for example (see McDaniel *et al.*, 2010; McKee, *et al.*, 2006). Alternatively, we may wish to investigate how surface constructions known to be complex in their processing demands, such as embedded clauses, affect the relative fluency of output. Finally, if the two languages of a bilingual differ in their realization of constituent ordering or complexity of marking, will this have an impact on a speaker's fluency profiles? Other well-known speech production variables, such as lexical frequency and phonological neighborhood characteristics of words, are already being explored in English-speaking PWS, and might be fruitful ways to contrast patterns of fluency in bilinguals (see Anderson, 2007).

Such concerns go well beyond others that we actually know are likely to impact analysis of bilingual speakers' samples. How large a language sample is required to get an accurate estimate of typical fluency profiles? With what kind of interlocutor? How do we estimate the actual proficiency of the speaker in his or her two languages, and how can we relate estimates of the 'native-like' qualities of their speech to the ease of the encoding processes that produced it?

In most cultures, we are more likely to find sequential bilinguals in the older population, rather than young children. However, we already know that language formulation demands are much more evident in the fluency and stuttering profiles of children, rather than adults. Adults are better language users, and seem less susceptible to language demand than are young children; additionally, a PWS develops learned reactions to an array of perceived or real fluency-disruptors that can vary from sound or word fears to much larger cognitive 'sets' that involve orientation to speakers, topics or other features of conversation. We would suggest, although it will be much harder to do, that future research make a special effort to examine fluency profiles in younger bilingual speakers. Such work could either greatly support or undermine what have come to be conventional views of the relationships between language demands and stuttering.

Acknowledgment

We thank Deanne Wayt for assistance with data collection.

Note

1. These background sections are primarily meant to establish context for our more specific discussions of language use in bilinguals. Because of the multiple studies conducted in each area discussed below, we will only provide exemplar citations for the sake of brevity. A more complete list of studies is available in Hall *et al.* (2007).

References

Abrahamsson, N. and Hyltenstam, K. (2009) Age of onset and nativelikeness in a second language: Listener perception versus linguistic scrutiny. *Language Learning* 59, 249–306.

Allum, P. and Wheeldon, L. (2007) Planning scope in spoken sentence production: The role of grammatical units. *Journal of Experimental Psychology: Learning, Memory, & Cognition* 33, 791–810.

Anderson, J. (2007) Phonological neighborhood and word frequency effects in the stuttered disfluencies of children who stutter. *Journal of Speech, Language, & Hearing Research* 50, 229–247.

Au-Yeung, J., Gomez, I.V. and Howell, P. (2003) Exchange of disfluency with age from function words to content words in Spanish speakers who stutter. *Journal of Speech, Language, & Hearing Research* 46, 754–765.

Berko Gleason, J. and Bernstein Ratner, N. (eds) (2008) *The Development of Language* (7th edn). Boston: Allyn & Bacon.

Bernstein, N. (1981) Are there constraints on childhood disfluency? *Journal of Fluency Disorders* 6, 341–350.

Bernstein Ratner, N. and Benitez, M. (1985) Linguistic analysis of a bilingual stutterer. *Journal of Fluency Disorders* 10 (4), 211–219.

Bernstein Ratner, N. and Sih, C.C. (1987) The effects of gradual increases in sentence length and complexity on children's dysfluency. *Journal of Speech & Hearing Disorders* 52 (3), 278–287.

Bloodstein, O. and Bernstein Ratner, N. (2008) *A Handbook on Stuttering* (6th edn). Clifton Park, NY: Thomson Delmar.

Bloodstein, O. and Gantwerk, B.F. (1967) Grammatical function in relation to stuttering in young children. *Journal of Speech & Hearing Research* 10, 786–789.

Bloodstein, O., and Grossman, M. (1981) Early stutterings: Some aspects of their form and distribution. *Journal of Speech & Hearing Research* 24, 298–302.

Boscolo, B., Bernstein Ratner, N. and Rescorla, L. (2002) Fluency characteristics of children with a history of Specific Expressive Language Impairment (SLI-E). *American Journal of Speech-Language Pathology* 11, 41–49.

Brown, R. (1957) Linguistic determinism and the parts of speech. *Journal of Abnormal & Social Psychology* 55, 10.

Brown, S.P. (1937) The influence of grammatical function on the incidence of stuttering. *Journal of Speech Disorders* 2, 207–215.

Buhr, A. and Zebrowski, P. (2009) Sentence position and syntactic complexity of stuttering in early childhood: A longitudinal study. *Journal of Fluency Disorders* 34, 155–172.

Dayalu, V.N., Kalinowski, J., Stuart, A., Holbert, D. and Rastatter, M.P. (2002) Stuttering frequency on content and function words in adults who stutter: A concept revisited. *Journal of Speech, Language, & Hearing Research* 45, 871–878.

Dworzynski, K., Howell, P., Au-Yeung, J. and Rommel, D. (2004) Stuttering on function and content words across age groups of German speakers who stutter. *Journal of Multilingual Communication Disorders* 2, 81–101.

Eisenson, J. and Horowitz, E. (1945) The influence of propositionality on stuttering. *Journal of Speech Disorders* 10, 193–197.

Ford, M. and Holmes, V. (1978) Planning units and syntax in sentence production. *Cognition* 6, 31–53.

Hahn, E.F. (1942) A study of the relationship between stuttering occurrence and phonetic factors in oral reading. *Journal of Speech Disorders* 7, 143–151.

Hall, N. (1996) Language and fluency in child language disorders: Changes over time. *Journal of Fluency Disorders* 21, 1–32.

Hall, N.E., Yamashita, T.S. and Aram, D.M. (1993) The relationship between language and fluency in children with developmental language disorders. *Journal of Speech & Hearing Research* 36, 568–579.

Hall, N., Wagovich, S. and Bernstein Ratner, N. (2007) Language considerations in childhood stuttering. In E. Conture and R. Curlee (eds) *Stuttering and Related Disorders of Fluency* (3rd edn) (pp. 153–167). New York: Thieme.

Hilton, H. (2008) The link between vocabulary knowledge and spoken L2 fluency. *Language Learning Journal* 36, 153–166.

Howell, P. (2010) *Recovery from Stuttering*. London: Psychology Press.

Howell, P., Au-Yeung, J. and Sackin, S. (1999) Exchange of stuttering from function words to content words with age. *Journal of Speech, Language, & Hearing Research* 42, 345–354.

Howell, P., Ruffle, L., Fernandez-Zuniga, A., Gutierrez, R., Fernandez, A.H., O'Brien, M.L., Au-Yeung, J. (2004) Comparison of exchange patterns of stuttering in Spanish and English monolingual speakers and a bilingual Spanish-English speaker. In A. Packman, A. Meltzer and H.F.M. Peters (eds) *Theory, Research and Therapy in Fluency Disorders. Proceedings of the 4th World Congress on Fluency Disorders* (pp. 415–422). Nijmegen: University of Nijmegen Press.

Jankelowitz, D.L. and Bortz, M.A. (1996) The interaction of bilingualism and stuttering in an adult. *Journal of Communication Disorders* 29, 223–234.

Janssen, D., Roelofs, A. and Levelt, W. (2002) Inflectional frames in language production. *Language & Cognitive Processes* 17, 209–236.

Jayaram, M. (1983) Phonetic influences on stuttering in monolingual and bilingual stutterers. *Journal of Communication Disorders* 16, 287–297.

Jayaram, M. (1984) Distribution of stuttering in sentences: Relationship to sentence length and clause position. *Journal of Speech & Hearing Research* 27, 338–341.

Kellenbach, M.L., Wijers, A.A., Hovius, M., Mulder, J. and Mulder, G. (2002) Neural differentiation of lexico-syntactic categories or semantic features? Event-related potential evidence for both. *Journal of Cognitive Neuroscience* 14, 561–577.

Levelt, W.J.M. (1989) *Speaking: From Intention to Articulation*. Cambridge, MA: MIT Press.

Levelt, W.J.M. and Maassen, B. (1981) Lexical search and order of mention in sentence production. In W. Klein and W.J.M. Levelt (eds) *Crossing the Linguistic Boundaries* (pp. 221–252). Dordrecht, the Netherlands: Reidel.

Li, C.N. and Thompson, S.A. (2003) *Mandarin Chinese: A Functional Reference Grammar*. Taipei: Crane Publishing Co.

Lim, V.P.C., Lincoln, M., Chan, Y.H. and Onslow, M. (2008) Stuttering in English-Mandarin bilingual speakers: The influence of language dominance on stuttering severity. *Journal of Speech, Language, & Hearing Research* 51, 1522–1537.

MacWhinney, B. and Osser, H. (1977) Verbal planning functions in children's speech. *Child Development* 48, 978–985.

Manning, W.H. (2009) *Clinical Decision Making in the Diagnosis and Treatment of Fluency Disorder* (3rd edn). Albany, NY: Delmar Publishing.

Marshall, C. (2005) The impact of word-end phonology and morphology on stuttering. *Stammering Research* 1, 375–391.

McDaniel, D., McKee, C. and Garrett, M.F. (2010) Children's sentence planning: Syntactic correlates of fluency variations. *Journal of Child Language* 37, 59–94.

McKee, C., McDaniel, D., Rispoli, M. and Garrett, M.F. (2006) The development of language production mechanisms. *Journal of Applied Psycholinguistics* 27, 1–7.

Meline, T., Stoehr, R.W., Cranfield, C. and Elliot, A. (2006) Stuttering and late bilinguals: What is the evidence to date? Poster presented at the Annual Convention of the American Speech-Language-Hearing Association, Miami, FL.

Melnick, K.S. and Conture, E.G. (2000) Relationship of length and grammatical complexity to the systematic and nonsystematic speech errors and stuttering of children who stutter. *Journal of Fluency Disorders* 25, 21–45.

Natke, U., Sandrieser, P., van Ark, M., Pietrowsky, R. and Kalveram, K.T. (2004) Linguistic stress, within-word position, and grammatical class in relation to early childhood stuttering. *Journal of Fluency Disorders* 29, 109–122.

Neville, H.J., Nicol, J.L., Barss, A., Forster, K.I. and Garrett, M.F. (1991) Syntactically based sentence processing classes: Evidence from event-related brain potentials. *Journal of Cognitive Neuroscience* 3, 151–165.

Ntourou, K., Conture, E.G. and Lipsey, M.W. (2009) *Language Abilities of Children who Stutter: A Meta-Analytical Review.* Manuscript submitted for publication.

Pechmann, T., Garrett, M. and Zerbst, D. (2004) The time course of recovery for grammatical category information during lexical processing for syntactic construction. *Journal of Experimental Psychology: Learning, Memory, & Cognition* 30, 723–728.

Pechmann, T. and Zerbst, D. (2002) The activation of word class information during speech production. *Journal of Experimental Psychology: Learning, Memory, & Cognition* 28, 233–243.

Perani, D., Paulesu, E., Galles, N.S., Dupoux, E., Dehaene, S., Bettinardi, V., Cappa, S.F., Fazio, F. and Mehler, J. (1998) The bilingual brain: Proficiency and age of acquisition of the second language. *Brain* 121, 1841–1852.

Quarrington, J., Conway, J. and Siegel, N. (1962) An experimental study of some properties of stuttered words. *Journal of Speech & Hearing Research* 5, 387–394.

Rispoli, M. (2003) Changes in the nature of sentence production during the period of grammatical development. *Journal of Speech, Language, & Hearing Research* 46, 813–830.

Roberts, P. (2002) Disfluency patterns in four bilingual adults who stutter. *Journal of Speech- Language Pathology & Audiology* 26, 5–19.

Roberts, P.M. and Shenker, R.C. (2007) Assessment and treatment of stuttering in bilingual speakers. In E.G. Conture and R.F. Curlee (eds) *Stuttering and Related Disorders of Fluency* (3rd edn) (pp. 183–209). New York: Thieme Medical Publishers.

Roll, M., Frid, J. and Horne, M. (2007) Measuring syntactic complexity in spontaneous spoken Swedish. *Language & Speech* 50, 227–45.

Schäfer, M. and Robb, M. (2008, November) Stuttering characteristics of German-English bilingual speakers. Presentation at the Annual Convention of the American Speech-Language and Hearing Association, Boston.

Shapiro, K., Pascual-Leone, A., Mottaghy, F., Gangitano, M. and Caramazza, A. (2001) Grammatical distinctions in the left frontal cortex. *Journal of Cognitive Neuroscience* 13, 713–720.

Shapiro, K.A., Mottaghy, F.M., Schiller, N.O., Poeppel, T.D., Fluss, M.O., Muller, H.W., *et al.* (2005) Dissociating neural correlates for nouns and verbs. *NeuroImage* 24, 1058–1067.

Sheehan, J., Hadley, R. and Gould, E. (1967) Impact of authority on stuttering. *Journal of Abnormal Psychology* 72, 290–293.

Siegel, G. and Haugen, D. (1964) Audience size and variations in stuttering behavior. *Journal of Speech & Hearing Research* 7, 381–388.

Silva-Pereyra, J., Conboy, B., Klarman, L. and Kuhl, P. (2007) Grammatical processing without semantics? An Event-related brain potential study of preschoolers using Jabberwocky sentences. *Journal of Cognitive Neuroscience* 19, 1050–1065.

Silverman, S. and Bernstein Ratner, N. (1997) Stuttering and syntactic complexity in adolescence. *Journal of Speech & Hearing Research* 40 (1), 95–106.

Smith, M. and Wheeldon, L. (2001) Syntactic priming in spoken sentence production – an online study. *Cognition* 78, 123–164.

Smith, M.C. and Wheeldon, L. (1999) High level processing scope in spoken sentence production. *Cognition* 73, 205–246.

Soderberg, G.A. (1967) Linguistic factors in stuttering. *Journal of Speech & Hearing Research* 10, 801–810.

Taft, M. (1984) Evidence for an abstract lexical representation of word structure. *Memory & Cognition* 12, 264–269.

Van Borsel, J., Maes, E. and Foulon, S. (2001) Stuttering and bilingualism: A review. *Journal of Fluency Disorders* 26, 179–205.

Yairi, E., Ambrose, N.G., Paden, E.P. and Throneburg, R. (1996) Predictive factors of persistence and recovery: Pathways of childhood stuttering. *Journal of Communication Disorders* 29, 51–77.

Young, M. (1980) Comparison of stuttering frequencies during reading and speaking. *Journal of Speech & Hearing Research* 23, 216–217.

Chapter 14

Treating Bilingual Stuttering in Early Childhood: Clinical Updates and Applications

ROSALEE C. SHENKER

Summary

The number of children speaking more than one language continues to increase, with at least 4.6 million bilingual children in US schools. Globalization has emphasized both the benefits of bilingualism and the need for better understanding of its impact on child development. Speech Language Pathologists are increasingly asked to treat bilingual children who stutter; however, few protocols or guidelines exist for assessment and/or treatment and there is a paucity of clinical trial evidence related to treatment of bilingualism and stuttering.

While the existing literature is limited to case study reports of small numbers of children, descriptions of clinical treatments are relevant to a better understanding of the clinical issues. This chapter focuses on those issues that are particular to bilingualism in preschool-aged and young children who stutter, with emphasis upon the author's experience within the context of linguistic and cultural diversity of Canada. Clinical case studies provide the methodology to explore some of the issues related to treatment of bilingual children who stutter. These include bilingualism as a factor in persistency of stuttering, treatment in one language or two, and treatment of stuttering in a language that is not spoken at home. The chapter will conclude with some recommendations to strengthen the work that will be done in the future in order to provide some guidelines for speech language pathologists.

1   Introduction

When children who stutter are bilingual, parents often ask about the effects of speaking two languages on fluency development. Ideally, the recommendations should be informed by current research about bilingualism. Unfortunately clinical findings are limited, restricted to small numbers of children, and the role of bilingualism as a potential risk factor in both prevalence and persistency continues to be debated. Despite this, clinicians are called upon to make decisions related to treatment.

Throughout most of the 20th century it was commonly assumed that when children have a communication disorder, bilingualism would be detrimental to their linguistic and intellectual development. As a result, families were frequently counseled to give up the second language in order to ensure that the communication disorder would not be aggravated by bilingualism (Roberts & Shenker, 2007; Van Borsel *et al.*, 2001). This can be difficult to implement and may have important consequences when it is recommended that the family's native language be removed.

Van Borsel *et al.* (2001) concluded that while bilingualism might contribute to the development of stuttering in some cases, other factors related to learning a second language at school entry such as being placed in a new situation, could play a role in its persistence as well. Some of these issues may be more pertinent to the concerns of second-language learning that arise when children from multicultural backgrounds are immersed in a second language at the start of school.

Globalization has re-emphasized the benefits of being bilingual, and the need for a better understanding of the impacts of bilingualism on all areas of development in children. The number of children speaking more than one language continues to steadily increase. There are at least 4.6 million bilingual children in US schools (Kindler, 2001). Throughout the European Union, about 10% of the school-aged population speaks a language that is different than that of the majority of the country in which they live (Siegel *et al.*, 2008).

The need for clinical protocols for clinicians who will be asked to treat bilingual children who stutter is crucial and must be framed by evidence about how exposure to more than one language impacts on the treatment of these children.

In a recent review of the literature, Roberts and Shenker (2007) concluded that much still remains to be done. The existing literature is extremely limited and future studies will require more rigorous methodologies and larger numbers of participants in order to better understand bilingualism and its impact on children who stutter.

In light of the dearth of clinical research to provide guidelines for assessment and treatment of bilingual children who stutter, descriptions of clinical experiences within the bilingual culture of Canada are relevant.

This chapter will concentrate on issues related to bilingualism in preschool-aged and young children who stutter, emphasizing treatment outcome within the context of the linguistic and cultural diversity of Canada. The questions that will be addressed include the following:

(1) Is bilingualism a risk factor for persistency of stuttering in young children?
(2) Can treatment of stuttering in children be successful without removing the child from bilingualism?

(3) In which language should treatment be given; one or both?
(4) Can treatment be successful if provided in a language different from the language spoken at home?
(5) Does bilingualism increase treatment time?

Although the number of multilingual speakers continues to grow, there is a dearth of literature on the effects of bilingualism on young children with communication disorders. Few treatment guidelines are provided for speech pathologists. The area of sequential bilingualism or second-language learning has not received as much attention as those related to spontaneous bilingualism. Because bilingualism is not well defined, subject selection within a single study may include children who are both spontaneous and sequential bilinguals. Certainly more studies that compare bilingual and monolingual treatment outcomes are needed before recommending switching to one language.

This chapter will describe clinical experiences in treatment of bilingual children who stutter that could inform clinical practice and provide some guidance for clinicians despite the lack of published studies.

The methodologies will primarily be drawn from the use of single case studies in the clinical experience of the author in treating stuttering in preschool-aged and young, school-aged children who speak both English and French, and using best practices to respond to the questions asked above.

2   Bilingualism in Canada

Much of the research related to the effect of bilingualism on children with communication and learning difficulties has been initiated in Canada (Genesee, 1989, 2008 Genesee & Nicoladis, 2007; Paradis *et al.*, 2003; Thordardottir, 2006) and mostly pertains to English-French bilinguals.

In 1969, the Official Languages Act of Canada recognized English and French as the official languages of all federal institutions. It is common practice for parents to voluntarily enroll English-speaking children in schools where instruction takes place in both English and French, and bilingualism is seen as desirable and beneficial. Not all Canadians are bilingual, but few would deny that linguistic and cultural diversity is fundamental to the Canadian landscape. Much of the research on bilingualism in the past decade has taken place in Canada, notably in the French-speaking province of Quebec, and is therefore a good reference point for discussion of the objectives of this chapter.

2.1   Raising children bilingually in Quebec

Quebec has a unique stature within North America, with many children growing up in households where two or more languages are commonly used in everyday life. As well as English and French, the languages spoken in Quebec also include those of its culturally-diverse population which derived from immigration, as well as Indigenous languages spoken by First Nations groups.

As a result of these demographics, bilingualism has become a fact of life in Quebec. While French is the language of the majority, the need to use English arises from the importance of the language within the North American context, which is dominated by English for purposes of commerce and culture. The prominence of English in Quebec has been so great that many felt the French language needed to be supported and sustained. This resulted in language laws issued to protect and foster French. The passing of Bill 101 in 1977 proclaimed French as the official language of Quebec, restricting English education mostly to those already in the system, their siblings, and those residing temporarily in Quebec or whose parents had themselves received an English elementary education in the province.

While some feel that the language laws have resulted in the erosion of bilingualism, and of the English language in Quebec, the fact is that Quebecers are now more bilingual than ever. French-speaking Quebecers increasingly visit other parts of the continent in greater numbers than ever, listen to English television, consume American cultural products, and interact with their Anglophone counterparts in the province.

In Quebec, 300,000 students study in French Immersion classrooms. Immersion is a form of bilingual education in which a child learns in his/her second language (L2). Most early immersion students start in kindergarten and do all their work in their second language with first language (L1) education gradually increased by Grade 6.

2.2 Definitions of bilingualism: Examples of different patterns

Some of the problems related to research in bilingualism stem from the use of the word 'bilingualism' to describe all types. For the purposes of this discussion, the term *early or simultaneous bilingual* will refer to children learning two languages simultaneously from birth or shortly after. *Later bilingual or sequential bilingual* refers to children who acquire two languages sequentially, and therefore may still be in the process of learning a second language (L2) (De Houwer, 1990; Mennen, this volume).

It is common practice in Quebec to evaluate children with both early and later patterns of bilingualism, resulting in the possibility of different implications for treatment based on the type of bilingualism. In Quebec the multicultural linguistic tableau offers opportunities to evaluate children who stutter, from a variety of cultural and linguistic backgrounds. Some of the difficulties noted might be more pertinent to concerns related to learning a second language that may arise when children from multicultural backgrounds are immersed in a new language at the start of school.

The following is a common example of *simultaneous bilingualism* in a case of early stuttering.

> David, a 4-year-old child with severe stuttering, presented at the clinic. David's mother always speaks to him in French, while his father speaks to him in English. David speaks to his parents in both languages, and sometimes mixes the two during one utterance, using a word that he does not know in one language, or to extend the length of a sentence. An example of this might be '**on met** all this one **en premier**' [we put all this one first]. He will begin his education in a school where he will study in English and French and will be introduced to a third language. His parents want to know if this educational plan is a bad idea, considering David's severe stuttering.

Early simultaneous bilingualism is also common in many communities elsewhere, including those in Belgium and Northern Italy, and could provide, along with the Quebec experience, unique opportunities for evaluating the relationship between early bilingualism and stuttering.

In contrast to later/sequential bilingualism, in many areas of Canada, the United States and Western Europe, monolingualism is the norm and families have the choice to introduce their children to a second language as part of a bilingual education. The second language can be introduced at the start of education or in the later grades. A case example of *sequential language learning* (L2) in early stuttering is described next:

> Emma, a 4-year-old English-speaking preschooler, who has stuttered for 1-1/2 years and has a history of persistent stuttering in her family, will begin her education in a school where early French Immersion is taught. Unambiguous stuttering is characterized by sound and syllable repetitions of 2–5 iterations per moment, audible sound prolongations and infrequent blocks. Until 3rd grade she will only receive a few hours a week of education in English. Up until this time she has had no introduction to French, and English is spoken at home. Her parents wonder if this will exacerbate her stuttering and if they should consider an English-only education.

In contrast, children who speak an L1 that is neither English nor French are the main source of population increase in Quebec. This reflects increases in immigration, as well as a demographic shift in immigration from countries where English is not the mother tongue, from 6.6% in 1971 to 10% of the immigrant population by 2001. According to a 2006 census report, speakers of languages other than French or English account for 20% of the population of Canada (2006 Census). In the USA, 47 million or 18% of the population speak a language other than English (Shin & Bruno, 2003). In

Montreal, the largest city in Quebec, 21.8% of the population is allophone, and in communities with the most vulnerable populations, as a result of poverty and lack of access to services, as much as 80% of the population speaks a language other than English or French as their home language. An example of *sequential (L2) language learning in a multicultural family* is cited as follows:

> Rana, a 5 ½ year old, presents with stuttering that is mostly char-acterized by multiple, frequent sound and syllable repetitions noted in both her home language and second language. While the home language is Arabic, Rana attends a French Kindergarten as the lan-guage of education. Neither parent is proficient in French, and Rana's mother speaks only Arabic. When using a second language, Rana's father speaks in English; however, they prefer to converse in Arabic at home. Rana is learning French as a second language in a school where no English is spoken. Rana's parents have been advised by the Speech-Language Pathologist to speak French at home in order to increase Rana's exposure to the language in which she will be educated, and that learning one language will be hard enough given the stuttering concerns. Is this a sensible or realistic recommendation for this family?

If some family members speak only one language, they could be cut off from communication with a child who has not learned their language. It is, therefore, critical for minority language children to learn the home language so that their parents can communicate easily with them. Lan-guage is integral to cultural identity and minority children risk becoming alienated from their community if they do not learn the home language (Wong-Filmore, 1991).

2.3 Benefits of bilingualism

There may be more children who grow up learning two or more languages than children who learn only one. The number of children from diverse linguistic backgrounds steadily increases, suggesting that dual language acquisition might be more common than monolingualism (Thordardottir, 2006). There are advantages to being bi- or multilin-gual. Bilinguals are noted to be better at problem solving, demonstrate greater creativity and express more tolerant attitudes toward each other (Bialystok & Martin, 2004; Genesee & Gándara, 1999).

There is no scientific reason to think that infant brains are equipped to learn only one language in early childhood or that developing two lan-guages is a cause of language impairment. There has been much research on infants and toddlers who learn two languages from birth, as in the case of David cited earlier. Evidence shows that bilingualism does not impair normal language development. The research shows that simultaneous bilingual children go through the same basic milestones in language development as monolingual children, and that they do it at the same rate, provided they are given an adequate learning environment (Genesee & Nicoladis, 2007). When members of the immediate or extended family speak different languages, it is beneficial for young children to learn those languages in order to be fully functioning members of the family. Such is the case with second language bilinguals such as Rana. Much less is known about children who begin to learn a second language after their first language is established (Genesee, 2008) as with Emma and Rana.

3   Treatment Outcomes with Young Bilingual Children Who Stutter

The literature search for this chapter failed to find any treatment outcome studies designed to compare bilingual with unilingual children. Few studies have provided data on the generalization of treatment gains across languages. Table 14.1 provides a summary of the descriptive case studies of bilingual children who stutter. In these studies data is provided for only 12 children. This includes studies of children speaking English and Arabic (Humphrey *et al.*, 2001; Roberts & Shenker, 2007); English and French (Harrison *et al.*, 2010; Rousseau *et al.*, 2005; Shenker *et al.*, 1998), and Baluchi and Persian (Bakhtiar & Packman, 2009). In all cases reviewed that evaluated treatment in children ranging from 3- to 11-years old, fluency increased in both languages spoken independsent of whether treatment was in one or both languages spoken by the child.

Humphrey *et al.* (2001) provided information on the transfer of fluency in a reading condition, using a combination of Fluency Shaping and Stuttering Modification techniques with 11-year-old twin girls. In this case study where the language of treatment was Arabic, fluency increased in Arabic reading and generalized to English reading in 11-year-old twin girls.

The case of a 13-year-old trilingual, Arabic, English and French, adolescent who received treatment that consisted of speech restructuring using prolonged speech (O'Brian *et al.* (2003) is described in Roberts & Shenker (2007)). Pre-treatment measures showed a range from 2.7% to 6.7%SS in English-speaking situations and 4.8%SS in an Arabic conversational sample. Stuttering was characterized by audible sound prolongations, multisyllabic unit repetitions and some nonverbal behaviors such as head movements that accompanied moments of stuttering. Therapy was provided in English by the clinician and in English and Arabic by the mother. Following the intensive treatment the %SS decreased to less than 1% in English and Arabic. It was necessary to do the follow-up with a distance monitored protocol that involved telephone calls. In a four-month post-treatment telephone follow-up session with the therapist, stuttering frequency in English was 1.1%SS and in an Arabic conversation with

Table 14.1 Treatment of stuttering in bilingual children: Review of studies in children 3–11-years old

Study	Subjects	Treatment	Pre-tx %SS	Post-tx %SS	Length of treatment
Shenker et al. (1998)	3-year-old girl; English/French from birth	Week 1–16 Indirect Treatment Week 17–30 Lidcombe Program initiated in English with French added at week 23. Both French and English spoken at home during all treatment	English – 13.5 French – 9.9	English – 2.8 French – 4.4	30 clinic sessions
Harrison et al. (2010)	5-year-old boy; English/French from birth	Lidcombe Program provided by mother (French) and father (English) both in clinic and at home	English 3.8–12.0 for clinic & home samples	English/French 0.4–1.4 for clinic & home samples	8 sessions over 12 weeks <1%SS in 1-year follow-up
Rousseau et al. (2005)	7-year-old boy; L1: French L2: English introduced at 5;6 years	Lidcombe Program was provided in French	English: 2–6%SS French: 2.5–5.5%SS Samples taken in and beyond clinic	English <1% French <1% for clinic and home samples	41 sessions over 51 weeks
Humphrey et al. (2001)	11-year-old identical twin girls L1: Arabic L2: English	Stuttering Modification, Fluency Shaping for reading only provided in Arabic Fluency increased in Arabic reading & generalized to English reading in both S1 and S2	S1: English – 29% S1: Arabic – 27% S2: English – 23% S2: Arabic – 18%	S1: English – 3% S1: Arabic – 2% S2: English – 1% S2: Arabic – 2%	21 sessions

Table 14.1 (Continued)

Study	Subjects	Treatment	Pre-tx %SS	Post-tx %SS	Length of treatment
Bakhtiar and Packman (2009)	8-year 11-month-old boy L1: Persian L2: Baluchi	Lidcombe Program provided in Persian in the clinic and Baluchi at home by the parent	Persian – 12% Baluchi – SR 5 SR 1 = mild, 10 = very severe stuttering	Persian – 0% Baluchi – 0%	12 sessions to Stage 2
Roberts and Shenker (2007)	6-year-old boy L1 – Arabic L2 – English introduced at 4;6 in school	Lidcombe Program (intensive format); followed through distance managed treatment	English – 5.8% Arabic – 8.0%	English – 2.4% Arabic – 1.4% 1.1% (English); 0.9% (Arabic) 4 months post treatment	1 month intensive treatment
Gutmann and Shenker (2006)	4-year 4-month-old boy; English/French from birth 5-year 3-month-old boy: English/French from birth 5-year 6-month-old boy; L1 English/L2 French 6-year 6-month-old boy: L1 English; L2 French	Lidcombe Program provided in English (Parents of S1 and S2 provided treatment in French at home)	L1: English – 12.5 L1: French – 7.8 L2: English – 3.8 L2: French – 3.2 L3: English – 2.8 L4: English – 2.6	L1: English – 0.2 L1: French – 1.1 L2: English – 1.6 L2: French – 0.8 L3: English – 0.9 L4: English – 0.8	Mean = 12 sessions to Stage 2; range 10–14
Roberts and Shenker (2007)	3-year 11-month-old boy; E/F from birth	Lidcombe Program: English for sessions 1–6; French introduced at session 7 with father.	English/French 5.6–9.8	English – 0.6 French – 0.9 maintained at 88 weeks following discharge from Stage 2	15 sessions over 23 weeks

340

the mother 1.5%SS. Severity ratings provided by the mother were 1 in both languages for the week prior to the follow-up call. (This indicates no stuttering on the 10-point perceptual scale described previously). The follow-up session needed to be done in this manner because the boy returned to Beruit from Montreal.

In one study of the treatment outcomes following intensive therapy in English, based on speech restructuring strategies for 6–8-year-old children, Druce *et al.* (1997) reported that the outcomes for six bilingual children were not significantly different from those of the nine unilingual English-speaking children. However, there are no details provided regarding the language histories of the bilingual children or the characteristics of the stuttering. Shenker *et al.* (1998), Roberts and Shenker (2007), and Rousseau *et al.* (2005) describe treatment with the Lidcombe Program in one language, with fluency transferring to the second language spoken by the child.

Case studies where treatment was input simultaneously in two languages are presented by Harrison *et al.* (2010), Roberts and Shenker (2007) and Gutmann and Shenker (2006).

With only a very small number of published papers that presented treatment effects or outcome, especially concerning the outcome of transfer of fluency in two languages, few resources are provided for the growing number of speech language pathologists who require guidance in treating bilingual children who stutter, although there is some support for the assumption that bilingualism may be a risk factor for persistent stuttering (Howell *et al.*, 2009).

These few studies support clinical observation that bilingual children who stutter may achieve fluency whether the treatment is provided in one or both languages that the children speak. However, there continues to be a lack of evidence-based treatment for stuttering in bilingual children reported in the literature. Some of the studies that have been reported fail to clearly describe the bilingual profile of the participants; the treatment and its outcomes are not well detailed; the assessment of stuttering varies between studies and is not always specified in detail. Druce *et al.* (1997) investigated the short- and long-term outcome for mono- and bilingual children by applying an intensive behavioral treatment program. In this study bilingualism was defined as 'the simultaneous acquisition of more than one language during the first 5 years of life.' The second language in addition to English for the six bilingual children was reported as Slovenian, German, Greek, Hindi, and Italian. Although no symptoms of stuttering are noted, the stuttering severity of the bilingual children ranged from mild to moderate pre-treatment and normal to severe post-treatment. They reported no significant difference between the %SS for the mono- and bilingual children either before treatment or after treatment and no significant association between bilingualism and treatment outcome. It is unclear whether speech fluency was transferred to both or all languages and in which language treatment was given.

A modification of a fluency shaping program described by Waheed-Kahn (1997) improved the outcome of bilingual children who stutter compared to their monolingual English-speaking peers. Although the second language of each of the bilingual children is not specified, the author refers to speakers of Spanish, Punjabi, and Persian in case descriptions. The modification included a 'speech helper' as co-therapist, if necessary an interpreter, inclusion of the cultural background of the client, and treatment offered in the dominant language. Before these modifications only 20% of the bilingual speakers achieved an increase of speech fluency in comparison to 85% of the monolingual speakers. After the modification 75% of the bilingual speakers achieved a fluent speech pattern. The methods of assessment and measurement of stuttering are not specified in this study. Aside from these studies, no others compare bilingual with unilingual children.

4 The Lidcombe Program with Bilingual Children Who Stutter

The majority of descriptive cases reviewed here have used the Lidcombe Program for Early Stuttering Intervention. The Lidcombe Program (Onslow *et al.*, 2003) is a behavioral treatment based on verbal response contingent stimulation. Stage 1 involves weekly parent and child clinic visits where parents are trained to provide daily verbal contingent responses to fluency and unambiguous stuttering in structured and unstructured conversations. In addition, parents collect daily perceptual severity ratings to show progress at home. These ratings are compared to the clinician's measure of percent stuttered syllables (%SS) in the clinic. The %SS measure relies on perceptual judgments of stuttering, since the listener judges each syllable as stuttered or not stuttered. Stuttering severity is measured by assigning a score on a 10-point scale where 1 indicates no stuttering, 2 indicates very mild stuttering, and 10 indicates very severe stuttering (Onslow *et al.*, 2003). This stage continues until the child reaches zero or near-zero levels of stuttering for three consecutive clinic visits, which are the criteria for entering Stage 2. The goal during Stage 2 is maintenance of zero or near-zero stuttering for at least 1 year. In Stage 2 the frequency of clinic visits and verbal contingencies are gradually decreased as long as the criteria for Stage 2 are met. These criteria are severity ratings for each day of the week as 1 or 2, with at least four of these being SR = 1, and %SS within the clinic below 1.0.

At the Montreal Fluency Centre children who are evaluated for early stuttering are classified as either early or later bilinguals. Assessment includes completion of bilingual history and proficiency case history, and language samples in all languages spoken. Although most children speak English and/or French in school, the languages of the homes represent the rich multicultural variety that make up the demographic of Montreal. Treatment of stuttering in young multilingual children is commonplace and it is from this background that the outcomes of treatment with bilingual children are examined.

4.1 Clinical applications

In a case of early bilingualim, Shenker *et al.* (1998) first introduced treatment with the Lidcombe Program in English only, adding treatment in French at week 23, in a 3-year-old girl. This study documented the treatment with the Lidcombe Program of a bilingual English/French 3-year-old girl and monitored gains in fluency to the untreated language, when treatment was initially provided only in English. Stuttering was initially treated in the language that was noted to be more linguistically complex, as determined from pretreatment analysis of a spontaneous language sample. Spontaneous conversational samples were videotaped in French and English. The average mean length of utterance (MLU) was computed in both languages. The number of complex sentences in each sample was computed manually. The preliminary language analysis indicated that English was the more complex language. Stuttering was assessed through a %SS of Stuttered Like Dysfluencies (SLD). Although the symptoms of the SLDs noted are not described, it is noted that analysis showed no significant difference between the loci of disfluencies occurring in English and French. During the course of treatment the less complex language (French) was monitored for changes in both stuttering and linguistic complexity. Although bilingualism was not discouraged at home, the parents were encouraged to speak in one language at a time, trying to avoid code-mixed utterances on input. Videotaped language samples were collected in both languages at the initial assessment, 1-week pretreatment and clinic session 30. The Lidcombe Program was introduced at week 16 of treatment after treatment based on the multifactorial model (Starkweather & Gottwald, 1999) failed to show a significant treatment effect. Treatment was provided in English only from week 16 to week 23, when stuttering decreased to <3%SS. At this point stuttering had begun to decrease in French and bilingual sessions were initiated so that both parents could participate in the treatment. Stuttering subsequently continued to decrease in both languages according to measures taken in and outside of the clinic. At clinic visit 30, the %SS had reduced from 13.5 to 2.8%SS in English and 9.9 to 4.4%SS in French. Parent severity rating (SR) for both languages spoken was reduced from 7 to 3.5 (1 = no stuttering, 2 = very mild stuttering, 10 = very severe stuttering). This single case study suggested that early stuttering could be successfully decreased in the presence of a bilingual language environment.

Another case study of simultaneous bilingualism in early stuttering is described in Roberts and Shenker (2007). In this case, treatment with the

Lidcombe Program was initiated at 3 years 11 months, after the child had been stuttering for more than 18 months. Exposed to English and French from birth, pre-treatment stuttering ranged from 5.6%SS to 9.8%SS in English and French samples of spontaneous conversation taken both in and outside clinic settings. Pre-treatment severity ratings were SR 8 (English) and SR 6 (French). The language of treatment was initially English with French treatment introduced at week 7 to allow the father to participate. After 15 sessions over 23 weeks, this child met the criteria for Stage 1 of the Lidcombe Program (<1%SS and Severity of mostly '1' over 3 consecutive weeks using the 10-point perceptual severity rating scale described earlier. Follow-up at 88 weeks following discharge from Stage 2 of the Lidcombe Program showed that fluency had been maintained in both English (0.6%SS) and French (0.9%SS) with severity ratings of '1' in both languages.

Harrison, Kingston and Shenker (in preparation) describe the case of a 5-year-old boy exposed to both English and French from birth. The Lidcombe Program was provided in both English and French from the initial session. Pre-treatment English and French ranged from 3.8% SS to 12%SS for spontaneous conversational samples both in and beyond clinic settings. Stuttering symptoms were sound and syllable repetitions of more than three iterations per moment, inaudible and audible sound prolongations that lasted for periods of up to 10 seconds per moment and frequent blocks. Post-treatment English and French ranged from 0.4%SS to 1.4%SS for both in and beyond clinic samples, with fluency maintained at <1%SS 12 months following discharge from Stage 2 in both languages. The criteria for Stage 1 of the Lidcombe Program were met in eight clinic visits over a period of 12 weeks.

Roberts and Shenker (2007) provided case study information for an early bilingual 6-year-old child treated in both English and Arabic over a one-month intensive treatment with the Lidcombe Program. In this case, treatment was provided in English by the clinician and in both English and Arabic by the parents in both in and out of clinic settings. In this treatment stuttering decreased in both English (pre-treatment 5; 8 to post-treatment 2.4%SS) and Arabic (pre-treatment 8; 0 to post-treatment 1.4%SS).

Other descriptions of successful clinical intervention with the Lidcombe Program with bilingual children have been documented by Rousseau *et al.* (2005) and Bakhtiar and Packman (2009).

Rousseau noted a simultaneous decrease of the stuttering rate in both English and French for a 7-year-old boy treated in French only with the Lidcombe Program in 41 clinic visits over a period of 51 weeks.

Most recently Bakhtiar and Packman (2009) reported treatment outcomes of the Lidcombe Program carried out in Baluchi and Persian with an 8-year 11-month-old boy who met the criteria for Stage 1 of the program in 12 sessions over 13 weeks and has continued to maintain the criteria for Stage 2 in both languages over 10 months. Stuttering was characterized by repeated syllables and fixed postures of the speech mechanism, consisting of vowel prolongations and some audible blocks in Persian. Conversational speech samples in Baluchi were recorded and replayed with presence/absence of stuttering confirmed by the therapist and parent. In this case, feedback was given in Baluchi, the first language of this child, in unstructured situations, by family members in the home, while feedback was given in Persian, the language introduced in school, in structured conversations when demonstrated by the clinician in weekly sessions. The criteria for Stage 1 of the Lidcombe Program (<1% Stuttered Syllables and severity ratings of mostly 1 suggesting no stuttering or extremely mild stuttering) were confirmed by recordings from in and beyond the clinic in both languages.

In an attempt to gather preliminary information regarding the relationship between language development, bilingualism and treatment outcomes, Gutmann and Shenker (2006) compared four children, two of whom were simultaneous bilinguals and two of whom were sequential language learners. This was assessed through case history interview with the parent that included a comprehensive history and proficiency description, as well as audio-recorded spontaneous conversational samples in both languages. Participants' ages at onset of therapy were 4 years 4 months; 5 years 3 months; 5 years 6 months, and 6 years 6 months. All children had been stuttering for at least 6 months prior to therapy. Pre-treatment measurements included a detailed linguistic proficiency questionnaire, spontaneous language samples taken both in the clinic and at home in English and French, the Expressive One Word Picture Vocabulary Test – Revised (EOWPVT-R) (Gardner, 1990), and the Clinical Evaluation of Language Fundamentals – Preschool (CELF-P) (Wiig *et al.*, 1998). Language samples in French and English were taken in the clinic and at home at weeks 6 and 12 of treatment with the Lidcombe Program. The results of the CELF-P showed a normal score for all four participants. Test results for all four participants showed expressive vocabulary ability within the average to high average range in relation to established norms for monolingual speakers. Based on SALT transcriptions of language samples in spontaneous conversation, all children showed a post-treatment increase in Mean Length of Utterance (MLU), Number of Different Words (NDW) and production of complex sentences. Treatment was provided in English in the clinic and either in English or French by the parent at home. In all cases fluency transferred to the untreated language. All children achieved the criteria for Stage 1 of the Lidcombe Program (<1%SS and Severity Ratings of at least four daily SR = 1 per week over a period of three consecutive weeks as previously stated) and were placed in Stage 2 in a mean 12 sessions (range 10–14) (see Table 14.2). Additionally, fluency

Table 14.2 Comparison of treatment outcomes with the Lidcombe program for simultaneous and sequentially bilingual preschool-aged children (adapted from Gutman & Shenker, 2006)

Subjects	%SS	NDW	MLU	% Complex utterances
Pre-treatment				
S1-French	7.8	62	3.98	–
S1-English	12.5	96	3.98	4
S2-French	3.2	81	6.5	–
S2-English	3.8	108	5	2
S3-English	2.8	132	9	18
S4-English	2.6	140	7	21
Week 12				
S1-French	1.1	104	5.75	–
S1-English	0.2	110	5.6	11
S2-French	0.8	161	7.2	–
S2-English	1.6	140	7.1	8
S3-English	0.9	185	12.7	25
S4-English	0.8	178	9.2	17

Note: Dashes indicate that Percentage of Complex Utterances was not estimated. From 'Achieving fluency in bilingual children with the Lidcombe Program,' by V. Gutmann and R.C. Shenker (2006), poster presented at the American Speech Language and Hearing Association, Miami, Florida. Reprinted with permission.

increased with no cost to language development. Sentence complexity was analyzed for both English and French samples for the two simultaneous bilingual children and in English only for the sequential bilinguals whose knowledge of French was not sufficient at these points to produce complex utterances. Two independent raters rescored three randomly selected samples for each child. The interjudge agreement for elements of the transcripts was 98.2%. An increase in both MLU and NDW were found post treatment. Results indicated that fluency increased in the presence of two languages and that the treatment times were not increased for either the early or the later bilingual children. In this study, treatment did not negatively influence the development of the second language and increases in fluency did not influence development of language complexity in the early bilinguals. This is consistent with the linguistic findings of Lattermann et al. (2005) for unilingual children. Neither the simultaneous or sequential bilinguals took longer to achieve fluency than their unilingual peers (Jones et al. 2000).

The results of these descriptive case studies suggest that fluency is achieved within the same time frame when the treatment is provided at home in a language that differs from the therapist's language in clinic. Additionally, the introduction of treatment in two languages did not influence treatment outcome. It must be noted, however, that the outcome of these studies are difficult to compare due to possible differences in definitions of bilingualism, methods of assessment of stuttering and its characteristics, and the small number of children comprising these case studies.

4.2 Treatment times

A retrospective file audit methodology has been used in two studies to evaluate treatment time to Stage 2 with the Lidcombe Program with unilingual children (Jones *et al.*, 2000; Kingston *et al.*, 2003). In both studies a median treatment time of 11 sessions was found. Findlay, Shenker and Matthews (2008) replicated this methodology to evaluate the effect of bilingualism on treatment time for stuttering using the Lidcombe Program. In this file audit, 56 children's case files were reviewed of children ranging in age from 2 years 9 months to 11 years 9 months. According to parent report during a case history interview that described linguistic proficiency in detail, 23 children were classified as French/English bilingual, having been spoken to and speaking two languages before age 4. Thirty-three children were classified unilingual, speaking only English or French before age 4. All children were treated with the researched version of the Lidcombe Program in the same clinic by clinicians who had received a two-day basic training in the program. The bilingual children had a %SS that ranged from 1.4 to 8.7 pre-treatment (median 4), and a post-treatment %SS of 1 to 1.9 (median 0.5). The unilingual children had a %SS that ranged from 2.1 to 11.8%SS pre-treatment (median 4.8) with a post-treatment %SS that ranged from 0 to 2.8 (median 0.9). The median treatment time for both the unilingual and bilingual children to Stage 2 was nine sessions, with no significant difference in median treatment time between bilingual and unilingual children and outcomes were consistent with Jones et al. and Kingston *et al.*'s findings. These preliminary findings indicate that early bilingualism does not affect treatment time in the Lidcombe Program (see Figure 14.1). It is noteworthy that this fairly large and reasonably homogeneous group was all treated at the same clinic by clinicians who had received basic training in the Lidcombe Program.

4.3 Follow-up

An important yardstick for any therapy is how well the gains achieved are maintained after discharge from treatment. This is equally relevant where children are bilingual.

Shenker and Roberts (2006) evaluated 14 bilingual children who had all completed the Lidcombe Program and were followed up from 2 to 7 years

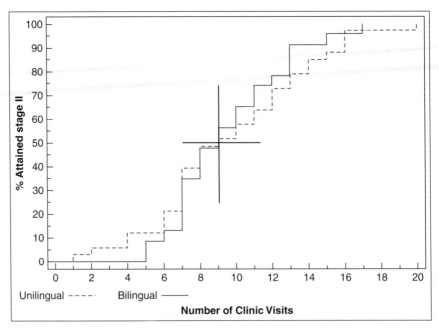

Figure 14.1 Treatment times with the Lidcombe program: Outcomes for bilingual children

Source: Adapted from Findlay *et al.* (2008)

after discharge from Stage 2. Ten children were classified as late bilinguals, having been introduced to a second language at age 4 or later (this criterion potentially masks a lot of individual variation). Four were classified as early bilinguals, having received input in two languages in the home from birth. Most rated their English as slightly better than their French, for both comprehension and oral expression. Each child was reassessed in a clinic setting by two therapists, one of whom they were unfamiliar with. All children completed three speaking tasks in each language; spontaneous conversation, monologue and story retell. Preliminary findings on the English conversation task found that 11/14 bilingual children had maintained a level of <1%SS. This was based on the number of SLDs and Normal Speech Disfluencies (NSD) per 100 syllables spoken. The SLDs noted were repetitions of one-syllable words, syllable and sound repetitions of 1–3 iterations per moment. There was only 1 audible sound prolongation in the 14 samples. Speaking rate on follow-up ranged from 170 to 215 syllables per minute (spm). Using the definitions of the Iowa Scale of Severity (Johnson *et al.*, 1963), these children were all classified as very mild or mild. Of the 14 children, 3 had a %SS of >1 (1.2%SS, 2.2%SS, 1.6%SS). Of the children who had failed to maintain the Stage 2 criteria, all had been classified as late bilinguals. Stuttering, when present, was characterized by whole-word repetitions of one iteration, short duration and very little perceived tension. Parents' response to a questionnaire giving feedback on their therapy experience noted that 96% of parents considered their child to be no longer stuttering. These results are similar to the findings of both Lincoln and Onslow (1997) and Miller and Guitar (2006) for a group of unilingual children.

Lincoln and Onslow (1997) followed 43 children 2–7 years after completing Stage 2 of the Lidcombe Program. Conversational samples were provided by each child in three situations, one of which was covert. In Group 1 (9 children who had participated in previous studies) all subjects achieved <1.5%SS in speech samples taken in the clinic and outside the clinic. The criteria for ending Stage 1 of the treatment is currently more stringent than what was followed in the Lincoln and Onslow study and reflects the revisions to the manual in 2003.

In Group 2, 34 children who had not participated in previous studies, the maximum stuttering rate was 1.9% SS, with most children well below that.

Miller and Guitar (2006) followed 15 monolingual children up to 58 months after completing Stage 2 of the Lidcombe Program. Spontaneous conversation samples with parents and with an unfamiliar conversational partner were collected in the child's home. This study found that 11 of 15 had zero levels of stuttering with four scored as mild or very mild on the SSI, indicating some residual stuttering. Two of the 15 children had scores that were >1%SS (3.6%SS and 2.6%SS). The authors used the Stuttering Severity Index (SSI-3; Riley, 1994) to describe changes in severity pre-treatment and at follow-up. The Pre-treatment SSI-3 score was 24.9 indicating moderate to very severe stuttering, while the follow-up score was 3.5 indicating normal fluency to mild stuttering. Additionally, 13/15 parents rated their children as completely fluent at follow-up.

The results of these case descriptions suggest some factors to consider in the treatment of young bilingual children who stutter. These preliminary case studies suggest that fluency increases can be achieved in bilingual children. Additionally, the Lidcombe Program appears to be a suitable treatment for young bilingual children. These findings suggest that (a) there is no need to reduce spoken languages to achieve fluency, (b) bilingual children who have been followed don't take longer to achieve fluency, (c) therapy with bilingual children doesn't influence language development in a negative way.

5 Summary and Conclusions: Future Needs

While we must be cautious in drawing conclusions from these data, preliminary case studies of young children indicate no need to reduce spoken languages to increase fluency. There are some encouraging results to indicate that bilingual children who were treated with the Lidcombe Program did not take longer to achieve fluency and that in these case description of bilingual children, fluency did not appear to increase at a cost to language development.

While the existing literature is based on single subject case studies, and retrospective file audits, future treatment research with bilingual children needs to increase the group sizes, and compare bilingual children who stutter with bilingual children who have never stuttered. Future studies that replicate these finings with more rigorous methodologies on larger numbers of children are critical to a better understanding of the relationship between bilingualism and stuttering. Clearly there is a need for more systematically controlled research in this area to answer questions related to order of acquirement of languages, the results of providing treatment in two languages simultaneously, and follow-up to show the long-term effect of early successful treatment on fluency and language development in two or more languages. There is also a need for research that considers the treatment outcomes when families have a multicultural background.

In conclusion, while the evaluation of treatment outcomes in bilingual as compared to monolingual stutterers is limited, the findings are encouraging showing that young bilingual stutterers can achieve fluency within the same treatment times as their unilingual peers. This information is limited to children following the Lidcombe Program and should be extended to evaluation of outcomes of other treatments for stuttering. It should be noted that the results of these case studies indicate that it is not necessary to ask parents of a child who is stuttering to stop exposing their child to two languages until there was good control over one language as a way of preventing stuttering, as had been historically recommended. There is a need for more studies to confirm these preliminary findings in a larger number of children. Other considerations must be given to evaluation of results when treatment is provided in all the languages that the child speaks, and whether the order of acquisition of languages has an effect on treatment outcome. Finally, all of these questions must be considered in children with multicultural/multilinguistic backgrounds in order to establish guidelines for clinical practice.

References

Bakhtiar, M. and Packman, A. (2009) Intervention with the Lidcombe program for a bilingual school-age child who stutters in Iran. *Folia Phoniatrica et Logopaedica* 61(5), 300–304.

Bialystok, E. and Martin, M. (2004) Attention and inhibition in bilingual children: Evidence from the dimensional change card sort task. *Developmental Science* 7, 325–339.

2006 Census: The evolving linguistic portrait, 2006 Census (2006, 2009-04-03) http://www12.statcan.ca/census-recensement/2006/as-sa/97–555/tables-tableaux-noteseng.efm.

De Houwer, A. (1990) *The Acquisition of Two Languages from Birth: A Case Study.* Cambridge: Cambridge University Press.

Druce, T., Debney, S. and Byrt, T. (1997) Evaluation of an intensive treatment program for stuttering in young children. *Journal of Fluency Disorders* 22 (3), 169–186.

Findlay, K. Shenker, R.C. and Matthews, S. (2008) Treatment time with the Lidcombe Program for bilingual children. Poster presented at the American Speech Language and Hearing Association. Chicago, Ill.

Gardner, M.F. (1990) *Expressive One-Word Picture Vocabulary Test-Revised.* Novato, CA: Academic Therapy.

Genesee, F. (1989) Early bilingual development: One language or two? *Journal of Child Language* 16, 161–179.

Genesee, F. (2008) Early dual language learning. *Zero to Three* (September), 17–23.

Genesee, F. and Gandara, P. (1999) Bilingual education programs: A cross-national perspective. *Journal of Social Issues* 55(4), 665–685.

Genesee, F. and Nicoladis, E. (2007) Bilingual acquisition. In E.H.M. Shatz (ed.) *Handbook of Language Development* (pp. 324–342). Oxford: Blackwell.

Gutmann, V. and Shenker, R.C. (2006) *Achieving Fluency in Bilingual Children with the Lidcombe Program.* Poster Presented at the American Speech Language and Hearing Association, Miami, Florida.

Harrison, E., Kingston, M. and Shenker, R.C. (2010) Case studies in evidence-based management of stuttering preschoolers. Manuscript submitted for publication.

Howell, P., Davis, S. and Williams, R. (2009) The effects of bilingualism on speakers who stutter during later childhood. *Archives of Disease in Childhood* 94, 42–46.

Humphrey, B., Al Natour, Y. and Amaryreh, M. (2001) *Does Treatment of Stuttering in Language 1 Generalize to Language 2: A Case Study.* Paper presented at the Florida Speech and Hearing Association (FLASHA).

Johnson,W., Darley, F. and Spriestersbach, D. (1963) *Diagnostic Methods in Speech Pathology.* New York: Harper & Row.

Jones, M., Onslow, M., Harrison, E. and Packman, A. (2000) Treating stuttering in young children: Predicting treatment time in the Lidcombe program. *Journal of Speech, Language and Hearing Research* 43, 1440–1450.

Kindler, A. (2001) *Survey of the states' LEP students 2000–2001 Summary Report.* Washington, D.C. National Clearinghouse for English Language Acquisition.

Kingston, M., Hubert, A., Onslow, M., Jones, M. and Packman, A. (2003) Predicting treatment time with the Lidcombe program: Replication and meta-analysis. *International Journal of Language and Communication Disorders* 38 (2), 165–177.

Koushik, S., Shenker, R.C. and Onslow, M. (2009) Follow-up of 6–10 year old children after Lidcombe Program Treatment. *Journal of Fluency Disorders* 34 (4), 279–290.

Lattermann, C., Shenker, R.C. and Thordardottir, E. (2005) Progression of language complexity with the Lidcombe Program for early stuttering intervention. *American Journal of Speech Pathology and Audiology* 14, 242–253.

Lincoln, M. and Onslow, M. (1997) Long-term outcome of early intervention for stuttering. *American Journal of Speech Language Pathology* 6, 51–58.

Miller, B. and Guitar, B. (2006) Long-term outcome of the Lidcombe Program of early stuttering intervention. *American Journal of Speech-Language Pathology* 18, 42–49.

O'Brian, S., Onslow, M., Cream, A. and Packman, A. (2003) The Camperdown program: Outcomes of a new-prolonged speech treatment model. *Journal of Speech, Language and Hearing Research* 46, 933–946.

Onslow, M., Packman, A. and Harrison, E. (2003) *The Lidcombe Program of Early Stuttering Intervention: A Clinician's Guide.* Austin, TX: Pro-Ed.

Paradis, J., Crago, M., Genesee, F. and Rice, M. (2003) Bilingual children with specific language impairment: How do they compare with their monolingual peers? *Journal of Speech, Language and Hearing Research* 46, 1–15.

Riley, G. (1994) *Stuttering Severity Instrument for Children and Adults* (3rd edn). Austin, TX: Pro-Ed.

Roberts, P.M. and Shenker, R.C. (2007) Assessment and treatment of stuttering in Bilingual speakers. In E.G. Conture and R.F. Curlee (eds) *Stuttering and Related Disorders of Fluency* (3rd edn). New York: Thieme Medical Publishers.

Rousseau, I., Packman, A. and Onslow, M. (2005) *Treatment of Early Stuttering in a Bilingual Child.* Paper presented at the 26th World Congress of the International Association of Logopedics and Phoniatrics. Brisbane, Australia.

Shenker, R., Conte, A., Gingras, A., Courcy, A. and Polomeno, L. (1998) The impact of bilingualism on developing fluency in a preschool child. In E.C. Healy and H.F. Peters (eds)*Proceedings of the 2nd World Congress of the International Fluency Association* (pp. 200–204). Nijmegen: Nijmegen University Press.

Shenker, R.C. and Roberts, P. (2006) Long-term outcome of the Lidcombe Program in Bilingual children. In J. Au-Yeung and M.M. Leahy (eds) *Proceedings of the International Fluency Association 5th World Congress* (pp. 431–436). Dublin: International Fluency Association.

Shin, H.B. and Bruno, R. (2003) Language Use and English-Speaking Ability: 2000. From http://www.census.gov/prod/2003pbus/c2kbr-29.pdf. Accessed June 2005.

Siegel, M., Iozzi, I. and Surian, L. (2008) Bilingualism and conversational understanding in young children. *Cognition* 110, 115–122.

Starkweather, C.W. and Gottwald, S.R. (1999) Stuttering prevention and early intervention: A multiprocess approach. In M. Onslow and A. Packman (eds) *Handbook of Early Stuttering Intervention* (pp. 53–82). San Diego, CA: Singular Publishing Group.

Thordardottir, E. (2006) Language intervention from a bilingual mindset. *The ASHA Leader* 11 (10), 20–21.

Van Borsel, J., Maes, E. and Foulon, S. (2001) Stuttering and bilingualism: A review. *Journal of Fluency Disorders* 26, 179–205.

Waheed-Kahn, N. (1997) Fluency therapy with multilingual clients. In E.C. Healey and H.F.M Peters (eds) *Proceedings of the Second World Congress on Fluency Disorders* (pp. 195–199). Nijmegen: Nijmegen University Press.

Wiig, E.H., Secord, W. and Semel, E. (1998) *Clinical Evaluation of Language Fundamentals-Preschool.* San Antonio, TX: The Psychological Corporation.

Wong-Filmore, L. (1991) When learning a second language means losing the first. *Early Childhood Research Quarterly* 6, 323–346.

Chapter 15
Methodology Matters

PATRICIA M. ROBERTS

Summary

How studies are designed is critical to the conclusions we can draw from them. In this chapter, two main issued are reviewed. First, describing participants as 'native speakers' is not adequate. Six of the many ways that bilingualism (in various degrees) affects the validity of a study are discussed. A set of four essential questions for describing the language background of all research participants is proposed. Second, authors need to be clearer about what disfluency behaviours they count and provide explicit definitions and counting rules. This is important to allow readers to understand the study (are 'stutters' defined perceptually or by the type of disfluency?) and to apply the results to their clinical work. Clear descriptions of participants and explicit definitions of disfluencies are also essential to allow much needed replications of each published study.

1 Introduction

There are exciting developments in our understanding of disfluencies and stuttering across a range of languages, as the other chapters of this book demonstrate. Researchers and clinicians are more and more aware of the issues in these relatively new fields of study and their importance for understanding stuttering and improving clinical services. Yet, within the already small field of fluency disorders, there are few clinicians and researchers who are able and willing to conduct the studies to document the symptom patterns (and the studies of disfluencies and speech in various languages), to examine assessment methods and to explore best treatment practices for speakers of different languages and for bilingual speakers. Studies are rarely replicated (an essential step to confirm the findings before accepting them or applying them to clinical practice). There may not even be other studies on the same topic for several years. These factors combine to make each contribution to the literature something very precious, and something that may stand, unchallenged, for several years. It is particularly important, therefore, for each of us to try to conduct the best possible studies.

Faced with something as interesting and as complex as bilingual stuttering, it can be difficult to design studies. Sometimes, our enthusiasm carries us in one direction while principles of research methodology point in another. The purpose of this chapter is to review some of the methodology issues and the impact of making small and relatively easy improvements to how studies are done.

I have chosen to not cite many published studies in this tutorial. There are two reasons for this. The first is to avoid (unfairly) singling out some studies, when others have omitted the same information or failed to control similar variables, but are not cited. It is impossible to review/critique every study. The second reason is to make this tutorial easier to read; to make the principles, not the references, the focus.

2   Defining and Recognising Bilingualism

2.1   Bilingualism as a continuum

The first thing to realise is that there are not two kinds of people in the world: monolingual and bilingual. Bilingualism is a continuum. There is no specific number of words or verbs or idiomatic expressions one must know to move from being monolingual to being bilingual. This definition of bilingualism is not new. It has been in the literature for decades (Hakuta, 1986; Mackey, 1962) (see Roberts & Shenker, 2007 for more on this point).

But the implications of this fact are often neglected in planning and reporting on research and when reading published studies. The fact that bilingualism and monolingualism are two end points on a continuum means that all speakers can/should be placed along it. Instead, the stuttering literature tends to pretend that all speakers are unilingual, except for the few who are studied by the small number of people doing research that explicitly targets 'bilingual stuttering'. In many studies, even the language of the testing/speaking samples is not stated.

Geography, immigration patterns and cultural factors ensure that, in many countries, most citizens know more than one language. Thus 'everyone' in the Netherlands, Belgium, Sweden and Germany, for example, falls towards the higher end of the bilingualism continuum. So do millions of native French speakers in Canada and the majority of Spanish speakers legally residing in the United States. In many regions of the world (e.g. India, the Middle East, South Africa), millions of people, across all education levels, use two or more languages in their daily lives.

2.2   Consequences of not identifying the level of bilingualism of participants

People who are not interested in bilingualism often assume that it is not part of their studies, and that it will not affect their results. Often, these two assumptions are false. Because researchers (and readers of the studies)

Table 15.1 Consequences of hidden bilingual participants

Noise in the data – lower power
Harder to identify real differences – Type II errors more likely
Stimuli not perceived or processed as intended
Harder to replicate studies
Disenchantment with research – it is all too confusing!

are not looking for bilingualism and do not ask any questions about it, they do not recognise its presence in their sample or its effect on their results. When people with various levels of (unidentified) bilingualism participate in a study, there are several important consequences – all of them negative (listed in Table 15.1).

2.2.1 Noise in the data

Ideally, in a study that compares groups, the groups differ only on the 'thing' being studied (the independent variable). For example, in studies of the symptoms of stuttering and studies of treatment, one group receives treatment and the other does not but the groups are supposed to be, in all other respects, similar. Or, in a study of spontaneous recovery, one group of children has a known family history of stuttering while the other does not. Having relatively bilingual and relatively unilingual participants in unknown proportions in the two groups introduces a confound, uncontrolled factor that could influence the results. While the authors may conclude that their independent variable (the treatment, or the family history, in these two examples) is the reason why one group changed/recovered and the other did not, the differing levels of bilingualism have had unknown and unmeasured effects on the results.

2.2.2 Statistical power

A statistically significant result is less likely if researchers fail to ensure their groups have equal levels of bilingualism. This is due to the variability that bilingualism introduces into the data. What if 5% or 20% (or more) of the variability we think of as being 'just part of stuttering . . .' is, in fact, due to a failure to identify bilingual speakers in some studies? Jones *et al.* (2002a, 2002b) have recently reminded us about the importance of adequate statistical power and pointed out how often studies of stuttering are under-powered. To increase power, one can increase the number of participants. This is hard to do, especially in studies that focus on a specific age group or time frame such as 'within 6 months of the onset of stuttering' or 'those who successfully completed treatment and attended all 3 follow-up appointments'. By partnering with colleagues in other centres, it is possible to increase the number of available participants over what is feasible in a single city/clinic/university.

A second, often neglected way to increase power is to increase the homogeneity of each group of participants. Screening out participants with specific levels of bilingualism or grouping them together into subgroups based on reported language proficiency are relatively simple ways to increase power by decreasing between-subject variability.

2.2.3 Stimulus properties

Stimuli do not have the properties the researchers think they do if there are people with knowledge of more than one language in their study. There are many studies (relatively speaking) of bilingual speakers showing that both languages are always active, to some degree, and showing that processing strategies, word frequencies and phonological neighbours (including cognates) from one language influence performance in the other language even when the speaker is not aware of it (e.g. Costa *et al.*, 2006; Van Heuven *et al.*, 2008). An example of phonological neighbours: if a bilingual French-English speaker hears the word *six* in French (the number 6), it activates words that rhyme in English, such as *peace, niece* or *lease*. In a unilingual French speaker, none of these words would be activated, since, in French, *paix, nièce* and *bail* do not rhyme with *six*. Interlingual homographs can also affect performance on lexical processing tasks, slowing down response time. This has been documented in several tasks across several pairs of languages. For example, the word *four* is an interlingual homograph in English/French. In French, it means *oven*. The two meanings are completely unrelated, but historical accident has created identically spelled words in the two languages. Although participants are not aware of having to search through and discard phonological neighbours from their other language, between-language interference occurs, nonetheless, and varies in strength and direction depending upon many factors currently being explored, including level of proficiency in each of the two languages. This cross-language influence is especially apparent on tasks that measure reaction time in milliseconds, such as lexical decision, grammaticality and phonological judgements.

In some studies, it is important to control for the age of acquisition of the nouns. There is no way to do this for bilingual speakers, where language acquisition is domain-/context-specific and there is no uniform sequence or method of language acquisition. Including participants who regularly use more than one language means that the frequency of occurrence of many words will be quite different for these participants compared to the more unilingual ones (e.g. Lehtonen & Laine, 2003) and may be unknowable (Roberts *et al.*, 2002).

Syntactic processing in each language is influenced by knowledge of the other. There is a series of studies on the production, comprehension and grammaticality judgements by bilingual speakers (e.g. Argyri & Sorace, 2007; Montrul, 2006) showing that underlying syntactic trees or argument structures in one language affect performance in the other language(s). Very common verbs such as 'to telephone' and 'to listen' have different argument structures (direct object or indirect object) in English and in French, for example. So do many reflexive verbs in Spanish compared to their equivalents in English. Even the brain regions involved in different language production and processing tasks are influenced by bilingualism (e.g. Videsott *et al.*, 2010) in ways that could skew studies comparing the neural activation patterns in people who stutter compared to those who do not.

There is a body of literature on auditory perception by stuttering and non-stuttering adults and children. Recent work shows that bilingualism influences performance on at least some of these types of tasks (e.g. Golestani *et al.*, 2009; Rogers *et al.*, 2006). One cannot help but wonder if some of the 'noise' in the conflicting results across studies of auditory processing in stuttering could have been filtered out by the creation of more homogeneous (more unilingual) groups.

There are many studies comparing groups of people who stutter and non-stutterers on measures of phonological processing, and language comprehension and production (Bloodstein & Bernstein Ratner, 2007; Hennessey *et al.*, 2008). Results from one study often contradict or fail to support previous results. This has generally been interpreted as meaning that differences between stuttering and non-stuttering groups in processing speed and accuracy are subtle and difficult to pin down. The conflicting results may be, at least partly, due to non-declared bilingual speakers in this body of work.

Similar questions arise concerning the studies of speech sound production and perception in stuttering and non-stuttering groups and individuals. There are studies of speech production by bilinguals (e.g. Baker *et al.*, 2008; Flege, 1991) examining many of the features that are the focus of studies in the speech science of stuttering: vowel length, plosive consonants, formant transitions etc. and the ways in which speech production is different in monolinguals and in proficient bilingual speakers. These differences often varying with the level of proficiency of the speaker's two languages.

Most studies of lexical, phonological and auditory processing and of speech production are careful to demonstrate that the experimental and control groups are similar in age and education (using a t-test) and similar in the numbers of males and females. This is an essential step to allow interpretation of the eventual results: the presence or absence of between group differences. But these studies fail to report on the level of bilingualism of the participants. Until researchers routinely report and control for level of bilingualism, we cannot rule out 'covert bilinguals' as one of the reasons for the results.

2.2.4 Replication

It is difficult to confirm findings by replication when unknown numbers of participants know more than one language. When another researcher does a similar study, they, in turn, will have unknown numbers of relatively bilingual participants in their groups, perhaps differently distributed across the groups than those in the original study, or different pairs of languages than in the original study (more similar to each other or less similar). They may use the same or different stimuli. If the two studies obtain different results, this is mistakenly interpreted as showing that the results from the first study are weak or inconclusive, since they could not be replicated.

2.2.5 Disenchantment with research

Studies reporting contradictory results are confusing, especially for students and those new to the field. Studies that fail to find a statistically significant result are often rejected by journals, leading to discouraged authors who become less and less willing to conduct studies on fluency and disfluency if the data do not align in some kind of orderly, comprehensible pattern.

2.2.6 Important results not published

The rejection of studies with null results also skews the available information (a problem often referred to as 'the file drawer problem'). The bias against publishing studies that find no statistically significant results slows down progress in understanding some complex phenomena, because important information is not made part of the public conversation in scholarly journals.

2.3 Solutions

2.3.1 Avoid 'are you bilingual?' and 'what is your native language?'

These two questions yield very unreliable answers. In the past 5 years or so, more studies are describing participants as 'native speakers of ___'. This is only a very small improvement over not mentioning language background at all. *Bilingual* means very different things to different people and some extremely proficient speakers who routinely use two languages in their daily lives will not identify themselves as bilingual if one language is even slightly weaker than the other.

Similarly, *native language* is a very unclear concept – both in research and in the minds of the general public. Many people have more than one native language but will fail to mention this. There is no consensus among researchers as to what the cut-off age is for 'native'. Some authors count all languages begun by 3 years of age as native languages while for others, any language learned after 1 month of age is a second (i.e. not a native) language (e.g. Håkansson *et al.*, 2003). New studies have set the ultimate cut-off point as prior to birth, showing that babies develop a preference for certain prosodic features of the language heard while in the womb (Byers-Heinlein *et al.*, 2010; Mampe *et al.*, 2009). The consequences of different patterns of acquisition are still being explored (e.g. Clahsen & Felser, 2006).

2.3.2   A quick set of questions for most studies

For group studies, authors should provide enough information to situate participants along the bilingual-unilingual continuum. As part of the routine demonstration that groups are equivalent in age, education, time post-onset and other variables, use a non-parametric test such as a Mann-Whitney U Test to compare the mean levels of bilingualism, using self-ratings. Some authors would recommend using a t-test for self-ratings, but others argue that this type of rating scale, although it does have a meaningful zero point, does not meet all requirements for ratio level of measurement. (Caveat: further research on the accuracy of self-ratings is needed; they are an estimate, not an exact measure of level of proficiency across modalities).

For single case studies, simply describing each participant this way will allow readers to better understand who is being studied. For designs where participants are matched, add self-ratings of bilingualism to the typical criteria of age and education used in finding appropriately matched pairs of people.

If the study is about relatively broad features of speech, disfluencies or stuttering, adequate description of participants can be a short set of questions similar to those in Table 15.2. Adding these to the demographic information sheet takes little time in relation to the very significant benefits. For studies that focus on bilingualism, or that measure response time to a controlled set of stimuli to measure lexical, syntactic or auditory processing or for studies of speech production features such as formants, transitions between phonemes, articulatory movements during plosive consonants, more rigourous screening of participants and more detailed descriptions of bilingualism are needed (see Dunn & Fox Tree, 2009; Roberts & Shenker, 2007; Van Borsel, this volume).

2.3.3   Lobby journals and granting agencies to value replications

If researchers fear there is little chance of publication, they will be unwilling to undertake replications of their own work or of published studies by others. Some fields such as psychology and second-language teaching have asked that journals designate replications as a category of articles or as a section within the journal to encourage more submissions

Table 15.2 Essential questions for describing all participants

(1) What language(s) did you speak with your family when you were a child?
(2) List all the languages you have been exposed to at home, as subjects in school, travelling and in movies and using the internet.
(3) For each of these languages, rate yourself on a scale of 1–7, where 1 means very little ability, hardly at all and 7 means at the level of the typical person your age who ONLY knows that one language.
Understanding what people say (auditory comprehension): ____
Expressing yourself, saying what you want to say: ____
Reading – understanding what you read and speed: ____
(4) In your daily life, in a typical month, what languages do you use (including internet/computer use)?

of this type of article. Granting agencies need to appreciate the essential role replications play in the self-correcting scientific process and be willing to award funding to proposals that include a replication – both self-replication within a single submission (in a separate study, or by including multiple groups in a single study) and replications of previously published work – in the same language and in new languages.

3 Defining What is Being Counted

Different studies count different types of behaviour. The issue of what is considered to be stuttering has been addressed in several chapters in this volume and elsewhere (Howell *et al.*, 2010). This will not be repeated here. Instead, we will look at the importance of defining what is counted and the need to consider that differences between languages can make applying systems developed in English problematic/invalid in other languages.

Two commonly reported types of overt behaviour are percent syllables stuttered and stuttering-like disfluencies. We will consider each of them in turn to illustrate the point: define what you counted and how you counted it. This chapter takes no position on whether these are appropriate measures, or on whether one is preferable to the other The focus is primarily on these two measures because of their widespread use in published studies.

3.1 What does 'Percent syllables stuttered' mean?

Percent syllables stuttered (%SS) has several definitions. As originally proposed by Onslow and colleagues in the context of the Lidcombe Program, each instance of disfluency produced is judged to be either unambiguously stuttered or not: 'In contrast to definition-based measures of stuttering, the measure of %SS records the number of speech events thought by an experienced clinician to be unambiguous stuttering' (Harris *et al.*, 2002:. 208). This way of counting disruptions to the flow of speech has the advantage that it is applicable to any language. It is not tied to the distribution of pauses, the prosody, the syntactic roles or the frequency of one-syllable words in one language compared to another. On the other hand, it also involves making a judgement, introducing an element of subjectivity into the counts.

3.2 What are stuttering-like disfluencies?

'Stuttering-like disfluencies' (SLD) is a label grouping several types of disfluency: monosyllabic word repetitions, part-word repetitions, dysrhythmic phonation (which includes prolongations, and blocks). Yairi has convincingly demonstrated that these disfluencies (taken together) are more frequent in the speech of preschool, American, English-speaking children who stutter than they are in the speech of similar, non-stuttering children (Yairi & Ambrose, 1992, 1995). SLDs also occur but fairly rarely in the speech of English-speaking adults (e.g. Roberts, Meltzer, & Wilding, 2009). Both SLDs and the very similar classifications of 'within-word disfluency' (Conture, 1990; Conture & Kelly, 1991) and 'less typical' (of normal speech) are now routinely used in the assessment and diagnosis of early stuttering, despite concerns about the basis for these terms (e.g. Cordes & Ingham, 1995; Einarsdottir & Ingham, 2005). The SLD label appears to be more widely used than the other two.

It is important to remember that SLD was developed by observing patterns of disfluencies in English-speaking children. There are studies that report the numbers of SLDs in the speech of adults in languages other than English. Again, each of these needs to be verified by replication (e.g. de Oliviera Martins & de Andrade, 2008; Roberts & Meltzer, 2004). There are a number of studies showing that SLDs (or within-word disfluencies) have low frequency of occurrence in the speech of non-stuttering children who speak other languages. Some results are very similar to those for English-speaking children. These include at least one study in Dutch (Boey *et al.*, 2007), German (Natke *et al.*, 2006), and Spanish (Carlo & Watson, 2003). As is always the case, each of these studies needs to be replicated before firm conclusions can be drawn.

A very large study by de Oliviera Martins and de Andrade (2008) used a variant of typical/less typical groupings to analyse the speech of Brazilian speakers of Portuguese. It is unclear from the definitions whether repetitions of one-syllable words counted as more typical (of normal speech) or less typical disfluencies. They appear to be in the 'typical disfluencies' group. Despite this modification, which reduces the number of less typical disfluencies by removing one-syllable word repetitions, the means for 4 of the 12 age groups tested, including preschoolers, were above 3 disfluencies per 100 syllables (intended syllables only or all syllables produced?)

Counting SLDs in languages other than English can be problematic, and, for some languages, may be impossible. Different syllable structures, the fact that one-syllable words may play different roles (function words vs content words) with different syllable structures in various languages and even the relative frequency of one-syllable words in some languages (compared to English) may lead to different frequencies of occurrence of repetitions of one-syllable words by far the largest (and the most controversial) component of SLDs in the speech of non-stuttering children and adults, in English.

In Vietnamese, for example, including repetitions of one-syllable words in a category that is typical of stuttered speech would be inappropriate. Wikipedia says the longest word in Vietnamese is seven letters long, compared to the longest words in most other languages that range from 25 to 40 letters long (http://en.wikipedia.org/wiki/Longest_words). One could imagine, therefore, that the contrast between one-syllable words (the most frequently occurring word length) and words of two syllables or longer does not function in the same way in Vietnamese as it does in English. The category of one-syllable words will be quite different in Vietnamese than in English. In contrast, in some languages, one-syllable words are very rare (see Jujihira, this volume, on Japanese).

The idea of a one-syllable word may vary a great deal from one language to another. In languages such as Turkish, Finnish and Greek, morphemes that would be stand-alone words in many languages are added onto a root word, making the definition of 'word' different than it is for languages where this process does not exist. In Arabic, function and content words can be merged to form a single word, making comparison to data on the contrasting locations of stutters in English impossible (Abdalla *et al.*, 2010).

3.3 Confusion between the two terms

Counting syllables judged to be unambiguous moments of stuttering is not at all the same thing as counting occurrences of certain types of disfluencies and explicitly NOT judging whether each instance is stuttered or not. As Yairi has repeatedly pointed out 'stuttering-like' is NOT synonymous with stuttering. Yairi did not intend it to become a synonym for 'stutters'. For example, he wrote (1996): 'Although not an ideal label, it (SLD) reflects the special relations of these disfluencies to stuttering while *recognizing that they are not exclusive to it*' (p. 403, added italics not in original). In other words, these types of disfluencies are produced by people who do not stutter and each time they occur in the speech of someone who stutters, they are not necessarily stuttered. It is all about probabilities: these types of disfluencies – taken together – are statistically more likely than other types to be overt moments of stuttering, in the speech of young, English-speaking, American children (as are within-word disfluencies and less-typical disfluencies, in the two other common classification systems).

It is unfortunate that over the last 8 to 10 years, more and more authors have begun, incorrectly, using %SS as a synonym for SLDs, often without offering an explicit definition.

It is even more unfortunate that reviewers allow this into published papers. Each author should define what they mean by %SS (or SLDs or any other type of behaviour that is the focus of the study), provide a reference for this definition (as defined by . . .) and this definition should be part of the published paper. Without this information, papers violate a basic principle in research report writing: publications should provide enough information to allow others to replicate the study. This is only possible if the meaning of key terms like 'what we counted' is crystal clear.

Interestingly, in a footnote to his original definition of SLDs, Yairi said: 'We are currently exploring better labels for SLD, attempting to avoid the word 'stuttering' (Yairi, 1996: 403). A different label might have reduced this drift towards confusing all SLDs with moments of stuttering.

As outlined elsewhere (Roberts, 2007; Roberts & Shenker, 2007), the many problems with the rules for defining and counting disfluencies need to be addressed, including whether to use all syllables uttered, or only intended, meaningful syllables in calculating percentages or ratios.

The credibility of the field, our ability to replicate studies and compare results across studies, and even the reliability of measurements from one clinician to another and one clinic to another are all diminished by confusing, ill-defined terminology and by the incomplete information in many published studies explaining how disfluencies or stutters were counted. As more studies are done of normal disfluencies, stuttering and treatment outcomes in different languages, comparisons of unclear counts of poorly defined disfluencies across languages will only compound the confusion.

4 The Missing Link – Replications

All research textbooks point out the importance of repeating studies in order to confirm their findings, to protect the discipline against research fraud (cooking or outright inventing the data), honest mistakes that affect the results, and the statistical possibility that the result obtained was from the 5 times out of 100 or 1 time out of 100 that the observed result would occur purely by chance.

Replication is the key to the support of any worthwhile theory. Replication involves the process of repeating a study using the same methods, different subjects, and different experimenters. It can also involve applying the theory to new situations in an attempt to determine the generalizability to different age groups, locations, races, or cultures. [. . .] Replication, therefore, is important for a number of reasons, including (1) assurance that results are valid and reliable; (2) determination of generalizability or the role of extraneous variables; (3) application of results to real world situations; and (4) inspiration of new research combining previous findings from related studies. (http://allpsych.com/researchmethods/replication.html)

4.1   Why replications are essential

Much of what we know about bilingual stuttering and disfluencies in various languages other than English comes from either a single study or a set of studies from a single author. Furthermore, studies in our field often have a small number of participants. The three most recent issues of the *Journal of Fluency Disorders* (at time of writing) contained studies with groups of 12, 24, 18, 17, 7, 15 and 16 participants. In such small groups, the inclusion of even two people with different language backgrounds can be enough to move the group average up or down. There are also problems with using %SS as the dependent variable in studies with fewer than 20 participants (Jones *et al.*, 2006). Before accepting any of these findings, it is essential to test the results obtained by doing replications – with different participants and/or in a different centre.

This is true of all research. Many research textbooks in psychology, for example, state that a finding is not 'true', does not become part of the knowledge base of the field until a second (or third, or fourth) study is done confirming the result (e.g. McBurney & White, 2009). Confirmation also usually requires that someone other than the original author do a study that finds the same result. Despite the mantra of evidence-based practice, few studies in the field of fluency disorders are replicated. This means that what is taken to be 'evidence' is shaky, at best, as a foundation for understanding and treating stuttering, especially bilingual stuttering.

There are several plausible reasons for this. They include (1) the small number of researchers in this field; (2) the even smaller number of researchers with proficiency in languages other than English; (3) the time and labour required to do most types of studies about stuttering, including treatment outcome studies and those that require transcribing samples and then counting disfluencies or analysing syntactic properties; (4) training in research methods teaches us how to plan and conduct single studies, not a group of studies; (5) 'statistical methods mostly focus on how to analyze a single set of data ("Is the result significant?"), rather than how to handle and interpret many sets of data ("Does the result generalize?")' (Lindsay & Ehrenberg, 1993); (6) the desire of most professors to do original work, not check someone else's hypothesis; granting agencies value original work over the mundane but essential step of direct and systematic replications; and finally, (7) journal editors and reviewers often reject replications with comments such as 'Other than applying the same protocol to a new set of participants, this replication adds nothing to the field'.

The field of stuttering is not alone in not doing the required replications of studies. It is a common problem in several social sciences. Neuliep's (1991) interdisciplinary book demonstrated the existence of a bias against publishing replications in a number of fields within psychology, communication and other areas of the social sciences. As many authors have pointed out in this often-quoted work and in subsequent years, the self-correcting nature of science can only work if replications are conducted. In the years since then, it appears that more replications are being done (although not always identified as being replications) and some have argued that replications are, perhaps, now viewed by journals and reviewers more favourably than in the past, at least in some fields (de Vaney, 2001; Neuliep & Crandall, 1993; Polio & Gass, 1997).

4.2 Consequences of so few replications

People tend to accept a single study at face value. There is no follow-up study to critique its methodology and improve on the reliability, the sample size, the selection criteria for participants, etc. Clinicians (and other researchers) fall into the trap of thinking 'if it is published, it must be true' and/or 'This author does good work, so I accept these results as true'.

Some findings that are not true are accepted as true, for too long. Clinicians and other researchers act upon the findings, incorporate them into the knowledge base and thus make decisions that do not result in the best possible assessment and treatment of children and adults who stutter. Many would cite the very sad impact of Wendell Johnson's Diagnosogenic Theory in this context: an idea that gained tremendous force because of the esteem its author was held in, despite a glaring lack of supporting data, especially the lack of studies by his contemporaries testing/challenging his theory.

The impact and value of replications is partly a function of their timing. Given the small number of people in the field of bilingual stuttering, delays between initial publication and a replication are likely to be longer than in areas with a larger number of active researchers. As noted above, this makes it especially important to strive to meet high methodological standards in each study. If a study is published and widely promoted at conferences, causing large numbers of people to accept its findings as 'true', it is embarrassing to have a replication fail to find the same result many years later. People may be so accustomed to reading and repeating the false finding that the replication has little impact. A long delay between the original study and its replication(s) harms the credibility of the field if the results of the new study and the original one differ.

On the other hand, if a study is followed one or two years later by a replication that obtains different results, this is more likely to be seen as part of the self-correcting mechanism of science, the ongoing conversation between colleagues trying to understand a complex phenomenon. The findings can be compared, debated, and further studies done before many cohorts of students and clients have come and gone, having been – mistakenly – taught the results of the original study.

4.3 Strategies for the future

It is important to provide the best possible description of participants. The literature on bilingualism has identified a number of characteristics that can influence performance of children and/or adults on various tasks. As our knowledge of bilingualism expands, studies in bilingual stuttering need to change to take the new discoveries into account.

Studies in past decades may not have provided all of the relevant information, but, in light of what we now know, it seems time to change the standards for describing participants in a study. As more and more studies on bilingual stuttering are done, it is important to be able to compare results across studies and the current muddles diminish the usefulness of each published study. More uniformity in the rating scales and background information provided will allow us to make progress faster. For example, if one study finds that bilingual Mandarin-English speakers produce more disfluencies in Mandarin, or more of some types of disfluencies, but a second study fails to find the same pattern, we can develop hypotheses about why this is so *if and only if* we have sufficient and similar information about the language background and proficiency levels of participants in the two studies.

4.4 Summary of recommendations

(1) For all studies, not just those explicitly about bilingual speakers, avoid using 'native speaker' or a dichotomy of bilingual/unilingual to describe participants.

(2) Use the questions in Table 15.2 (as a minimum) as part of intake questionnaires.

(3) Ensure that groups are equivalent in their level of knowledge of languages by reporting self-rated levels of proficiency and by statistical comparisons of the group means.

(4) To avoid the chronic problem of underpowered studies common in stuttering, increase the number of participants through collaboration with colleagues AND maximise the linguistic homogeneity of groups (similar participants).
(5) Define all terminology clearly, especially the definitions of disfluencies and rules for how they were counted.
(6) Do replications of your own studies and those of colleagues, preferably as soon as possible following the original study.
(7) Encourage granting agencies, journal editors and colleagues who review manuscripts to accept replications as essential contributions to the literature.

References

Abdalla, F., Robb, M.P. and Al-Shatti, T. (2010) Stuttering and lexical category in adult Arabic speakers. *Clinical Linguistics & Phonetics* 24, 70–81.

Argyri, E. and Sorace, A. (2007) Crosslinguistic influence and language dominance in older bilingual children. *Bilingualism: Language and Cognition* 10, 79–99.

Baker, W., Trofimovich, P., Flege, J.E., Mack, M. and Halter, R. (2008) Child-adult differences in second-language phonological learning: The role of cross-language similarity. *Language and Speech* 51, 317–342.

Byers-Heinlein, K., Burns, T.C. and Werker, J.F. (2010) The roots of bilingualism in newborns. *Psychological Science*. doi: 10.1177/0956797609360758. Published online 29 January 2010.

Bloodstein, O. and Bernstein Ratner, N. (2007) *Handbook on Stuttering* (6th edn). Toronto: Delmar.

Boey, R.A., Wuyts, F.L., Van de Heyning, P.H., De Bodt, M.S. and Heylen, L. (2007) Characteristics of stuttering-like disfluencies in Dutch-speaking children. *Journal of Fluency Disorders* 32, 310–329.

Carlo, E.J. and Watson, J.B. (2003) Disfluencies of 3- and 5-year old Spanish-speaking children. *Journal of Fluency Disorders* 28, 37–53. document doi:10.1016/S0094-730X(03)00004-4.

Clahsen, H. and Felser, C. (2006) How native-like is non-native processing? *Trends in Cognitive Science* 10, 564–570. doi:10.1016/j.tics.2006.10.002.

Conture, E.G. (1990) *Stuttering* (2nd edn). Englewood Cliffs, NJ: Prentice-Hall.

Conture, E.G. and Kellly, E.M. (1991) Young stutterers' nonspeech behaviors during stuttering. *Journal of Speech and Hearing Research* 34, 1041–1056.

Cordes, A.K. and Ingham, R.J. (1995) Stuttering includes both within-word and between-word disfluencies. *Journal of Speech and Hearing Research* 38, 382–386.

Costa, A., La Heij, W. and Navarrete, E. (2006) The dynamics of bilingual lexical access. *Bilingualism: Language and Cognition* 9, 137–151. doi:10.1017/S1366728906002495.

De Oliviera Martins, V. and de Andrade, C.R.F. (2008) Speech fluency developmental profile in Brazilian Portuguese speakers. *Pro Fono Revista de Atualização Científica* 20(1), 7–12. doi: 10.1590/S0104-56872008000100002.

De Vaney, T.A. (2001) Statistical significance, effect size, and replication: What do the journals say? *Journal of Experimental Education* 69, 310–320 URL: http://www.jstor.org/stable/20179992.

Dunn, A.L. and Fox Tree, J.E. (2009) A quick, gradient bilingual dominance scale. *Bilingualism: Language and Cognition* 12, 273–289. doi:10.1017/S1366728909990113.

Einarsdottir, J. and Ingham, R.J. (2005) Have disfluency-type measures contributed to the understanding and treatment of developmental stuttering? *American Journal of Speech-Language Pathology* 14, 260–273. doi: 10.1044/1058-0360(2005/026).

Flege, J.E. (1991) Age of learning affects the authenticity of voice-onset time (VOT) in stop consonants produced in a second language. *Journal of the Acoustical Society of America* 89, 395–411.

Golestani, N., Rosen, S. and Scott, S.K. (2009) Native-language benefit for understanding speech-in-noise: The contribution of semantics. *Bilingualism: Language and Cognition* 12, 385–392. doi:10.1017/S1366728909990150.

Håkansson, G., Salameh, E.K. and Nettelbladt, U. (2003) Measuring language development in bilingual children: Swedish-Arabic children with and without language impairment. *Linguistics* 41, 255–288.

Hakuta, K. (1986) *Mirror of Language: The Debate on Bilingualism.* New York: Basic Books.

Harris, V., Onslow, M., Packman, A., Harrison, E. and Menzies, R. (2002) An experimental investigation of the impact of the Lidcombe Program on early stuttering. *Journal of Fluency Disorders* 27, 203–214. doi:10.1016/S0094-730X(02)00127-4.

Hennessey, N.W., Nang, C.Y. and Beilby, J.M. (2008) Speeded verbal responding in adults who stutter: Are there deficits in linguistic encoding? *Journal of Fluency Disorders* 33, 180–202. doi:10.1016/j.jfludis.2008.06.001.

Howell, P., Bailey, E. and Kothari, N. (2010) Changes in the pattern of stuttering over development for children who recover or persist. *Clinical Linguistics and Phonetics* 24, 556–575. doi:10.3109/02699200903581034.

Jones, M., Gebski, V., Onslow, M. and Packman, A. (2002a) Statistical power in stuttering research: A tutorial. *Journal of Speech, Language, and Hearing Research* 45, 243–255.

Jones, M., Gebski, V., Onslow, M. and Packman, A. (2002b) Statistical power in stuttering research: A tutorial. Erratum. *Journal of Speech, Language, and Hearing Research* 45, 493.

Jones, M., Onslow, M., Packman, A. and Gebski, V. (2006) Guidelines for statistical analysis for percentage of syllables stuttered. *Journal of Speech, Language, and Hearing Research* 49, 867–878. doi:10.1044/1092-4388(2006/062).

Lehtonen, M. and Laine, M. (2003) How word frequency affects morphological processing in monolinguals and bilinguals. *Bilingualism: Language and Cognition* 6, 213–225. doi: 10.1017/S1366728903001147.

Lindsay, R.M. and Ehrenberg, A.S.C. (1993) The design of replicated studies. *The American Statistician* 47(3), 217–228. URL: http://www.jstor.org/stable/2684982.

Mackey, W.F. (1962) The description of bilingualism. *Canadian Journal of Linguistics* 7, 51–85.

Mampe, B., Friederici, A.D., Christophe, A. and Wermke, K. (2009) Newborns' cry melody is shaped by their native language. *Current Biology* 19, 1994–1997. doi:10.1016/j.cub.2009.09.064.

Montrul, S. (2006) On the bilingual competence of Spanish heritage speakers: Synatx, lexical-semantics and processing. *International Journal of Bilingualism* 10, 37–69. doi: 10.1177/13670069060100010301.

McBurney, D.H. and White, T.L. (2009) *Research Methods* (7th edn). Belmont, CA: Wadsworth Publishing.

Natke, U., Sandrieser, P. Pietrowsky, R. and Kalveram, K.T. (2006) Disfluency data of German preschool children who stutter and comparison children. *Journal of Fluency Disorders* 31, 165–176. document doi:10.1016/j.jfludis.2006.04.002.

Neuliep, J.W. (ed.) (1991) *Replication Research in the Social Sciences*. Washington: Sage Publications.

Neuliep, J.W. and Crandall, R. (1993) Everyone was wrong: There are lots of replications out there. *Journal of Social Behavior and Personality* 8, 1–8.

Polio, C. and Gass, S. (1997) Replication and reporting. *Studies in Second Language Acquisition* 19, 499–508. doi:10.1017/S027226319700404X.

Roberts, P.M. (2007) Stuttering in bilinguals. In A. Ardila and E. Ramos (eds) *Speech and Language Disorders in Bilinguals* (pp. 131–149). New York: Nova Science Publishers.

Roberts, P.M., Garcia, L.J., Desrochers, A. and Hernandez, D. (2002) English performance of proficient bilingual adults on the Boston Naming Test. *Aphasiology* 16, 635–645.

Roberts, P.M. and Meltzer, A. (2004) Normal rates and disfluencies in French and English. In A. Packman, A. Meltzer and H.F.M. Peters (eds) *Theory, Research and Therapy in Fluency Disorders: Proceedings of the Fourth World Congress of Fluency Disorders* (pp. 389–395). Nijmegen: Nijmegen University Press.

Roberts, P.M., Meltzer, A. and Wilding, J. (2009) Disfluencies in non-stuttering adults across sample lengths and topics. *Journal of Communication Disorders* 42, 414–427.

Roberts, P.M. and Shenker, R. (2007) Assessment and treatment of stuttering in bilingual children and adults. In R.F. Curlee and E.G. Conture (eds) *Stuttering and Related Disorders of Fluency* (3rd edn) (pp. 183–209). New York: Thieme Medical Publishers.

Rogers, C.L., Lister, J.J., Febo, D.M., Besing, J.M. and Abrams, H.B. (2006) Effects of bilingualism, noise, and reverberation on speech perception by listeners with normal hearing. *Applied Psycholinguistics* 27, 465–585. doi:10.1017.S014271640606036X.

Van Borsel, J. (this volume) Review of research on the relationship between bilingualism and stuttering.

Van Heuven, W.J.B., Schriefers, H., Dijkstra and Hagoort, P. (2008) Language conflict in the bilingual brain. *Cerebral Cortex* 18, 2706–2716. doi:10.1093/cercor/bhn030.

Videsott, G., Herrnberger, B., Hoenig, K., Schilly, E., Grothe, J., *et al.*, (2010) Speaking in multiple languages: Neural correlates of language proficiency in multilingual word production. *Brain and Language* 113, 103–112. doi:10.1016/j.bandl.2010.01.006.

Yairi, E. (1996) Applications of disfluencies in measurements of stuttering. *Journal of Speech and Hearing Research* 39, 402–404.

Yairi, E. and Ambrose, N. (1992) A longitudinal study of stuttering in children: A preliminary report. *Journal of Speech and Hearing Research* 35, 755–760.

Yairi, E. and Ambrose, N. (1995) *Early Childhood Stuttering: For Clinicians by Clinicians*. Austin, TX: Pro-Ed.

Part 4

Conclusions

Chapter 16

Fluency Disorders and Language Diversity: Lessons Learned and Future Directions

PETER HOWELL AND JOHN VAN BORSEL

Summary

Some potential directions for future research and implications for practical work are considered.

1 Introduction

Our initial aims when planning this volume were summarized in the preface. The chapters that were written met our expectations and, in many ways, they have brought up new topics to be considered as well as rekindled some older issues that have been debated in the wider literature. It is not the intention to recap here what has been said in the previous chapters. Rather, we aim to address the following goals: (1) comment briefly on the state of the art in cross-lingual work, bilinguals and stuttering; (2) highlight some of the prominent disputes in the language and fluency domains; (3) offer our point of view on these issues as they pertain to stuttering; (4) see what impact these disputes have on interpretation of results; (5) identify some areas where questions remain in one domain or the other (bilingualism, cross-lingual work or stuttering); and (6) examine ways in which issues in one domain (e.g. stuttering) could usefully include information from the other domains (across language groups and bilingualism).

2 Assessment Issues (Bilingualism and Stuttering)

Not all chapters were about bilingualism and stuttering. However, some comments about common concerns across these areas concerning definitions of these states are appropriate. The issues of perceptual definition of fluency problems, full documentation of symptoms and so on feature in all parts of this book. These same concerns apply to bilingualism. Additional considerations relevant to definitions arose too when considering bilingualism. For instance, in the opening chapter De Houwer made the point that a child who does not produce speech in two languages may, nevertheless, be regularly hearing them both and that this is a form of bilingual input. Clearly this calls for precise examination of exposure to use of language by children and would apply when considering the impact of bilingualism on stuttering (an example of a study on stuttering where languages heard and produced were assessed is Howell *et al.*, 2009).

2.1 Definitions

The definitions of both bilingualism and stuttering are fraught with difficulties. As pointed out in this book, probably the majority of the people in the world speak a language other than their native one, to some degree. The questions when defining bilingualism are where to draw the dividing lines between being and not being bilingual, and how to specify the criteria sufficiently objectively so that other people can adopt them or adapt them to their needs. De Houwer's and Mennen's chapters each offered us an indication of two widely used sets of criteria used in bilingualism. Some of the issues that have dominated stuttering over the years apply to bilingualism as well.

When examining bilingualism and stuttering together, there are additional considerations that people need to be aware of. For example, there needs to be compatibility between methods for assessing the two. Thus, if bilingualism is referred to in a way that rules out certain fluency symptoms (e.g. De Houwer, this volume when talking about bilingual studies), then you cannot subsequently examine stuttering in bilingual groups that includes these symptoms.

The argument has been made that some of the findings about bilingualism and stuttering may be due to allowing whole-word repetitions to be used as an indication of stuttering. What is necessary is to ensure compatibility between how fluency is specified in bilingual and stuttering work. Inconsistent positions (e.g. De Houwer who considers that whole-word repetitions should not be considered as symptoms of stuttering versus Lim and Lincoln, this volume, and Shenker, this volume, who consider they should) are mutually incompatible. Whilst the issues raised here may be debated in the bilingualism field as they are in stuttering, it would be useful to openly recognize alternative positions and to encourage clear statement of the exact procedures required and the position taken on these dimensions.

The issue just raised, of whether whole-word repetitions should be considered as stuttering or not has repeatedly surfaced in this volume in different ways. Roberts' methodology chapter notes that different authors include or exclude this symptom, and there is similar discussion in Howell and Rusbridge. With respect to stuttering in general, opinion seems to be split roughly 50/50 as to whether these should be considered features of stuttering. Whole-word repetitions are prevalent in typically developing children's speech, so counting them as stutters may bias toward diagnosing too many cases of typically developing speech as stuttering. Another compelling argument for the view that whole-word repetitions may not be appropriate for characterizing stuttering is in the chapter by Ujihira. He noted that Japanese has little scope for allowing whole-word repetition because of its structural features. Consequently this symptom class is not involved in diagnosis of stuttering in his country. He noted that the recovery rate of children who stutter in Japan is lower than the 80% and higher values commonly reported in the West, he has interpreted this as a direct consequence of excluding whole-word repetitions and suggests that excluding them may be the appropriate thing to do in general. Another domain where whole-word repetitions tend to be used in identifying stuttering is in early intervention. As Shenker (this volume) notes, reports do not always make clear whether or not this class of symptoms was considered as stuttering or not.

2.2 Expert judgment

This and the next section raise issues specifically about assessment of stuttering. Here the concern is about the use of perceptual definitions of stuttering. Clinicians sometimes claim that they are able to make expert judgments and that these are reliable. It is well-known, however, that experts do not agree about whether a speaker is a stutterer or not (Kully & Boberg, 1988) and so expert judgment is a subjective opinion, not an objective benchmark. It has already been seen that there is no agreed decision about whether whole-word repetition is considered a sign of stuttering or not. A perceptual definition does not solve this problem, it just disguises it. Claims that judgments were made by experts can lead to procedures not being fully documented. That said, generally speaking most studies on stuttering do not claim expert judges made decisions.

2.3 Mild stuttering

There is also empirical work in this volume that shows that there may be particular difficulties when cases of mild stuttering have to be assessed (Watson *et al.*, this volume). Watson *et al.* observed that some fluent speakers show higher stuttering counts than speakers considered (on other grounds) to stutter. This points to the limitation of using symptoms alone. Considerations like these led Riley (1994) to develop the stuttering severity instrument (SSI-3), which specifies what symptoms should be counted to obtain %SS and includes the ancillary measures of duration of stuttered events and physical concomitants. Researchers often use different ways of counting stuttered syllables to those specified in the manual; for example, Miller and Guitar (2009) used perceptually defined stutters that were discussed in Section 2.1. The use of perceptually defined stuttering in conjunction with SSI-3 preclude use of the norms, so it is not clear what is achieved with this hybrid form of SSI-3, nor how duration of three longest stuttering events can be made. It is possible that stuttering classified perceptually by experts plus physical concomitants improve classification of mild cases, but that remains to be demonstrated empirically. It is worth repeating that translation of SSI-3 into other languages does not automatically mean that the published norms can be applied (renorming is necessary), but before that is attempted other features of SSI-3 need to be considered (Howell, 2010). Discussion of some of these follows:

3   Thresholds and Assessment Procedures

An issue that is inherently tied up with what symptoms should be considered as signs of stuttering is what threshold value should be applied. That is, should a child who shows 3% stuttered syllables or syllable-like disfluencies be considered to stutter? The way that this and, indeed, any proposed threshold is related to the issue of what symptoms should be considered as signs of stuttering can be illustrated by considering some implications of applying this threshold with stuttering-like disfluencies (SLD). SLD includes whole-word repetitions and commonly uses the 3% threshold. Therefore, it is possible that a child might repeat a whole monosyllabic word every 33 words and be designated a stutterer using this criterion alone. A further thing to be wary about when considering threshold values is that these give different values when different procedures are employed (Howell *et al.*, 2010). Thus, depending on what assessment procedures are used, a child may be designated as stuttering or not according to the same numerical threshold.

4   Selecting Representative Samples of Bilingual Speakers and Speakers Who Stutter for Studies

A major concern that has arisen is whether the participant groups used in studies in stuttering and bilingualism are representative of the population as a whole (only then can the results be generalized to the population). Any biases may affect interpretation of the outcome of studies. Studies investigating childhood stuttering recruit cases via academic communities and their contacts (Yairi & Ambrose, 2005). Such children are likely to have a richer verbal environment in the family home and show advanced language relative to the population at large.

A similar bias occurs in another study on stuttering by Reilly *et al.* (2009). They assessed educational status of the mothers. At follow-up there was a significant increase in mothers who had degree-level education or higher. Thus, this sample is biased towards families where the mother was educated to degree standard or above. This would be expected to lead to higher verbal performance. Thus the bias in the sample could lead to apparent better language development being associated with stuttering, which was one finding reported in the study and is one which may be artefactual. Similar biases may operate in experimental studies that recruit participants from undergraduates. This is ameliorated to some extent by carefully matching control groups of participants on factors that are salient to performance.

In terms of bilingualism, the same type of bias may operate. For instance, diary studies by parents who are academics obviously lead to children who are biased toward rich language environments. Additionally, the form of bilingualism may not be similar to that acquired in more naturalistic settings. One study has attempted to avert such biases by excluding children who do not necessarily have to use multiple languages in the home, which would exclude middle-class academic parents who seek to teach their children additional languages for social, educational and cultural advancement (Howell *et al.*, 2009). An additional feature of that study was that control groups who did not stutter were carefully matched to the children who stuttered.

De Houwer also raised the question of whether a clinical sample is appropriate to address issues associated with developmental stuttering in bilingual speakers (Reilly *et al.*, 2009). The implication appears to be that a clinical sample will have some preselection of cases who are or are not (this is not explicit) likely to respond to treatment. The clinicians we work with indicate that they do not do this and would consider this unethical. If selection by speech-language therapists did take place, then most of the work on risk factors for stuttering, not just that to do with bilingualism, would be wasted effort, yet several groups have indicated their motivation for conducting such studies: For example, the Illinois group in their early work stated:

> The ability to make accurate predictions could have a revolutionary impact on the long-term objective of cost-effective selective treatment for stuttering children. It is not practical, possible, or necessary to put every child who stutters into therapy. Economic conditions and emerging health policies, in fact, may make this option more difficult. For any child who appears likely to continue to stutter, treatment should not be delayed. But it may be advantageous to defer treatment for children with few or no risk factors and/or mild stuttering that does not cause concern for either child or parents. (Yairi *et al.*, 1996: 74)

Reilly *et al.* (2009) in their original paper say:

> Particularly pressing is the need to identify children in whom stuttering is and is not likely to persist, so that differing advice (watchful

waiting versus recommending treatment) can be correctly targeted. (Reilly *et al.*, 2009: 271)

The motivation of each of these pieces of work would be seriously hampered by the biases mentioned earlier in this section (e.g. towards higher socio-economic families).

5 Bilingualism and Risk for Stuttering

The review chapter by Mennen looked at lower order phonological factors. Here some indications were seen that bilingualism affects phonological or phonetic properties of sounds and, as such, could potentially support such factors interacting with children prone to stuttering that then leads to actualization of the problem. Dworzynski's chapter described how environmental factors (which would include language circumstances in the home) could result in different degrees of penetrance of stuttering. Watkins and Klein worked through the common neural pathways involved in bilingual speech and stuttering that would also permit bilingualism to adversely affect stuttering.

The work on genetics, brains, reviews of the influence of specific languages and some studies in treatment all allow knowledge of second language to affect stuttering. The effects may be small but this is true of many other medical interventions that can influence risk for allied disorders. De Houwer's work might suggest that co-influences between bilingualism and stuttering at higher level cognitive-linguistic factors are immune from such influences, but this remains to be explored.

Howell *et al.* (2009) have claimed that risk for stuttering is slightly increased in bilingual speakers for reasons discussed in the previous two sections. At least two of the chapters imply that Howell *et al.*'s study is the only one which shows that bilingualism poses a higher risk for stuttering (De Houwer, Shenker). There is older work on this topic, reviewed in the chapter by Van Borsel. This work has some methodological limitations. It is notable that bilingualism was not included as a risk factor in the Reilly *et al.* (2009). However, there is one recent study that is methodologically sound (limitations are stated explicitly in the paper) that pointed clearly to bilingualism being a risk factor for stuttering:

Ajdacic-Gross *et al.* (2009) used logistic regression and path analysis in a study intended to establish what factors predicted risk of stuttering in a cohort of adult army conscripts, which would not be biased with respect to socio-economic group. Ajdacic-Gross *et al.* (2009) reported an analysis of risk factors for stuttering on this database that had self-reported information about whether the respondents stuttered or not. Fourteen thousand one hundred and fifty seven conscripts aged 18–20 years underwent intensive screening by psychiatrically trained personnel. Individuals who had incomplete or erroneous records were excluded, leaving 11,905 cases. Cases with high psychiatric scores were excluded (it is stated that these were mainly malingerers), leaving 9814 records. Four hundred and eight men (4.2% of the 9814) reported having stuttered in childhood (those who recovered and those who persisted were not distinguished). This is comparable with other estimates for incidence.

The main analyses looked at 17 variables identified as risk factors. Logistic regression and path analyses were reported on these variables. Six variables that were significant predictors in the logistic regression after adjustments were identified as risk factors. These were: (1) incubator; (2) restless and fidgety in school (which they suggested may reflect ADHD); (3) alcohol abuse of mother; (4) alcohol abuse of father; (5) obsessive-compulsive disorder (OCD) in family members; and (6) having a parent from a foreign country. In their discussion, Ajdacic-Gross *et al.* attributed factor 6 to bilingualism being a risk factor for stuttering. The strengths of this study are the large sample size, that there was no bias to higher socio-economic groups, all cases were thoroughly examined by trained personnel and the group conducted sophisticated and appropriate statistical analysis. The main limitation in this study is that stuttering was self-referred, although the fact that the incidence rates are close to those reported in other studies (Howell, 2010) suggests that cases were correctly identified by the interviewers. Also, self- or parent-referral is common in this area (for instance, parental referrals were made in Reilly *et al.*, 2009). Taking all these observations together, the claim that bilingualism poses a risk factor for stuttering should not be dismissed lightly.

6 The Link between Language, Bilingualism, Stuttering and Age-dependent Language Milestones

The consensus in the literature seems to be that monolingual children speaking different languages reach language milestones across languages at similar ages (Newman & Newman, 2008) although the milestones are crude. De Houwer reported that bilingual children without fluency problems reached age-dependent language milestones at or before monolingual children (see however comments made earlier about socio-economic class biases, suggest these factors may have affected the results). Mennen's chapter showed that speech production skills show subtle deviations from the norm. There is then, a difference of opinion about whether bilingualism affects speech-language development. This may be partly to do with whether higher cognitive-linguistic skills or speech skills are being considered.

Mennen gives some indication in her chapter about the stages of language development in bilingualism and how fluency is affected with regards to speech-related skills. This is less true of De Houwer's chapter, and many of the studies in the latter involve children who are well beyond the age at which stuttering starts. The studies probably have few implications about stuttering *onset* although they may have some bearing on how stuttering develops subsequently.

Considerable empirical and theoretical work has been undertaken on how stuttering is linked to early developmental milestones in language acquisition. The broad details of empirical work in monolingual speakers are reasonably well accepted: The average child starts to stutter at about age three, there is a period where children may show patterns indicative of recovery (which last up to about teenage), after teenage additional changes occur which may be associated with pragmatic or emotional changes in the individual. Needless to say, the theoretical interpretation of this work is often debated. Two important issues concern diagnosis, which was discussed earlier (whether using different symptoms might lead to different conclusions about stuttering) and which language factor or factors may be involved in the development of stuttering. The latter has not been discussed so far in this chapter, but it discussed in the chapters by Howell and Rusbridge and Tsai *et al.*

In the research literature, some assessment of stuttering as a speech disorder is usually deemed necessary. As we have said earlier, this is not to deny that there are other associated features, such as meta-linguistic and socio-emotional influences, that arise at later ages. An example of this is seen in Tsai *et al.*'s chapter, where the authors suggest that pragmatic conversational factors, use of the speaker's own name etc. feature in later development. If such influences occur, they would be of less interest to researchers interested in developmental stuttering, as they occur at the period after most stuttering development is complete. For example, the issue of whether stuttering will persist or recover is usually considered to be complete by teenage and, for this reason, many authors interested in developmental stuttering cease their studies at this age.

Most of the chapters have focused on stuttering that started in childhood. Speakers who continue to stutter beyond childhood and those who start to stutter in adulthood may differ form those who recover and, conceivably this could relate to language acquisition (whether of a single language or more than one). We do not want to give the impression that stuttering in childhood is all that is important. Some authors are interested in adult stuttering (Plexico *et al.*, 2009a, 2009b) and would see teenage or beyond as the starting point, rather than the end-point of their investigations. It is probably fair to say that stuttering in adulthood is more variable than that in childhood (even stuttering in childhood is heterogeneous and a difficult topic to investigate).

There are a number of reasons why stuttering in adults may be more variable/heterogenous. One is that adults in the course of the years they have stuttered may or may not have sought treatment to control the disorder and improve speech fluency. If they have sought treatment, it may have been more or less successful depending on factors such as availability and quality of resources, motivation, family support, financial support, the existence of local support groups for people who stutter and so on. Another possible reason is that, depending to some extent on personality and success in various domains of life (family, professional life, etc.), the speech disorder may or may not have been an issue in an individual's life. Furthermore, and in direct relationship to the overall topic of this volume, individuals may differ considerably with regard to their 'language development' beyond the childhood period. For some individuals language and communication plays a very important role in their life. This relates not only to the use of spoken and written language in daily activities but also includes the learning and use of foreign languages. For other individuals, language and communication are less important.

The proposal Tsai *et al.* make in their chapter that new language factors that influence stuttering arise at the end of the period of language development is likely to raise debate itself. Thus other authors consider emotional, rather than language, influences emerge during adolescence. The debate over whether emotional or language factors are predominant from adolescence onwards has relevance for treatment and service delivery issues. Are clients happy to have emotional concomitants of stuttering treated or do they want to see reductions of language symptoms? More consultation with stutterers themselves would provide valuable input here.

There are other fluency disorders to consider as well, many of which might be more important after teenage when a lot of recovery from developmental stuttering has occurred. One group of disorders to take into account is that of acquired stuttering. Van Riper (1971) pointed out that the fact that stuttering usually begins in childhood is 'one of the few solid bits of information we have about stuttering' (p. 62). In recent years evidence is accumulating, however, that stuttering or at least forms of disfluent speech closely resembling stuttering may appear also for the first time later in life, beyond the typical childhood period (see Van Borsel, 1997). These include disfluency due to brain damage, often called neurogenic stuttering, disfluency associated with a psychological problem or an emotional trauma, known as psychogenic stuttering, dysfluency resulting from the use of drugs, called drug-induced or pharmacogenic stuttering, and malingered stuttering. Certainly, not everybody would agree with labeling the disfluency patterns observed in these cases as stuttering. Culatta and Leeper (1988) for instance, in a letter to the editors of the *Journal of Speech and Hearing Disorders* suggested that 'the label "stuttering" be restricted to describe that well-defined and researched developmental dysfluency, the causes of which remain unknown.' And according to Curlee (1995), in a comment pertaining to acquired stuttering of neurogenic origin '... it may not be informative to label such dysfluencies as stuttering until there is better evidence that their superficial similarities have etiologic, diagnostic, or treatment significance'. On the other hand, these various clinical pictures sometimes resemble each other quite closely, to the extent that even for experienced clinicians, it may be difficult to distinguish between them (Van Borsel & Taillieu, 2001). As already pointed by Van Riper (1971), in cases of acquired stuttering there is always the suspicion that the disfluency is a recurrence of previously existing (childhood) stuttering that the stutterer had outgrown. Furthermore some persons who start to stutter for the first time in adulthood may have been interiorized stutterers who under great stress could no longer hide their disorder. In both cases the stuttering is actually of developmental origin and not acquired.

The picture becomes even more complex if one has a closer look at the disfluencies that are demonstrated in individuals with certain genetic syndromes, such as Down syndrome, fragile-x syndrome, Prader-Willi syndrome, Tourette syndrome, Neurofibromatosis type I and Turner syndrome. All of these list disfluency as a characteristic of that particular syndrome (Van Borsel & Tetnowski, 2007), and in many studies the disfluency has been characterized as stuttering. However, the disfluency patterns in these various syndromes are far from similar. Some of these genetic syndromes even show patterns of disfluency that may be indicative of only that syndrome (or similar syndromes). On the other hand, it should be stressed that the diagnosis in these cases becomes increasingly difficult with increasing severity of the impairment, perhaps because other, possibly more severe, speech and language disorders are more likely to occur which blur and complicate the picture (Boberg *et al.*, 1978).

Clearly, then, the identification of stuttering may not be as straightforward as is sometimes claimed. As far as defining stuttering is concerned, until the demarcation between the different types of fluency problems (developmental and acquired stuttering, cluttering, covert stuttering, disfluency associated with a genetic syndrome) has become clearer, it may be wise to adopt the position taken by the World Health Organization (2001), that the term 'stuttering' refers to 'disorders [plural] in the rhythm of speech in which the individual knows precisely what he or she wishes to say but at the time is unable to say it because of an involuntary repetition, prolongation or cessation of a sound'.

7 Cultural Aspects

Although this book is about multilingualism (linguistic diversity) and stuttering, it should be recalled that language and culture always go together and that speakers of two languages also are participants of two cultures. Evidently such cultural differences or diversity may impact upon both the diagnosis and treatment of stuttering. A reference to this was found for instance in the chapter by de Britto Pereira, where she stated that the treatment approaches for stuttering that are currently available in Brazil and which are almost always developed in the United States and Europe. At times cultural differences may be so overwhelming that any linguistic differences are swamped out. The chapter by Simon describing traditional treatment practices for stuttering in Sub-Saharan Africa clearly illustrates this point. An animism perspective on stuttering regards the disorder in such a different way than in the West that it would seem that stuttering is hardly a speech disorder. One practical lesson to learn from a chapter like this is that one should never forget that the cultural background of clients should always be incorporated in assessment and treatment. The chapter by Simon further seems to support Shames' (1989) statement that much remains to be learned about the interactions between cultures and stuttering.

8 Concluding Remarks

The relationship between language and stuttering in general and between bilingualism and stuttering in particular remains a challenging topic. The various chapters in this volume raised several issues that researchers may want to take into account in their future work. Among the most important things to remember, in our opinion, is that many of the research findings and ensuing conclusions are determined by how stuttering and bilingualism are defined. It would further seem that with increasing knowledge from other languages, definitions that now prevail will no longer be acceptable. The differences between languages make comparison between stuttering in different languages and the study of stuttering in individuals who speak more than one language a complex endeavor. The task is even more difficult to the extent to which cultural differences enter the stage. Certainly, our knowledge of stuttering and language diversity has grown in recent years, but it also becomes increasingly clear that great care is necessary when designing studies or drawing conclusions from them. Careful and detailed description of the population studied, of what we did and how we did it, are mandatory. We could extend and refine Haugen's (1953) well-known statement and conclude that the main lessons learned are that the only common thing about people who stutter is that they are not fluent and that the only thing bilinguals have in common is that they are not monolingual.

References

Ajdacic-Gross, V., Vetter, S., Muller, M., Kawohl, W., Frey, F., Lupi, G., Blechschmidt, A., Born, C., Latal, B. and Rossler, W. (2009) Risk factors for stuttering: A secondary analysis of a large data base. *European Archives of Psychiatry and Clinical Neuroscience* 260, 279–286.

Boberg, E., Ewart, B., Masson, G., Lindsay, K. and Wynn, S. (1978) Stuttering in the retarded. *Mental Retardation Bulletin* 6, 67–76.

Culatta, R. and Leeper, L. (1988) Dysfluency isn't always stuttering. *Journal of Speech and Hearing Disorders* 53, 486–487.

Curlee, R.F. (1995) Comments on 'neurogenic stuttering: An analysis and critique'. *Journal of Medical Speech-Language Pathology* 3, 125–127.

Harris, V., Onslow, M., Packman, A., Harrison, E. and Menzies, R. (2002) An experimental investigation of the impact of the Lidcombe Program on early stuttering. *Journal of Fluency Disorders* 27, 203–214.

Haugen, E. (1953) *The Norwegian Language in America: A Study in Bilingual Behavior.* Philadelphia: University of Pennsylvania Press.

Howell, P. (2010) *Recovery from Stuttering.* New York: Psychology Press.

Howell, P., Davis, S. and Williams, R. (2009) The effects of bilingualism on speakers who stutter during late childhood. *Archives of Disease in Childhood* 94, 42–46.

Howell, P., Davis, S. and Williams, R. (2009) Stuttering and bilingualism: A reply to Packman, Onslow, Reilly, Attansioand Shenker. *Archives of Disease in Childhood.*

Howell, P., Soukup-Ascencao, T., Davis, S. and Rusbridge, S. (2010) Comparison of alternative methods for obtaining severity scores from the speech of people who stutter. *Clinical Linguistics and Phonetics* xx, xx–xx.

Kully, D. and Boberg, E. (1988) An investigation of interclinic agreement in the identification of fluent and stuttered syllables. *Journal of Fluency Disorders* 13, 309–318.

Miller, B. and Guitar, B. (2009) Long-term outcome of the Lidcombe Program for early stuttering intervention. *American Journal of Speech-Language Pathology* 18, 42–49.

Newman, B. M. and Newman, P. (2008) *Development through Life: A Psychosocial Approach.* Belmont, CA: Wadsworth Publishing Company.

Plexico, L., Manning, W. and Levitt, H. (2009a) Coping responses by adults who stutter: I. Protecting the self and others, *Journal of Fluency Disorders* 34, 87–107.

Plexico, L., Manning, W. and Levitt, H. (2009b) Coping responses by adults who stutter: II. Approaching the problem and achieving agency. *Journal of Fluency Disorders* 34, 108–126.

Reilly, S., Onslow, M., Packman, A., Wake, M., Bavin, E.L., Prior, M., Eadie, P., Cini, E., Bolzonello, C. and Ukoumunne, O.C. (2009) Predicting stuttering onset by the age of 3 years: A prospective, community cohort study. *Pediatrics* 123, 270–277.

Riley, G.D. (1994) *Stuttering Severity Instrument for Children and Adults (SSI-3)* (3rd edn). Austin, TX: Pro Ed.

Shames, G.H. (1989) Stuttering: An RFP for a cultural perspective. *Journal of Fluency Disorders* 14, 67–77.

Van Borsel, J. (1997) Neurogenic stuttering: A review. *Journal of Clinical Speech and Language Studies* 7, 6–33.

Van Borsel, J. and Taillieu, C. (2001) Neurogenic stuttering versus developmental stuttering: An observer judgement study. *Journal of Communications Disorders* 34, 385–395.

Van Borsel, J. and Tetnowski, J. (2007) Fluency disorders in genetic syndromes. *Journal of Fluency Disorders* 32, 279–296.

Van Riper, C. (1971) *The Nature of Stuttering.* Englewood Cliffs, NJ: Prentice-Hall.

World Health Organization. (2001) *The International Classification of Functioning, Disability, & Health.* Geneva: World Health Organization.

Yairi, E. and Ambrose, N.G. (2005) *Early Childhood Stuttering.* Austin, TX: Pro-Ed.

Yairi, E., Ambrose, N.G., Paden, E.P. and Throneburg, R. (1996) Predictive factors of persistence and recovery: Pathways of childhood stuttering. *Journal of Communication Disorders* 29, 51–77.

Index

Authors

Subject index